Cellular and Molecular Mechanisms of Nephropathic Cystinosis

Cellular and Molecular Mechanisms of Nephropathic Cystinosis

Editor

Elena N. Levtchenko

MDPI • Basel • Beijing • Wuhan • Barcelona • Belgrade • Manchester • Tokyo • Cluj • Tianjin

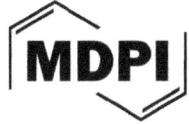

Editor
Elena N. Levtchenko
Pediatrics & Development and Regeneration
University Hospitals Leuven & KU Leuven
Leuven Belgium

Editorial Office
MDPI
St. Alban-Anlage 66
4052 Basel, Switzerland

This is a reprint of articles from the Special Issue published online in the open access journal *Cells* (ISSN 2073-4409) (available at: https://www.mdpi.com/journal/cells/special_issues/nephropathic_cystinosis).

For citation purposes, cite each article independently as indicated on the article page online and as indicated below:

LastName, A.A.; LastName, B.B.; LastName, C.C. Article Title. *Journal Name* **Year**, *Volume Number*, Page Range.

ISBN 978-3-0365-4568-4 (Hbk)
ISBN 978-3-0365-4567-7 (PDF)

© 2022 by the authors. Articles in this book are Open Access and distributed under the Creative Commons Attribution (CC BY) license, which allows users to download, copy and build upon published articles, as long as the author and publisher are properly credited, which ensures maximum dissemination and a wider impact of our publications.

The book as a whole is distributed by MDPI under the terms and conditions of the Creative Commons license CC BY-NC-ND.

Contents

About the Editor vii

Preface to "Cellular and Molecular Mechanisms of Nephropathic Cystinosis" ix

Jerry Schneider and Elena Levtchenko
A Personal History of Cystinosis by Dr. Jerry Schneider
Reprinted from: *Cells* **2022**, *11*, 945, doi:10.3390/cells11060945 1

Katharina Hohenfellner, Ewa Elenberg, Gema Ariceta, Galina Nesterova, Neveen A. Soliman and Rezan Topaloglu
Newborn Screening: Review of its Impact for Cystinosis
Reprinted from: *Cells* **2022**, *11*, 1109, doi:10.3390/cells11071109 9

Francesco Emma, Giovanni Montini, Marco Pennesi, Licia Peruzzi, Enrico Verrina, Bianca Maria Goffredo, Fabrizio Canalini, David Cassiman, Silvia Rossi and Elena Levtchenko
Biomarkers in Nephropathic Cystinosis: Current and Future Perspectives
Reprinted from: *Cells* **2022**, *11*, 1839, doi:10.3390/cells11111839 21

Dieter Haffner, Maren Leifheit-Nestler, Candide Alioli and Justine Bacchetta
Muscle and Bone Impairment in Infantile Nephropathic Cystinosis: New Concepts
Reprinted from: *Cells* **2022**, *11*, 170, doi:10.3390/cells11010170 33

Aude Servais, Jennifer Boisgontier, Ana Saitovitch, Aurélie Hummel and Nathalie Boddaert
Central Nervous System Complications in Cystinosis: The Role of Neuroimaging
Reprinted from: *Cells* **2022**, *11*, 682, doi:10.3390/cells11040682 45

Ahmed Reda, Koenraad Veys and Martine Besouw
Fertility in Cystinosis
Reprinted from: *Cells* **2021**, *10*, 3539, doi:10.3390/cells10123539 57

Pang Yuk Cheung, Patrick T. Harrison, Alan J. Davidson and Jennifer A. Hollywood
In Vitro and In Vivo Models to Study Nephropathic Cystinosis
Reprinted from: *Cells* **2022**, *11*, 6, doi:10.3390/cells11010006 69

Koenraad Veys, Sante Princiero Berlingerio, Dries David, Tjessa Bondue, Katharina Held, Ahmed Reda, Martijn van den Broek, Koen Theunis, Mirian Janssen, Elisabeth Cornelissen, Joris Vriens, Francesca Diomedi-Camassei, Rik Gijsbers, Lambertus van den Heuvel, Fanny O. Arcolino and Elena Levtchenko
Urine-Derived Kidney Progenitor Cells in Cystinosis
Reprinted from: *Cells* **2022**, *11*, 1245, doi:10.3390/cells11071245 89

Elena Sendino Garví, Rosalinde Masereeuw and Manoe J. Janssen
Bioengineered Cystinotic Kidney Tubules Recapitulate a Nephropathic Phenotype
Reprinted from: *Cells* **2022**, *11*, 177, doi:10.3390/cells11010177 111

Elizabeth G. Ames and Jess G. Thoene
Programmed Cell Death in Cystinosis
Reprinted from: *Cells* **2022**, *11*, 670, doi:10.3390/cells11040670 129

Laura Rita Rega, Ester De Leo, Daniela Nieri and Alessandro Luciani
Defective Cystinosin, Aberrant Autophagy—Endolysosome Pathways, and Storage Disease: Towards Assembling the Puzzle
Reprinted from: *Cells* **2022**, *11*, 326, doi:10.3390/cells11030326 137

Mohamed A. Elmonem, Koenraad R. P. Veys and Giusi Prencipe
Nephropathic Cystinosis: Pathogenic Roles of Inflammation and Potential for New Therapies
Reprinted from: *Cells* **2022**, *11*, 190, doi:10.3390/cells11020190 157

Stephanie Cherqui
Hematopoietic Stem Cell Gene Therapy for Cystinosis: From Bench-to-Bedside
Reprinted from: *Cells* **2021**, *10*, 3273, doi:10.3390/cells10123273 173

Thomas Quinaux, Aurélia Bertholet-Thomas, Aude Servais, Olivia Boyer, Isabelle Vrillon, Julien Hogan, Sandrine Lemoine, Ségolène Gaillard, Candide Alioli, Sophie Vasseur, Cécile Acquaviva, Olivier Peyruchaud, Irma Machuca-Gayet and Justine Bacchetta
Response to Cysteamine in Osteoclasts Obtained from Patients with Nephropathic Cystinosis: A Genotype/Phenotype Correlation
Reprinted from: *Cells* **2021**, *10*, 2498, doi:10.3390/cells10092498 187

Anna Taranta, Mohamed A. Elmonem, Francesco Bellomo, Ester De Leo, Sara Boenzi, Manoe J. Janssen, Amer Jamalpoor, Sara Cairoli, Anna Pastore, Cristiano De Stefanis, Manuela Colucci, Laura R. Rega, Isabella Giovannoni, Paola Francalanci, Lambertus P. van den Heuvel, Carlo Dionisi-Vici, Bianca M. Goffredo, Rosalinde Masereeuw, Elena Levtchenko and Francesco Emma
Benefits and Toxicity of Disulfiram in Preclinical Models of Nephropathic Cystinosis
Reprinted from: *Cells* **2021**, *10*, 3294, doi:10.3390/cells10123294 203

About the Editor

Elena N. Levtchenko

Elena Levtchenko is the division chief of Pediatric Nephrology in the University Hospitals Leuven and a full professor of Medicine at the Katholieke Universiteit (KU) Leuven. She started to study cystinosis as a Ph.D. student supervised by Prof. Leo Monnens in Radboud University Medical Centre, The Netherlands. Since then, Dr. Levtchenko devoted her carrier to unraveling the disease mechanisms, finding new treatment, and improving the clinical care of patients with cystinosis.

Preface to "Cellular and Molecular Mechanisms of Nephropathic Cystinosis"

Cystinosis has much to offer as a model disease – multisystem involvement, disease progression, fascinating histopathology, definitive diagnostics, symptomatic and directed therapies involving small molecules and other interventions, unsolved cell biological mysteries, robust clinical and basic research, substantial academic interest and financial support, numerous active advocacy groups, and a rich history of investigations. It is no wonder that a Special Issue of *Cells* is devoted to this intriguing lysosomal storage disease.

It is also most appropriate to dedicate this issue to the father of cystinosis research, Jerry Schneider, MD. Jerry identified the lysosomal location of cystine storage, trained a generation of clinical and basic investigators, fostered the formation of advocacy groups, and formed a community dedicated to the advancement of our understanding and treatment of cystinosis. He would beam with pride to see the articles in this issue elucidating the natural history of muscle, bone, central nervous system, and testicular involvement; model systems and biomarkers to study renal tubular dysfunction; mechanisms of cell death, autophagy, and inflammation; therapeutic benefits of cysteamine; and the potential for gene therapy. Perhaps the most impactful contribution will be the introduction of molecular-based newborn screening for cystinosis, which would bring current and future therapies to cystinosis patients shortly after birth, before significant kidney damage ensues. This is the yield of Jerry's early work, the harvest of the seed he sowed.

William A. Gahl
National Institute of Health
Bethesda, USA

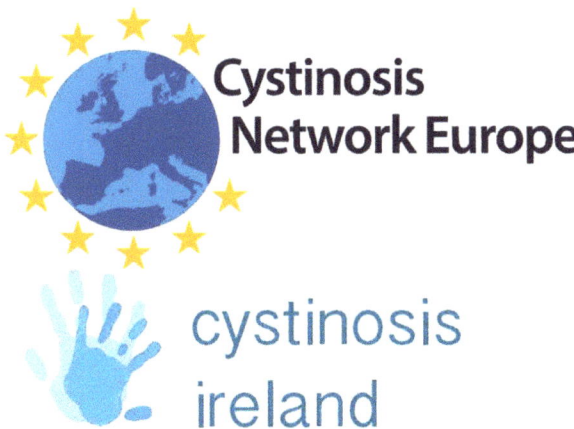

Acknowledgements

The Guest Editor and the authors are grateful for the financial support of Cystinosis Network Europe (CNE) and Cystinosis Ireland that was indispensable for this Special Issue.

The Special Issue is endorsed by the European Reference Kidney Network (ERKNet).

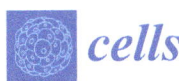

Editorial

A Personal History of Cystinosis by Dr. Jerry Schneider

Jerry Schneider [1] and Elena Levtchenko [2,3,*]

[1] Department of Pediatrics, School of Medicine, University of California San Diego, La Jolla, CA 92093, USA; jschneider@ucsd.edu
[2] Department of Development and Regeneration, Katholieke Universiteit (KU) Leuven, 3000 Leuven, Belgium
[3] Department of Paediatrics, Division of Nephrology, University Hospitals Leuven, 3000 Leuven, Belgium
* Correspondence: elena.levtchenko@uzleuven.be; Tel.: +32-16-34-13-62

Abstract: Cystinosis is a rare lysosomal storage disease that is tightly linked with the name of the American physician and scientist Dr. Jerry Schneider. Dr. Schneider (1937–2021) received his medical degree from Northwestern University, followed by a pediatrics residency at Johns Hopkins University and a fellowship in inherited disorders of metabolism. He started to work on cystinosis in J. Seegmiller's laboratory at the National Institutes of Health (NIH) and subsequently moved to the UC San Diego School of Medicine, where he devoted his entire career to people suffering from this devastating lysosomal storage disorder. In 1967, Dr. Schneider's seminal *Science* paper 'Increased cystine in leukocytes from individuals homozygous and heterozygous for cystinosis' opened a new era of research towards understanding the pathogenesis and finding treatments for cystinosis patients. His tremendous contribution transformed cystinosis from a fatal disorder of childhood to a treatable chronic disease, with a new generation of cystinosis patients being now in their 40th and 50th years. Dr. Schneider wrote a fascinating 'Personal History of Cystinosis' highlighting the major milestones of cystinosis research. Unfortunately, he passed away before this manuscript could be published. Fifty-five years after his first paper on cystinosis, the 'Personal History of Cystinosis' by Dr. Schneider is a tribute to his pioneering discoveries in the field and an inspiration for young doctors and scientists who have taken over the torch of cystinosis research towards finding a cure for cystinosis.

Keywords: cystinosis; lysosomal storage disorder; history; treatment strategies for cystinosis

Citation: Schneider, J.; Levtchenko, E. A Personal History of Cystinosis by Dr. Jerry Schneider. *Cells* **2022**, *11*, 945. https://doi.org/10.3390/cells11060945

Received: 21 February 2022
Accepted: 23 February 2022
Published: 10 March 2022

Publisher's Note: MDPI stays neutral with regard to jurisdictional claims in published maps and institutional affiliations.

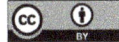

Copyright: © 2022 by the authors. Licensee MDPI, Basel, Switzerland. This article is an open access article distributed under the terms and conditions of the Creative Commons Attribution (CC BY) license (https://creativecommons.org/licenses/by/4.0/).

1. Introduction

When people write about the history of cystinosis, they usually start with Emil Abderhalden, who in 1903 described cystine crystals in the liver and spleen at the autopsy of a 21-month-old child [1]. For the next 30 years, physicians reported occasional cases of "cystine storage diseases" in children. It is not possible to know which of these patients actually had cystinosis because of the confusion between cystinosis and cystinuria at that time.

In cystinosis, cystine accumulates within cells [2], while in cystinuria, the cystine content of cells is normal, but the cystine concentration is elevated in the urine to such a degree that cystine can come out of solution and form cystine stones within the urinary tract [3]. Cystine was first discovered in renal stones from patients with cystinuria. These stones were found to be a unique compound by a British doctor, William Hyde Wollaston, who first called them "cystic oxide", cystic because the word cyst sometimes referred to the bladder in those days and oxide because Wollaston guessed they contained oxygen [4]. In fact, they did not contain oxygen, and the name was changed to cystine. Cystinuria is about ten times more common than cystinosis, but because the names of these conditions are so similar, people often get them confused.

2. Unravelling the Cellular Basis of Cystinosis

I saw my first cystinosis patient in 1965 at the National Institutes of Health (NIH) where I spent two years studying cystinosis in J. Seegmiller's laboratory. At that time, we knew that cystinosis patients had cystine crystals in most of their tissues. They also had delayed growth, very large urine volume, developed rickets and excreted excessive glucose and protein in their urine. We also knew it was an inherited disorder, but no one knew its cause. These patients had normal intelligence and, if treated symptomatically, would do relatively well for several years. Symptomatic treatment meant replacing orally what they lost in their urine. However, by 9–10 years of age, they were in end-stage kidney failure. At this time, neither renal dialysis nor transplantation was available for them. Since then, much has been learned about cystinosis, both the basic defect that causes this disorder and its treatment. I believe that each advance in our understanding of cystinosis is always followed new technology, often developed by scientists who have never heard of this disease. I will also discuss why it repeatedly took a long time to evaluate new potential treatments.

Early investigators had been stymied by the lack of a good method to measure cystine. I was very lucky that ion-exchange chromatography had just been developed to measure small amounts of amino acids [5]. Furthermore, there was an amino acid analyzer at the NIH that I could use. A visiting scientist at the NIH, John Crawhall, had just developed a better method to measure cystine with this analyzer and was eager to help me [6]. In addition, the company that manufactured this analyzer had just increased its sensitivity ten-fold. Without all of this help, my studies never would have succeeded.

When I looked at bone-marrow aspirates from cystinosis patients, I saw huge clumps of cystine crystals (Figure 1) [6]. I wondered if the crystals were inside or outside the cells. If the crystals were inside the cells, was the cystine concentration so great in these cells that the crystals formed intracellularly, or had the crystals formed extracellularly and been phagocytized (ingested) by the cells?

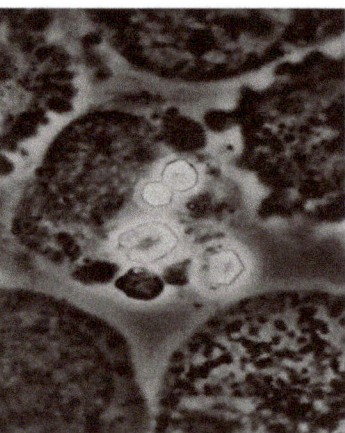

Figure 1. Cystine crystals seen in an unstained bone marrow aspirate obtained from a child at 10 weeks of age. (Phase Optics. ×1280) [6].

I also found that the solubility of cystine in human plasma at 37° and at physiological pH was about 50 times higher than the plasma cystine concentration in cystinosis patients. This proved to me that the cystine crystals must have formed intracellularly. I later found that a pathologist in Birmingham, England had come to the same conclusion by careful study of pathological sections from cystinosis patients.

I isolated leukocytes in small volumes of blood from cystinosis patients and found that the amount of soluble cystine in these cells was 50–100 times higher than in leukocytes isolated from individuals who did not have cystinosis [7]. We also performed the same measurements in cultured fibroblasts grown from skin biopsies of cystinosis patients and from normal controls. Although we never saw cystine crystals in cystinotic fibroblasts, once again the cystine content was 50–100 times higher in cells from cystinosis patients than in non-cystinotic control cells [8].

My two-year assignment in Seegmiller's lab was coming to an end and I performed one more experiment that excited me. I wondered if there was an enzyme that reduced cystine to cysteine ("half-cystine") that might be defective in cystinotic tissue. I decided to develop an essay for glutathione reductase and compare the activity of this enzyme in cystinotic compared to normal tissue. The idea was that glutathione reductase might indirectly reduce cystine to cysteine. In normal tissue, the cystine would be reduced to cysteine and be further metabolized, whereas in cystinotic tissue, the cystine would not be metabolized and would accumulate and form crystals. Sure enough, I found no glutathione reductase activity in the cystinotic tissue, but high amounts of glutathione reductase activity in the normal control tissue. I was very excited by this finding; fortunately, I decided to conduct control studies. I added cystine to normal tissue, and the activity of glutathione reductase disappeared. I dialyzed the cystinotic tissue for a long period with large volumes of solution to remove the cystine, and the activity of this enzyme returned to normal. It was obvious that cystine inhibited the activity of glutathione reductase. Some reading in the library informed me that cystine inhibits many common intracellular enzymes that are necessary for the normal life of cells. Just before leaving the NIH for further training in other areas of science, I conducted a brief experiment that demonstrated that cystine was somehow compartmentalized in the cell so that it did not inhibit the activity of important cellular enzymes.

The next physician who studied cystinosis in Seegmiller's laboratory was Joe Schulman. He found that the excess cystine in cystinotic tissue was located in the lysosomes of the cells. The Belgian scientist Christian de Duve shared the 1974 Nobel Prize in Physiology or Medicine for his discovery of lysosomes, an intracellular organelle that "digests" proteins and other cellular molecules [9]. Another Belgian investigator, Henri Géry Hers, later found that a defective lysosomal enzyme was the cause of a rare condition called Pompe Disease [10]. We now know that many other rare diseases result from the lack of a specific lysosomal enzyme. However, no lysosomal enzyme is known to metabolize cystine. At this point, we knew that cystine accumulated in cystinotic lysosomes, presumable from protein degradation, but did not understand why it accumulated in cystinotic and not in normal lysosomes.

Seegmiller moved to the University of California San Diego (UCSD) in 1969, and Schulman took over his NIH laboratory. In 1970, Seegmiller recruited me to UCSD, where I was able to establish my own laboratory in the Department of Pediatrics. Schulman and I were friends and decided we would both continue to study cystinosis. I decided the major problem we had in these studies was how time consuming and difficult it was to assay cystine. Since each assay took 8 h, we could only perform three cystine assays a day on our one amino acid analyzer (I had to come to the laboratory each evening at midnight to start the third measurement.) Fortunately, I learned that a biochemist (Clement Furlong) at the University of California Riverside was isolating proteins from the bacteria E. coli that had the property of specifically binding small molecules and that there was a cystine-binding protein. I thought this might allow us to develop a sensitive assay for cystine. I called Furlong and asked if he could help me isolate this protein. He told me he was preparing some of these proteins later that week and he thought he knew where the cystine-binding protein came off the column he used to prepare these proteins. He invited me to visit and take some of this material. I had a new post-doctoral fellow (Robert Oshima) who had just arrived and we drove to Riverside later that week (90 min drive). We returned that evening with a beaker full of solution that we hoped contained the cystine-binding protein. I went home for dinner and sleep. Oshima was too excited to sleep and worked all night with the material we obtained and the next morning told me he was certain it would work. We submitted a paper to the Journal of Biological Chemistry two months later describing the use of this cystine-binding protein to measure small amounts of cystine [11]. For many years this assay was the "gold standard" for measuring intracellular cystine.

3. Discovery of Cysteamine Treatment

Before I continue describing our laboratory studies, I must discuss some of the attempts to find a specific treatment for cystinosis. It is never easy to find a successful treatment for any disease, but in some cases it quickly becomes obvious that the treatment works. Of course, you have to be certain the treatment is not harmful, but at least you know if it works. For instance, if you develop an antibiotic for a certain bacterial infection, you soon learn if the antibiotic kills that bacteria. Cystinosis is much more difficult. The kidney damage we were attempting to arrest progresses very slowly, and our methods of measuring kidney function in children were not very exacting. We assumed that the cystine was causing the kidney damage, but we could not be certain. It was always possible that whatever was causing the storage of cystine was also causing the kidney damage, and that the two processes were not related. Fortunately, this was not to be the case, and measurement of leukocyte cystine proved to be an excellent marker of whether any particular drug was effective in treating cystinosis.

Over the years many approaches were tried to specifically treat cystinosis and they all seemed to work! I will discuss two treatments that did not work and one that did. Horst Bickel directed the first treatment I will discuss. Dr. Bickel trained in pediatrics from 1947 to 1949 at the University Children's Hospital in Zurich with Professor Fanconi. He then worked as a research fellow at the University Children's Hospital in Birmingham, England from 1949 to 1954. While in Birmingham, Bickel developed the successful treatment for another inherited metabolic disease, phenylketonuria (PKU). This condition was treated with a specific diet very low in the amino acid phenylalanine [12]. It was reasonable for Dr. Bickel to attempt a diet low in cystine and other sulfur-containing substances for the treatment of cystinosis. Initially, this diet seemed so successful that it was made and distributed by a major company. The children felt better, their schoolteachers and parents thought they were better, etc. I was still working at the NIH and started several cystinosis patients on this diet. I found that their plasma cystine concentration, which was normal to start, decreased significantly, but their leukocyte cystine content remained elevated. Years later, Dr. Bickel obtained data on all the patients who received this diet and learned that they had died sooner than expected. Apparently, the diet caused liver damage. The fact that they all felt the diet was working is called a "placebo effect".

Our group tried another treatment that did not work. A German post-doctoral fellow working in my lab (Wolfgang Kroll) found that adding fresh ascorbic acid (Vitamin C) to the culture media in which cystinotic fibroblasts were growing lowered the cystine content of the cells by over 50%. He was very eager to publish this finding. I thought we should try to understand why this occurred before submitting a paper for publication. Dr. Kroll was relentless in insisting we publish the finding even though we did not understand it. Furthermore, he wanted to submit it to the very prestigious journal, *Science*. I finally agreed to submit the paper being certain it would be promptly rejected and Dr. Kroll would learn to trust his mentor. To my astonishment, the paper was promptly accepted [13]. I was concerned that when this publication appeared every cystinotic patient in the world would be started on a high dose of Vitamin C, and it would take years before we knew if it worked. I promptly organized a placebo controlled, masked study. Sixty-four patients entered the study; half received high doses of Vitamin C and half received a placebo. They all were certain they were receiving the actual drug because they all felt better. They saw their physicians every 4 months for routine tests of kidney function, and the results were sent to a committee at the NIH who knew which patients were receiving the drug and which the placebo. After about 18 months, I received an emergency phone call from the committee telling me to stop the study at once because the patients receiving a high dose of Vitamin C were doing worse than the patients receiving the placebo. This study was published in the New England Journal of Medicine [14].

John Crawhall, the scientist who helped me at the NIH, began the study that did work. He was then working in Montreal but came to UCSD for a sabbatical and decided to add a variety of compounds to the media in which cystinotic cells were growing to see if any had an effect on the cystine content of these cells. The only compound that seemed to have such an effect was cysteamine (Figure 2). By the time we saw this result, Crawhall had returned to Montreal, and I assigned the project to a new post-doctoral fellow, Jess Thoene.

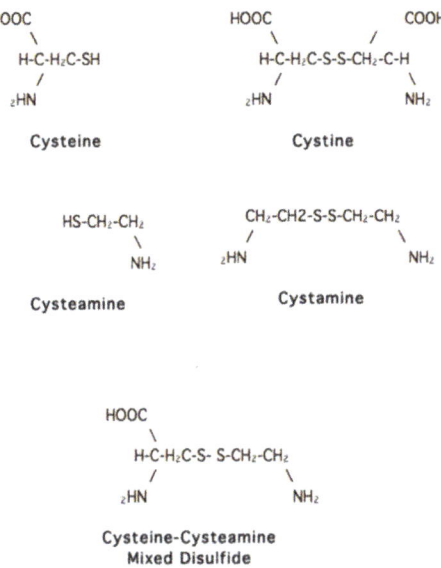

Figure 2. Structures of compounds mentioned in this article. The two compounds shown on the upper left are sulfhydryls because they have a -SH group. The compounds to their right are disulfides. The compound at the bottom is a mixed disulfide of two different compounds.

Cysteamine occurs naturally in humans, but at very low concentrations [15]. It was being used successfully in Europe as an antidote for an overdose of acetaminophen (called paracetamol in Europe and usually Tylenol in the USA). Experiments were also being conducted for its use as a radio-protective agent. Thoene found that cysteamine not only removed cystine from cystinotic cells in culture, but also removed the cystine from leukocytes in a cystinosis patient when given either intravenously or orally [16]. He worked out the proper dose to use orally, and this is essentially the same dose used today.

We joined with the NIH group of Joe Schulman, his post-doctoral fellow Bill Gahl and biostatistician James Schlesselman to start a large study. Many physicians contributed patients, including Michel Broyer in Paris and William van't Hoff in London. In 1987, we reported the success of cysteamine in treating cystinosis [17]. At first, we used cysteamine hydrochloride. It had to be distributed as a liquid and had a horrible smell and taste. We next used phosphocysteamine. In its pure form it was odorless, but we could not obtain this chemical in the pure form in the quantities required. It was somewhat better than cysteamine hydrochloride, but still difficult for patients to take and could not be manufactured in a way that regulatory agencies would ever approve.

4. Cystinosis as a Treatable Lysosomal Storage Disease

Meanwhile, we continued to search for the metabolic defect in cystinosis. We all agreed that the most likely cause was a transport defect in the lysosomal membrane. As proteins are digested in the lysosomes, individual amino acids are released. Specific transporters exist in the lysosomal membrane that carry specific amino acids from the lysosome to the cytoplasm of the cell. Could the transporter for cystine be missing in cystinosis lysosomes? None of us knew how to test this idea. Eric Harms visited our laboratory from Germany and helped us isolate excellent preparations of lysosomes, but we still did not know how to study transport in the lysosomes. The breakthrough came when Frank Tietze, a biochemist at the NIH, saw a paper in the Journal of Biological Chemistry and pointed it out to Drs. Schulman and Gahl at the NIH. This paper described a method of loading lysosomes with a specific amino acid [18]. Thus, we could study the egress of this amino acid from the lysosome. Dr. Schulman pointed out this paper to my post-graduate fellow, Adam Jonas, and me. We decided that the NIH group would study this method in cystinotic leukocytes, and the UCSD group would use cultured cystinotic fibroblasts. At UCSD, we were greatly helped by the contributions of Drs. Margaret Smith and Alice Greene. Both groups found that the lysosomal transport of cystinosis was defective in cystinotic cells (Figure 3) [19,20].

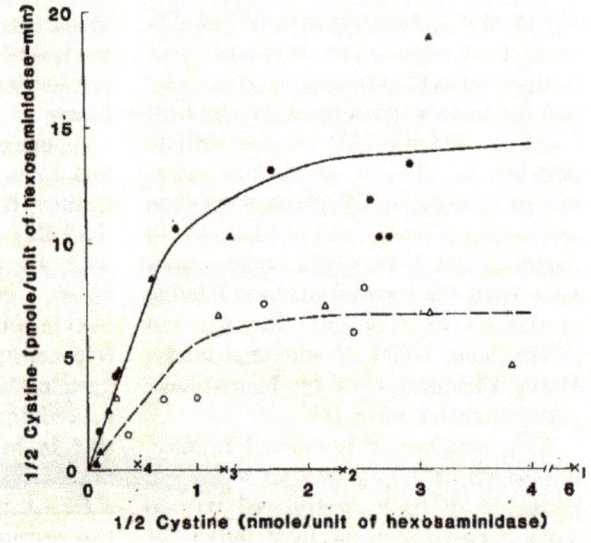

Figure 3. Lysosomes from cystinosis patients (x), their parents (open symbols) and normal controls (filled symbols) were loaded with cystine, and the initial velocity of cystine egress was compared [20].

The groups at the NIH and the University of Michigan (Jess Thoene, Halvor Christensen and Ron Pisoni) found that cysteamine works in the cystinotic lysosome by "attacking" the cystine molecule and forming a "mixed disulfide" of half cystine and cysteamine. This "mixed disulfide" resembles the amino acid lysine and exits the lysosome via the alternative transporting system that is normal in cystinotic lysosomes [21]. Finally, Corinne Antignac's group in Paris found that the defective gene in cystinosis is located on chromosome 17 and encodes the lysosomal cystine transporter cystinosin [22].

In the 1980s, we began to use cysteamine bitartrate to treat cystinosis. Although this drug is also difficult to synthesize, a company in Italy was producing it. The drug was stable as a solid and more acceptable for patients. In 1994, the United States Food and Drug Administration (FDA) approved cysteamine bitartrate for the treatment of cystinosis. Although this formulation of cysteamine was very effective in removing cystine from cystinotic cells, it still had several problems as a drug for cystinosis. It has a very bad smell and taste, and must be taken every 6 h to be completely effective. Elena Levtchenko, in Belgium, showed that if a patient went 8 h between doses, for instance while sleeping, the leukocyte cystine content went unacceptably high in the last two hours [23]. For acceptable treatment, neither the patient nor his/her caregivers ever had a full night sleep. A pediatric gastroenterologist Ranjan Dohil performed careful studies of cysteamine uptake by the intestine and developed a way to package cysteamine so that it would be easier for patients to take and would only have to be taken every 12 h [24]. Recently, the FDA and EMA approved this new extended-release form of cysteamine.

If started early in life, cysteamine bitartrate slows the progression of kidney glomerular but not kidney tubular damage. Studies from both the NIH and Hôpital Necker Enfants-Malades in Paris found that, even if started at an older age, cysteamine delays the progression of hypothyroidism, diabetes and neuromuscular disorders [25,26]. However, this is not a cure for cystinosis. Stephanie Cherqui, one of Antignac's students, moved to San Diego, and using a mouse model of cystinosis that she had developed in Antignac's laboratory, used hematopoietic stem cell (HSC) gene therapy to essentially correct the cystinosis defect in the mouse organs [27]. Currently, a clinical trial is underway to test the effect of gene-corrected autologous HSC in cystinosis patients [28].

5. Conclusions

Jerry Schneider devoted his whole career to unraveling the disease mechanisms and finding a curative therapy for cystinosis. His work transformed cystinosis from a fatal condition of childhood into a treatable disease with which patients can now reach advanced adult age. Dr. Schneider inspired several generations of clinicians and researchers to take over the torch of cystinosis research and to find cure for this devastating disorder. Fifty fine years after the first pioneering paper on cystinosis in *Science* 1967, the Special Issue of Cells is devoted to cystinosis and to the tremendous contribution of Dr. Schneider as a pioneer and founder of cystinosis research.

Conflicts of Interest: J. Schneider was a consultant for Raptor Pharmaceutical Company, the manufacturer of the new form of cysteamine. E. Levtchenko performs consultancy for Recordati, Chiesi, Kyowa Kirin and Advicenne and was supported by a research grant of Horizon Pharma.

References

1. Aberhalden, E. Familiäre Cystindiathese. *Z. Physiol. Chem.* **1903**, *38*, 557–561. [CrossRef]
2. Gahl, W.A.; Thoene, J.G.; Schneider, J.A. Cystinosis. *N. Eng. J. Med.* **2002**, *347*, 111–121. [CrossRef]
3. Dello Strologo, L.; Laurenzi, C.; Legato, A.; Pastore, A. Cystinuria in children and young adults: Success of monitoring free-cystine urine levels. *Pediatr. Nephrol.* **2007**, *22*, 1869–1873. [CrossRef] [PubMed]
4. Wollaston, W. On cystic oxide: A new species of urinary calculus. *Philos. Trans. R. Soc. Lond.* **1810**, *100*, 223–230. [CrossRef]
5. Crawhall, J.C.; Scowen, E.F.; Thompson, C.J.; Watts, R.W.E. The renal clearanc of amino acids in cystinuria. *J. Clin. Investig.* **1967**, *46*, 1162–1171. [CrossRef] [PubMed]
6. Schneider, J.A.; Wong, V.; Seegmiller, J.E. The early diagnosis of cystinosis. *J. Pediatr.* **1969**, *74*, 114–116. [CrossRef]
7. Schneider, J.A.; Bradley, K.; Seegmiller, J. Increased cystine in leukocytes from individuals homozygous and heterozygous for cystinosis. *Science* **1967**, *157*, 1321–1322. [CrossRef] [PubMed]
8. Schneider, J.A.; Rosenbloom, F.M.; Bradley, K.H.; Seegmiller, J.E. Increased free-cystine content of fibroblasts cultured from patients with cystinosis. *Biochem. Biophys. Res. Commun.* **1967**, *29*, 527–531. [CrossRef]
9. De Duve, C. The significance of lysosomes in pathology and medicine. *Proc. Int. Med. Chic.* **1966**, *26*, 73–76.
10. De Barsy, T.; Jacquemin, P.; Devos, P.H.H. Rodent and human acid -glucosidase. Purification, properties and inhibition by antibodies. Investigation in type II glycogenosis. *Eur. J. Biochem.* **1972**, *31*, 156–165. [CrossRef]
11. Oshima, R.G.; Willis, R.C.; Furlong, C.E.; Schneider, J.A. Binding assays for amino acids. The utilization of a cystine binding protein from Escherichia coli for the determination of acid-soluble cystine in small physiological samples. *J. Biol. Chem.* **1974**, *249*, 6033–6039. [CrossRef]
12. Bickel, H. The effects of a phenylalanine-free and phenylalanine-poor diet in phenylpyruvic oligophrenis. *Exp. Med. Surg.* **1954**, *12*, 114–118.
13. Kroll, W.; Schneider, J. Decrease in free cystine content of cultured cystinotic fibroblasts by ascorbic acid. *Science* **1974**, *186*, 1040–1042. [CrossRef]
14. Schneider, J.; Schlesselman, J.; Mendoza, S.; Orloff, S.; Thoene, J.; Kroll, W.; Godfrey, A.; Schulman, J. Ineffectiveness of ascorbic acid therapy in nephropathic cystinosis. *N. Eng. J. Med.* **1979**, *300*, 756–759. [CrossRef]
15. Coloso, R.; Hirschberger, L.; Dominy, J.; Lee, J.; Stipanuk, M. Cysteamine dioxygenase: Evidence for the physiological conversion of cysteamine to hypotaurine in rat and mouse tissues. *Adv. Exp. Med. Biol.* **2006**, *583*, 25–36.
16. Thoene, J.G.; Oshima, R.G.; Crawhall, J.C.; Schneider, J.A. Cystine depletion of cystinotic cells by aminothiols. *Proc. R. Soc. Med.* **1977**, *70* (Suppl. S3), 37–40. [CrossRef]
17. Gahl, W.A.; Reed, G.F.; Thoene, J.G.; Schulman, J.D.; Rizzo, W.B.; Jonas, A.J.; Denman, D.W.; Schlesselman, J.J.; Corden, B.J.; Schneider, J.A. Cysteamine therapy for children with nephropathic cystinosis. *N. Eng. J. Med.* **1987**, *316*, 971–977. [CrossRef]
18. Reeves, J.P. Accumulation of amino acids by lysosomes incubated with amino acid methyl esters. *J. Biol. Chem.* **1979**, *254*, 8914–8921. [CrossRef]

19. Jonas, A.J.; Greene, A.A.; Smith, M.L.; Schneider, J.A. Cystine accumulation and loss in normal, heterozygous, and cystinotic fibroblasts. *Proc. Natl. Acad. Sci. USA* **1982**, *79*, 4442–4445. [CrossRef]
20. Gahl, W.; Bashan, N.; Tietze, F.; Bernardini, I.; Schneider, J. Cystine transport is defective in isolated leukocyte lysosomes from patients with cystinosis. *Science* **1982**, *217*, 1263–1265. [CrossRef]
21. Pisoni, R.L.; Thoene, J.G.; Christensen, H.N. Detection and Characterization of Carrier-mediated Cationic Amino Acid Transport in Lysosomes of Normal and Cystinotic Human Fibroblasts. *J. Biol. Chem.* **1985**, *260*, 4791–4798. [CrossRef]
22. Town, M.; Jean, G.; Cherqui, S.; Attard, M.; Forestier, L.; Whitmore, S.A.; Callen, D.F.; Gribouval, O.; Broyer, M.; Bates, G.P.; et al. A novel gene encoding an integral membrane protein is mutated in nephropathic cystinosis. *Nat. Genet.* **1998**, *18*, 319–324. [CrossRef]
23. Levtchenko, E.N.; van Dael, C.M.; de Graaf-Hess, A.C.; Wilmer, M.J.; van den Heuvel, L.P.; Monnens, L.A.; Blom, H.J. Strict cysteamine dose regimen is required to prevent nocturnal cystine accumulation in cystinosis. *Pediatr. Nephrol.* **2006**, *21*, 110–113. [CrossRef]
24. Brodin-Sartorius, A.; Tête, M.J.; Niaudet, P.; Antignac, C.; Guest, G.; Ottolenghi, C.; Charbit, M.; Moyse, D.; Legendre, C.; Lesavre, P.; et al. Cysteamine therapy delays the progression of nephropathic cystinosis in late adolescents and adults. *Kidney Int.* **2012**, *81*, 179–189. [CrossRef]
25. Nesterova, G.; Gahl, W. Nephropathic cystinosis: Late complications of a multisystemic disease. *Pediatr. Nephrol.* **2008**, *23*, 863–878. [CrossRef]
26. Dohil, R.; Fidler, M.; Gangoiti, J.A.; Kaskel, F.; Schneider, J.A.; Barshop, B.A. Twice-Daily Cysteamine Bitartrate Therapy for Children with Cystinosis. *J. Pediatr.* **2010**, *156*, 71–75.e3. [CrossRef]
27. Syres, K.; Harrison, F.; Tadlock, M.; Jester, J.V.; Simpson, J.; Roy, S.; Salomon, D.R.; Cherqui, S. Successful treatment of the murine model of cystinosis using bone marrow cell transplantation. *Blood* **2009**, *114*, 2542–2552. [CrossRef]
28. Rocca, C.J.; Cherqui, S. Potential use of stem cells as a therapy for cystinosis. *Pediatr. Nephrol.* **2019**, *34*, 965–973. [CrossRef] [PubMed]

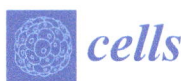

Review

Newborn Screening: Review of its Impact for Cystinosis

Katharina Hohenfellner [1,*], Ewa Elenberg [2], Gema Ariceta [3], Galina Nesterova [4], Neveen A. Soliman [5] and Rezan Topaloglu [6]

1. Department of Pediatric Nephrology, RoMed Clinis, Pettenkoferstr. 10, 83022 Rosenheim, Germany
2. Department of Pediatrics, Texas Children's Hospital, Baylor College of Medicine, 6701 Fannin Street 11th Floor, Houston, TX 77030, USA; exelenbe@texaschildrens.org
3. Department of Pediatric Nephrology, University Hospital Vall d' Hebron, University Autonomous Barcelona, Passeig de la Vall d'Hebron, 119-129, 08035 Barcelona, Spain; gariceta@vhebron.net
4. Cystinosis Research Network, Medical Advisory Committee, Chicago, IL 60045, USA; gnesterova@hotmail.com
5. Department of Pediatrics, Center of Pediatric Nephrology and Transplantation (CPNT), Kasr Al Ainy Faculty of Medicine, Cairo University, 99 El-Manial Street, Cairo 11451, Egypt; neveenase@yahoo.com
6. Department of Pediatric Nephrology, Hacettepe University School of Medicine, Ankara 06610, Turkey; rezantopaloglu@hacettepe.edu.tr
* Correspondence: Katharina.Hohenfellner@ro-med.de

Abstract: Newborn screening (NBS) programmes are considered to be one of the most successful secondary prevention measures in childhood to prevent or reduce morbidity and/or mortality via early disease identification and subsequent initiation of therapy. However, while many rare diseases can now be detected at an early stage using appropriate diagnostics, the introduction of a new target disease requires a detailed analysis of the entire screening process, including a robust scientific background, analytics, information technology, and logistics. In addition, ethics, financing, and the required medical measures need to be considered to allow the benefits of screening to be evaluated at a higher level than its potential harm. Infantile nephropathic cystinosis (INC) is a very rare lysosomal metabolic disorder. With the introduction of cysteamine therapy in the early 1980s and the possibility of renal replacement therapy in infancy, patients with cystinosis can now reach adulthood. Early diagnosis of cystinosis remains important as this enables initiation of cysteamine at the earliest opportunity to support renal and patient survival. Using molecular technologies, the feasibility of screening for cystinosis has been demonstrated in a pilot project. This review aims to provide insight into NBS and discuss its importance for nephropathic cystinosis using molecular technologies.

Keywords: newborn screening; infantile nephropathic cystinosis; clinical course; *CTNS*-pathogenic variants; newborn screening for cystinosis

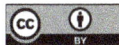

1. Introduction

Newborn screening programmes (NBS) aim to identify presymptomatic newborns with rare serious or fatal disorders that can be successfully treated, thereby achieving a significant reduction in morbidity and mortality [1]. NBS programmes are now implemented in more than 50 countries worldwide [1].

NBS represents a mostly underestimated, complex process involving different representatives of the public healthcare system to enable sample collection, analysis, communication of the result and, if necessary, coordination of treatment initiation, within a narrow time window [2,3]. Accordingly, there are high demands on the process quality of an NBS programme in terms of communication, logistics, analysis, and evaluation.

NBS programmes are country-specific and dependent on their respective healthcare systems, with their associated socio-economic, cultural, ethical, and legal requirements [1,4–7]. Before introducing screening or adding another target disease, the benefits (reduction in morbidity and mortality), harms (overdiagnosis, false positives, false negatives), and costs incurred during the screening process (implementation of screening and subsequent treatment costs) have to be assessed, taking into account available resources (human, analytics, information systems) and ethical aspects [2,8–11].

The history of NBS is closely linked to the fate of Dr Robert Guthrie. In the early 1950s, Horst Bickel demonstrated that the implementation of a low-phenylalanine diet from an early age could prevent the mental retardation associated with phenylketonuria (PKU) [12]. While the diagnosis of PKU in the early 1960s utilized the presence of phenylpyruvic acid in the urine, the sensitivity of this method was not sufficient enough to identify patients prior to the development of irreversible brain damage [13]. Following bacteriological tests used in cancer research, Dr Guthrie developed a test that could be used as a screening method for PKU [14]. In 1961, the first screening of newborns began, and by 1965 all newborns had been screened for PKU in the USA [15]. In the following years, a programme of NBS concerning PKU was established in other countries and was successively extended to include other diseases, due to the availability of newer technologies (radioimmunoassay, colorimetric and fluorometric assays, and enzymatic, isoelectric focusing, high-performance liquid-chromatography) [16]. The methodological limitation of NBS in the mid-1990s was the number of individual tests required for the various diseases. With the introduction of tandem mass spectrometry (MS/MS), which enables the cost-effective simultaneous identification of up to 50 metabolic conditions from amino acid metabolism, organic acid metabolism, and fatty acid degradation from a single blood spot, this limitation could be overcome [17]. Several new additions to NBS programmes, such as those for cystic fibrosis [18], severe combined immunodeficiency (SCID) [19], and spinal muscular atrophy (SMA) [20], have been possible following the introduction of molecular technologies.

The screening framework was formulated by Wilson and Jungner in 1968 under the auspices of the World Health Organization (WHO) and is still valid today in an adapted form [21,22]. According to these principles, each target disease requires clarification of sufficient available knowledge, and it needs to represent a relevant health problem for the individual/population group which cannot be diagnosed clinically with certainty in the neonatal period. In addition, appropriate therapy must be available, with early initiation of treatment resulting in reduced morbidity and mortality. The screening test procedure should display high sensitivity and specificity, be cost-effective, and any benefit/harm assessment of test must be on the side of 'benefit' [21] (Table 1).

Table 1. Principles of screening by Wilson and Jungner (1968).

1.	The condition sought should be an important health problem.
2.	There should be an accepted treatment for patients with recognized disease.
3.	Facilities for diagnosis and treatment should be available.
4.	There should be a recognizable latent or early symptomatic stage.
5.	There should be a suitable test or examination.
6.	The test should be acceptable to the population.
7.	The natural history of the condition, including development from latent to declared disease, should be adequately understood.
8.	There should be an agreed policy on whom to treat as patients.
9.	The cost of case finding (including diagnosis and treatment of patients diagnosed) should be economically balanced in relation to possible expenditure on medical care as a whole.
10.	Case finding should be a continuing process and not a "once and for all" project.

NBS involves examining a large population of clinically inconspicuous newborns in order to identify very few affected children [3,23,24]. Of note, 99.9% of all children examined in NBS programmes are found to be without any noticeable finding [3,23,24]. As such, this necessitates the use of a subsequent stepwise analytical approach. The initial analytical test method must have a high sensitivity and specificity and should be able to identify or exclude the disease with the highest possible certainty (Figure 1) [23]. If the screening result is positive, the individual is not necessarily ill, but does require a more disease-specific workup. The recall rate describes the percentage of control examinations due to a conspicuous finding in the initial screening. The positive predictive value indicates the probability of actually having the disease in the case of a positive test result, depending on the prevalence of the target disease and the specificity of the chosen method.

Test results	Positive	Negative
Child with disease	Real positive	False negative
Child without disease	False positive	Real negative

Sensitivity = $\dfrac{\text{real positive}}{\text{real positive + false negative}}$

Specificity = $\dfrac{\text{real negative}}{\text{real negative + false positive}}$

Positive predictive value (PPV) = $\dfrac{\text{real positive}}{\text{real positive + false positive}}$

Negative predictive value = $\dfrac{\text{real negative}}{\text{real negative + false negative}}$

Recall rate = Requested repeat examinations due to abnormal findings (recall)

Figure 1. Test results and quality parameters in neonatal screening. Sensitivity: Ability of the test to accurately identify those individuals with a specific condition/disease. Specificity: Ability of the test to accurately identify those individuals without the condition/disease. Positive predictive value (PPV): Probability that the person tested has the disease when the test is positive. Negative predictive value: Probability that the person does not have the disease, when the test is negative.

From a diagnostic perspective, the aim of NBS is to increase the specificity of the analysis and to identify individuals with mild phenotypes, i.e., carriers not requiring treatment, thus reducing costs and the psychological burden on the parents caused by unnecessary further examinations. The notification of a positive finding always causes a high burden for the family [25,26]. Parents of children with a false-positive screening result for a metabolic genetic disease have a 23% higher stress level [25], while a 143% increase in depressive mood has been reported in parents with false-positive results for cystic fibrosis [26].

So far, NBS programmes have demonstrated both substantial benefits and deficits, preventing the full benefit of NBS from being achieved [27,28]. Only a few screening programmes, such as those in Sweden or the German state of Bavaria, include matching with a birth registry and allow completeness of coverage to be verified [29]. In addition, despite considerable effort and expense at all levels, tracking systems that follow up positive screenings to verify that controls and/or confirmation diagnostics have been performed and therapy has been initiated are not available in most countries. Long-term systematic monitoring (clinical and laboratory parameters) of diagnosed patients identified by screening is also not ensured [30]. The lack of feedback from or recording of those patients not identified during the screening process remains largely unregulated, preventing any valid and robust statement being made on the sensitivity of NBS. Considering the rarity of most diseases in any newborn panel, there is an ongoing need to combine all available data to provide a clearer clinical picture on confirmed genotype/phenotype correlation and the different expression of the diseases, age of disease onset, and treatment response.

Regarding the target diseases, there are significant differences even within Western countries [5,31]. NBS programmes in European Union (EU) member states differ significantly in terms of target diseases, among other factors [5]. NBS in France, Germany, and Austria includes 9, 17, and 26 target diseases, respectively [5]. There are no current policy recommendations or direct NBS overview at a European level as the sole responsibility for setting health policy and managing health/medical care, including financing of services and overall scope, lies with the respective member states. Harmonization of NBS programmes for target diseases at a European level is a current request of the European patient organization EURORDIS [32,33]. Central efforts to standardize NBS have been underway in the USA since 2000 [34–36]. With the help of the American Academy of Pediatrics Task Force, the Advisory Committee on Heritable Disorders in Newborn and Children (ACHDNC) was established. The American College of Medical Genetics (ACMG) created an evidence-based core screening panel in 2005, which was subsequently adopted as the recommended uniform screening panel by the ACHDNC and recommended by the Secretary of Human Services [31,37]. This screening panel contains 35 core conditions and 29 secondary conditions (differential diagnostic features) which have been adopted and implemented by almost all US states.

2. Cystinosis

Cystinosis is a rare autosomal recessive systemic disease with high morbidity and mortality caused by pathogenic variants in the *CTNS* gene that encodes the lysosomal cystine transporter cystinosin, leading to accumulation of cystine within the lysosome [38,39]. Life-long cystine-depleting therapy with oral cysteamine, the only specific therapy for cystinosis, along with the availability of renal replacement therapy in childhood, has dramatically improved patient outcomes [40]. There is robust evidence that early initiation and sustained therapy with cysteamine are both essential for delaying progression to chronic kidney disease (CKD) and end-organ damage [41].

Infantile nephropathic cystinosis is the most common cause of renal Fanconi syndrome in children and is a hallmark of the disease [42]. Renal Fanconi syndrome presents with proximal renal tubular acidosis along with a generalized dysfunction of the proximal tubule, characterized by the presence of polyuria, glycosuria, phosphaturia, tubular proteinuria, growth retardation, and rickets; later glomerular involvement leads to progressive kidney failure. The proximal tubular cells (PTCs) are first to be affected [43]. However, evidence from mouse models suggests that differentiation (structural changes) of PTCs starts prior to the accumulation of cystine crystals in both PTCs and the interstitium, leading to a loss of their brush border, flattening and thickening of tubular basement membrane, and the eventual development of the characteristic swan-neck deformity [44]. These changes progress to tubular atrophy and, in addition, heavy inflammatory cell infiltrates can be observed in the renal interstitium. Glomerular involvement with multinucleated podocytes and focal segmental glomerulosclerosis lesions can be seen in renal biopsies [42]. While the defect in cystine transport by cystinosin is the hallmark of cystinosis, it is not the only key player in the pathogenesis of renal Fanconi syndrome; cystinosin has additional roles, including regulation of autophagy, mTOR signalling, lysosomal biogenesis, and vesicle trafficking in proximal tubular epithelial cells.

Early diagnosis of cystinosis enables treatment with cysteamine, the only specific therapy for the disease, which should be administered as early as possible and continued throughout the life of the patient [38]. It is well accepted that early treatment with cysteamine improves patient outcome, delays progression to renal failure with a mean age of 9 years when starting dialysis, and prevents or attenuates end-organ damage [41,45–49]. Initiation of cysteamine before 3, 2.5, or even <2 years of age has been associated with preservation of renal function in patients with cystinosis [40,45–47,50–52]; thus, patient age at initiation of cysteamine therapy appears to be a major predictive factor of renal survival. In a large international contemporary cohort of 453 patients with cystinosis, cysteamine was initiated in 89% of patients at a median age of 1.6 years, and a near linear relationship between the age of cysteamine initiation and renal function was observed [47]; patients treated before the age of 1 year exhibited the best renal outcome. All these findings provide the rationale to develop NBS to diagnose cystinosis as early as possible, ideally before the development of clinical manifestations and irreversible PTC damage prior to cystine crystal accumulation. Table 2 summarizes published evidence (in chronological order) of the impact of early treatment with cysteamine on renal outcome in patients with cystinosis [53].

Table 2. Impact of early initiation of oral cysteamine.

First Author, Year	Study Description	Impact of Early Initiation of Cysteamine on Renal Function	Impact of Early Initiation of Cysteamine on Extra-Renal Manifestations
Kleta, 2004 [40]	Family case report of two siblings (children)	A non-symptomatic child, identified after an affected brother who initiated cysteamine at 2 months of age, achieved and maintained normal renal function at 8 years of age. Patient's brother had CKD stage II at similar age despite treatment with cysteamine from 2 years of age	NR
Broyer, 2008 [50]	Necker Enfants-Malades Hospital series; patients born before 1988; aged 20–39 years (n = 56)	Initiation < 3 years of age vs. later delayed ESRD onset (mean age at onset 17.4 vs. 9.6 years)	Initiation < 3 years of age vs. later: Improved linear growth and visual acuity Reduced rates of glucose intolerance, thyroxine requirements, myopathy, cerebellar/pyramidal symptoms or mental deterioration, and hepatosplenic disorders
Greco, 2010 [45]	Italian single-centre study; patients diagnosed at 3–60 years of age; median follow-up 17.6 years (n = 23)	Initiation < 2.5 years of age vs. later improved evolution of renal function ($p = 0.006$), and decreased risk of CKD stage III	Patients treated more recently (initiated < 2.5 years of age) had improved linear growth curves vs. older children
Vaisbich, 2010 [51]	Brazilian multicentre nephropathic study; patients aged 1.3–29 years enrolled since 1999 (n = 102)	Initiation < 2 years of age vs. later reduced rate of CKD stage II–V (25% vs. 77.5%)	Initiation < 2 years of age vs. later: Improved growth (weight and height) parameters Reduced rates of hypothyroidism, diabetes, muscular weakness, hepatic dysfunction, CNS disorders, and swallowing dysfunction
Brodin-Sartorius, 2012 [46]	French study; adults (aged ≥15 years) diagnosed between 1961 and 1995 (n = 86)	Initiation < 5 years of age vs. later delayed ESRD onset (mean age at onset 13.4 vs. 9.6 years; $p < 0.05$)	Initiation < 5 years of age (vs. later or no treatment): reduced rates of hypothyroidism, diabetes, neuromuscular disorders, and death
Viltz, 2013 [54]	Children and adolescents (aged 3–18 years) [n = 46]	NR	Initiation < 2 years of age vs. later: improved cognitive function (verbal, performance, and full-scale IQ scores, and spatial-relations test), but not visual-motor performance scores
Bertholet-Thomas, 2017 [52]	Multinational study in children and adolescents from 41 centres and 30 nations (n = 213)	Earlier cysteamine treatment resulted in better renal outcome. Median renal survival increased up to 16.1 (12.5–/) years in patients treated at <2.5 years of age ($p = 0.0001$)	NR
Topaloglu, 2017 [49]	Multicentral study in children and adolescent from 26 centres [n = 136]	Patients in whom cysteamine treatment was initiated at age < 2 years old had delayed progression to renal failure compared to the patients in whom cysteamine treatment was initiated > 2 years ($p = 0.02$)	NR
Emma, 2021 [47]	Large international cohort of patients followed along five decades (n = 453)	A nearly linear relationship between the age at cysteamine initiation and renal survival was observed. Patients who started cysteamine aged < 1 year had delayed progression to renal failure in comparison with those who started aged 1–2 years old, and those who started cysteamine after 2 years of age (HR: 1.24; 95% CI: 1.9, 1.42; $p < 0.002$)	Initiation of cysteamine before the age of 1.5 years had a positive effect on growth with a gain of 0.57 SDSs in comparison with those who started cysteamine later.

CI, confidence interval; CKD, chronic kidney disease; CNS, central nervous system; ESRD, end-stage renal disease; HR, hazard ratio; NR, not referred; SDS, standard deviation score.

Progressive renal failure develops in most patients with nephropathic cystinosis [41,55]. Renal transplantation is the best therapeutic option for end-stage renal disease and improves both survival rate and quality of life [56]. More pre-emptive transplants in patients with cystinosis reflect temporal changes in paediatric transplantation practice [57]. Mortality in patients with cystinosis who undergo transplantation occurs at a late stage (10 years post-transplantation), frequently from extrarenal manifestations of cystinosis, and contrasts with a relatively good 5-year post-transplantation survival. Renal transplantation markedly improves the lifespan of patients with cystinosis, although cystine accumulation continues in non-renal organs [46]. While Fanconi syndrome does not recur in the transplanted organ, cysteamine therapy needs be continued for the lifetime of the patient to prevent extrarenal complications.

Beside time of diagnosis, adherence to cysteamine therapy is another critical factor for preservation of renal function [58]. The benefits of long-term cysteamine therapy are most evident in patients with good adherence to treatment.

3. Prenatal Testing and Preimplantation Genetic Diagnosis

Families known to be at risk of INC can consider options such as preimplantation genetic diagnosis or prenatal diagnosis [59]. There are two options for prenatal testing: biochemical testing and molecular genetic testing [59]. For pregnancies at risk of INC, prenatal diagnosis is possible biochemically, by measuring ^{35}S-labeled cystine accumulation in cultured amniocytes (14–16 weeks of gestation) or chorionic villi samples (CVS) (8–9 weeks of gestation) and by a direct measurement of cystine in uncultured CVS [60]. Once the *CTNS* pathogenic variants have been identified in an affected family member, for a pregnancy at increased risk and preimplantation genetic diagnosis for cystinosis are possible. Differences in perspective may exist among medical professionals and within families regarding the use of prenatal testing, particularly where this is being considered for the purpose of pregnancy termination rather than early diagnosis of a target disease. DNA analysis for detecting mutant alleles is currently the most frequently used antenatal screening method. While most clinical centres typically consider decisions regarding prenatal testing to be the parents' choice, discussion of any potential issues with the medical team remains important, together with the possible involvement of a genetic counsellor.

4. CTNS Pathogenic Variants in Different Countries

The *CTNS* gene for cystinosis, which encodes cystinosin, was identified by Town et al. in 1998 [39]. Since then, approximately 150 *CTNS* pathogenic variants have been described in patients with cystinosis worldwide [61]. The first pathogenic variant of the *CTNS* gene was reported as a large 57-kb deletion involving the first 9 exons and part of exon 10 of the *CTNS* gene, along with two upstream genes (*CARKL* and *TRPV1*). The 57-kb deletion is the most common pathogenic variant that causes cystinosis in Northern Europe and North America [62,63]. Germany is considered to be the country of origin for the 57-kb deletion which now accounts for 50–70% of the alleles in the USA and Northern Europe [63,64]. The frequency of the 57-kb deletion in patients with cystinosis is 22% in Mexico, 17% in Italy, and 0% in Turkey and Egypt [49,65–67].

A single-centre Turkish study and a Turkish national study based on the national registry of cystinosis confirmed that the most common allele (31%) in Turkey is c.681G>A (p.E227E), a missense pathogenic variant that causes a frameshift [49,68]. In Iran, the most common pathogenic variant is c.681G>A (p.E227E) [69]. Studies from Egypt show no patients with cystinosis having the 57-kb deletion, but they have confirmed that the c.829dup (p.T277NfsX19) is the most common *CTNS* pathogenic variant identified in a homozygous state among Egyptian patients with cystinosis [67]; this pathogenic variant has been reported only once in a heterozygous state in a European patient. The exclusive identification of c.681G>A (p.E227E) pathogenic variant, with variable frequencies, in the Middle Eastern population, along with its absence in European and American populations, suggests the existence of a possible founder pathogenic variant in this area.

c.1015G>A (G339R) has been identified as a founder pathogenic variant for cystinosis in the Ontario Amish Mennonite population in Canada [63]. This missense pathogenic variant has also been frequently observed in patients with cystinosis in Northern and Southern Italy, Spain, Turkey, and the Middle East [61,68]. Another possible founder pathogenic variant is c.971-12G>A which has been identified in the black population of South Africa [70]. A further pathogenic variant of interest is the nonsense stop codon pathogenic variant p.W138X, which accounts for 50% of cystinotic alleles in the French-Canadian population [71]. This novel stop codon pathogenic variant shows the possibility for read through in the presence of an aminoglycoside, which may enable a potential treatment.

The impact of the various types of *CTNS* pathogenic variants has been investigated and it is thought that individuals who harbour severe pathogenic variants, such as loss of function pathogenic variants on both alleles, have severe infantile cystinosis, while individuals homozygous or compound heterozygous for milder pathogenic variants have milder forms of the disease [41,63,72]. Homozygosity for the 57-kb deletion is associated with an increased risk of morbidity and mortality [41].

Of note, recent studies have shown that pathogenic variants appear to have no significant impact on either kidney function or progression to kidney failure in infantile cystinosis, whereas early initiation of cysteamine treatment has a significant impact on the preservation of renal function [47,49].

5. Newborn Screening for Cystinosis

The implementation of genetic testing in NBS was undertaken in Utah in 1998 for the detection of sickle cell disease [73]. Molecular biological methods have since been introduced as first tier, second tier, or third tier methods in NBS [74].

Currently, the diagnosis of cystinosis is based on the presence of elevated cystine levels in white blood cells [39]; this method is unsuitable for NBS. In 2018, as part of a pilot study, the existing German NBS programme was expanded to incorporate high-throughput first-tier molecular genetic screening for cystinosis and spinal muscular atrophy (SMA) [75,76]. Both congenital disorders are suitable for molecular-based NBS because they have known genetic causes and effective therapies are available. Based on the results of the pilot project, SMA screening has been successfully included as a regular part of NBS in Germany [77].

For cystinosis screening in Germany, the first tier involved multiplex PCR to detect the three most common *CTNS* pathogenic variants, i.e., a 57 kb deletion, c.18_21delGACT, p.T7Ffs*7, and c.926dupG, p.S310Qfs*55 [64]. Heterozygous samples were submitted to amplicon-based next-generation sequencing for 101 pathogenic *CTNS* pathogenic variants published at the time. A detection rate of 98.5% was subsequently predicted using this approach [75]. In 299,631 newborns, two patients with a homozygous 57-kb pathogenic variant and one patient with a 57-kb compound homozygous pathogenic variant were identified. A total of 805 patients with heterozygous pathogenic variants were identified, 655 with 57-kb pathogenic variant, 85 with c.18_21delGACT, p.T7Ffs*7, and 65 with c.926dupG, p.S310Qfs*55.

In the first patient identified with a homozygous 57-kb pathogenic variant and confirmed diagnosis by determining the leucocyte cystine level (2.82 nmol cystine/mg protein; normal, <0.2), treatment was initiated within the first month of life [78]. Even at the age of 3.5 years, the patient presented with normal physical development (height 20% percentile, weight 21% percentile) and without renal Fanconi syndrome or proteinuria. Apart from cysteamine treatment, the patient did not require any other pharmaceutical therapy. Unfortunately, the mother of the second patient with a homozygous 57-kb deletion initially refused NBS for cystinosis. At 8 months of age, the child was admitted to an intensive care unit with a severe electrolytic disturbance. In the course of the latter, a dried blood (DBS) card was re-sent to the screening laboratory and re-evaluated to include cystinosis, which yielded a positive test result. The patient then presented with the full clinical presentation of Fanconi syndrome and required high electrolyte replacement and growth hormone therapy in addition to cysteamine therapy. A third neonate, screened as heterozygous for the common 57-kb deletion, was found to harbour an additional promotor variant (c.-512G>C) in *CTNS* previously reported as being disease causing. However, according to current ACMG schemes, the respective promotor variant needs to be reclassified as a non-pathogenic change [78]. In fact, this infant showed no biochemical evidence of cystinosis, with a normal leucocyte cystine level, i.e., <0.2 nmol cystine/mg protein).

Detection rates estimate the known incidence of cystinosis at (1:150,000–1:200,000) [79]. False positive and false negative results did not occur until now. One key requirement of all NBS programmes is that they must provide direct clinical benefit [21]. Patients with cystinosis are generally diagnosed at 12–18 months of age, by which time significant renal tubular and glomerular damage has already occurred [58,80]. As previously described, early treatment with oral cysteamine has salutary effects on preservation of renal function, growth, and prevention of late complications of the disease [58]. For those few infants treated shortly after birth due to an older sibling already having cystinosis, even the renal tubular Fanconi syndrome that typically presents in the first months of life was ameliorated in these individuals [40].

Molecular screening for the 57-kb pathogenic variant can be combined with an existing NBS for severe combined immunodeficiency (SCID) and/or SMA. According to the results of the German pilot project, 655 of approximately 300,000 newborns carried a heterozygous 57-kb pathogenic variant, which required further screening with NGS for defined *CTNS*-pathogenic variants [78]. The feasibility of implementing NGS in a regular NBS programme has been demonstrated in Norway, where NBS was increased from 2 diseases to 25 in 2018 [24], using a second-tier strategy utilizing MS/MS methodologies and NGS for certain diseases. Thus, screening in Northern Europe and North America for the 57-kb pathogenic variant homozygous and heterozygous with downstream NGS, where the 57-kb allele accounts for 50–70% of the alleles, appears to be feasible [63,64]; this is further supported by the fact that also in other target diseases not all patients are identified (e.g., late-onset hypothyroidism and atypical adrenal hyperplasia).

Due to the heterogeneity of screening panels in different countries, the often slow and difficult implementation of additional target diseases, and the limited availability of genomic sequencing in public health and clinical settings, commercial laboratories have begun to offer genomic screening panels for newborns. Hopefully, these will not be as successful as the commercial tests already available from Ancestry, 23andMe, or MyHeritage, whose 2019 databases were estimated at 20 million, 12 million, and 2.5 million, respectively [81,82].

6. Conclusions

NBS programmes are secondary prevention measures in early childhood to prevent or reduce morbidity and/or mortality via early disease identification and subsequent initiation of therapy. Specific target diseases, and thus screening programs, may vary from country to country.

In cystinosis, both diagnosis and treatment at the earliest possible stage is the clinical goal. There is great hope that the use of neonatal testing to enable this early diagnosis and treatment, as discussed in this article, will provide a turning point in the natural history of cystinosis.

Given that more than 150 *CTNS* pathogenic variants have been described, countries/continents could implement NBS for the most commonly reported ones. For Northern Europe and North America, screening for the 57-kb deletion would prove useful and this could be augmented by other commonly reported pathogenic variants. However, this approach may not be possible in all countries, particularly those with limited resources and no known founder pathogenic variant.

In the future, we will have advanced packages for NBS, as early diagnosis and treatment of diseases will gain even more importance. In addition, other methods for early detection may be possible, such as preimplantation genetics and in vitro fertilization in families with known risks.

Author Contributions: K.H., E.E., G.A., N.A.S., G.N. and R.T. have written, reviewed, and edited the original draft. All authors have read and agreed to the published version of the manuscript.

Funding: Not applicable.

Conflicts of Interest: K.H., E.E., N.A.S. and G.N. have no competing interest. G.A. has received honoraria for lectures, presentations, or educational events from Alexion Pharmaceuticals, Recordati Rare Disease, Advicenne, Chiesi, Kyowa Kirim, support for attending meetings from Recordati Rare Disease, Kyowa Kirim, and Advicenne and for participating on Advisory Boards for Alexion Pharmaceuticals, Advicenne, Dicerna, and Alnylam. R.T. has received honorarium for lectures from Recordati and Alnylam.

References

1. Therrell, B.L.; Padilla, C.D.; Loeber, J.G.; Kneisser, I.; Saadallah, A.; Borrajo, G.J.; Adams, J. Current status of newborn screening worldwide: 2015. *Semin. Perinatol.* **2015**, *39*, 171–187. [CrossRef] [PubMed]
2. Cornel, M.; Rigter, T.; Weinreich, S.; Burgard, P.; Hoffmann, G.F.; Lindner, M.; Loeber, J.G.; Rupp, K.; Taruscio, D.; Vittozzi, L. Newborn Screening in Europe Expert Opinion. Available online: https://isns-neoscreening.org (accessed on 13 February 2022).
3. World Health Organization. Screening Programmes: A Short Guide. Available online: https://apps.who.int/iris/bitstream/handle/10665/330829/9789289054782-eng.pdf (accessed on 13 February 2022).
4. Therrell, B.L.; Lloyd-Puryear, M.A.; Ohene-Frempong, K.; Ware, R.E.; Padilla, C.D.; Ambrose, E.E.; Barkat, A.; Ghazal, H.; Kiyaga, C.; Mvalo, T.; et al. Empowering newborn screening programs in African countries through establishment of an international collaborative effort. *J. Community Genet.* **2020**, *11*, 253–268. [CrossRef] [PubMed]
5. Loeber, J.; Platis, D.; Zetterström, R.; Almashanu, S.; Boemer, F.; Bonham, J.; Borde, P.; Brincat, I.; Cheillan, D.; Dekkers, E.; et al. Neonatal Screening in Europe Revisited: An ISNS Perspective on the Current State and Developments Since 2010. *Int. J. Neonatal Screen.* **2021**, *7*, 15. [CrossRef] [PubMed]
6. McCandless, S.E.; Wright, E.J. Mandatory newborn screening in the United States: History, current status, and existential challenges. *Birth Defects Res.* **2020**, *112*, 350–366. [CrossRef]
7. Pollitt, R.J. Different Viewpoints: International Perspectives On Newborn Screening/Različita Gledišta: Međunarodne Perspektive U Vezi Sa Testiranjem Novorođenčadi. *J. Med. Biochem.* **2014**, *34*, 18–22. [CrossRef]
8. Alonso-Coello, P.; Schünemann, H.J.; Moberg, J.; Brignardello-Petersen, R.; Akl, E.A.; Davoli, M.; Treweek, S.; Mustafa, R.A.; Rada, G.; Rosenbaum, S.; et al. GRADE Evidence to Decision (EtD) frameworks: A systematic and transparent approach to making well informed healthcare choices. 1: Introduction. *BMJ* **2016**, *353*, i2016. [CrossRef]
9. Austoker, J. Gaining informed consent for screening. *BMJ* **1999**, *319*, 722–723. [CrossRef]
10. Ewart, R.M. Primum non nocere and the quality of evidence: Rethinking the ethics of screening. *J. Am. Board Fam. Pract.* **2000**, *13*, 188–196. [CrossRef]
11. Shickle, D.; Chadwick, R. The ethics of screening: Is "screenitis" an incurable disease? *J. Med. Ethics* **1994**, *20*, 8–12. [CrossRef]
12. Bickel, H.; Gerrard, J.; Hickmans, E. Preliminary Communication. *Lancet* **1953**, *262*, 812–813. [CrossRef]
13. Gonzalez, J.; Willis, M.S. Robert Guthrie, MD, PhD. *Lab. Med.* **2009**, *40*, 748–749. [CrossRef]
14. Guthrie, R.; Susi, A. A simple phenylalanine method for detecting phenylketonuria in large populations of newborn infants. *Pediatrics* **1963**, *32*, 338–343. [CrossRef] [PubMed]
15. MacCready, R.A.; Hussey, M.G. Newborn Phenylketonuria Detection Program in Massachusetts. *Am. J. Public Health Nations Health* **1964**, *54*, 2075–2081. [CrossRef] [PubMed]
16. Clague, A.; Thomas, A. Neonatal biochemical screening for disease. *Clin. Chim. Acta* **2001**, *315*, 99–110. [CrossRef]
17. Chace, D.H.; Millington, D.S.; Terada, N.; Kahler, S.G.; Roe, C.R.; Hofman, L.F. Rapid diagnosis of phenylketonuria by quantitative analysis for phenylalanine and tyrosine in neonatal blood spots by tandem mass spectrometry. *Clin. Chem.* **1993**, *39*, 66–71. [CrossRef]
18. Ranieri, E.; Ryall, R.G.; Morris, C.P.; Nelson, P.V.; Carey, W.F.; Pollard, A.C.; Robertson, E.F. Neonatal screening strategy for cystic fibrosis using immunoreactive trypsinogen and direct gene analysis. *BMJ* **1991**, *302*, 1237–1240. [CrossRef]
19. Chan, K.; Puck, J.M. Development of population-based newborn screening for severe combined immunodeficiency. *J. Allergy Clin. Immunol.* **2005**, *115*, 391–398. [CrossRef]
20. Chien, Y.-H.; Chiang, S.-C.; Weng, W.-C.; Lee, N.-C.; Lin, C.-J.; Hsieh, W.-S.; Lee, W.-T.; Jong, Y.-J.; Ko, T.-M.; Hwu, W.-L. Presymptomatic Diagnosis of Spinal Muscular Atrophy Through Newborn Screening. *J. Pediatr.* **2017**, *190*, 124–129.e1. [CrossRef]
21. Wilson, J.M.G.; Jungner, G.; World health Organization. Principles and Practice of Screening for Disease. 1968. Available online: https://apps.who/iris/handle/10665/37650 (accessed on 13 February 2022).
22. Andermann, A.; Blancquaert, I.; Beauchamp, S.; Dery, V. Revisting wilson and Jungner in the genomic age: A review of screening criteria over the past 40 years. *Bull. World Health Organ.* **2008**, *86*, 317–319. [CrossRef]
23. Lüders, A.; Blankenstein, O.; Brockow, I.; Ensenauer, R.; Lindner, M.; Schulze, A.; Nennstiel, U. Neonatal Screening for Congenital Metabolic and Endocrine Disorders. *Dtsch. Arztebl. Int.* **2021**, *118*, 101–108. [CrossRef]

24. Tangeraas, T.; Sæves, I.; Klingenberg, C.; Jørgensen, J.; Kristensen, E.; Gunnarsdottir, G.; Hansen, E.V.; Strand, J.; Lundman, E.; Ferdinandusse, S.; et al. Performance of Expanded Newborn Screening in Norway Supported by Post-Analytical Bioinformatics Tools and Rapid Second-Tier DNA Analyses. *Int. J. Neonatal Screen.* **2020**, *6*, 51. [CrossRef] [PubMed]
25. Gurian, E.A.; Kinnamon, D.D.; Henry, J.J.; Waisbren, S.E. Expanded Newborn Screening for Biochemical Disorders: The Effect of a False-Positive Result. *Pediatrics* **2006**, *117*, 1915–1921. [CrossRef] [PubMed]
26. Tluczek, A.; Koscik, R.L.; Farrell, P.M.; Rock, M.J. Psychosocial Risk Associated with Newborn Screening for Cystic Fibrosis: Parents' Experience While Awaiting the Sweat-Test Appointment. *Pediatrics* **2005**, *115*, 1692–1703. [CrossRef] [PubMed]
27. Hoffmann, G.F.; Lindner, M.; Loeber, J.G. 50 years of newborn screening. *J. Inherit. Metab. Dis.* **2014**, *37*, 163–164. [CrossRef]
28. Zimmer, K.-P. Newborn Screening: Still Room for Improvement. *Dtsch. Ärzteblatt Int.* **2021**, *118*, 99–100. [CrossRef]
29. Liebl, B.; Nennstiel-Ratzel, U.; von Kries, R.; Fingerhut, R.; Olgemöller, B.; Zapf, A.; Roscher, A.A. Expanded Newborn Screening in Bavaria: Tracking to Achieve Requested Repeat Testing. *Prev. Med.* **2002**, *34*, 132–137. [CrossRef]
30. Lajic, S.; Karlsson, L.; Zetterström, R.; Falhammar, H.; Nordenström, A. The Success of a Screening Program Is Largely Dependent on Close Collaboration between the Laboratory and the Clinical Follow-Up of the Patients. *Int. J. Neonatal Screen.* **2020**, *6*, 68. [CrossRef]
31. Recommended Uniform Screening Panel. Available online: https://www.hrsa.gov/advisory-committees/heritable-disorders/rusp/index.html (accessed on 13 February 2022).
32. Health. Supporting Public Health in Europe. Available online: https://european-union.europa.eu/priorities-and-actions/actions-topic/health_en (accessed on 13 February 2022).
33. EURORDIS Rare Disease Europe. Key Principles for Newborn Screening. Available online: https://www.eurordis.org/newbornscreening (accessed on 13 February 2022).
34. Brower, A.; Chan, K.; Hartnett, M.; Taylor, J. The Longitudinal Pediatric Data Resource: Facilitating Longitudinal Collection of Health Information to Inform Clinical Care and Guide Newborn Screening Efforts. *Int. J. Neonatal Screen.* **2021**, *7*, 37. [CrossRef]
35. Darby, E.; Thompson, J.; Johnson, C.; Singh, S.; Ojodu, J. Establishing a National Community of Practice for Newborn Screening Follow-Up. *Int. J. Neonatal Screen.* **2021**, *7*, 49. [CrossRef]
36. Lloyd-Puryear, M.; Brower, A.; Berry, S.A.; Brosco, J.P.; Bowdish, B.; Watson, M.S. Foundation of the Newborn Screening Translational Research Network and its tools for research. *Genet. Med.* **2019**, *21*, 1271–1279. [CrossRef]
37. Congress.gov. HR 1281-. Newborn Screening Saves Lives Reauthorization Act of 2014. Available online: https://www.congress.gov/bill/113th-congress/house-bill/1281 (accessed on 13 February 2022).
38. Gahl, W.A.; Thoene, J.G.; Schneider, J.A. Cystinosis. *N. Engl. J. Med.* **2002**, *347*, 111–121. [CrossRef] [PubMed]
39. Town, M.M.; Jean, G.; Cherqui, S.; Attard, M.; Forestier, L.; Whitmore, S.A.; Callen, D.F.; Gribouval, O.; Broyer, M.; Bates, G.; et al. A novel gene encoding an integral membrane protein is mutated in nephropathic cystinosis. *Nat. Genet.* **1998**, *18*, 319–324. [CrossRef] [PubMed]
40. Kleta, R.; Bernardini, I.; Ueda, M.; Varade, W.S.; Phornphutkul, C.; Krasnewich, D.; Gahl, W.A. Long-term follow-up of well-treated nephropathic cystinosis patients. *J. Pediatr.* **2004**, *145*, 555–560. [CrossRef]
41. Gahl, W.A.; Balog, J.Z.; Kleta, R. Nephropathic Cystinosis in Adults: Natural History and Effects of Oral Cysteamine Therapy. *Ann. Intern. Med.* **2007**, *147*, 242–250. [CrossRef] [PubMed]
42. Cherqui, S.; Courtoy, P.J. The renal Fanconi syndrome in cystinosis: Pathogenic insights and therapeutic perspectives. *Nat. Rev. Nephrol.* **2016**, *13*, 115–131. [CrossRef]
43. Chevalier, R.L.; Forbes, M.S.; Galarreta, C.I.; Thornhill, B.A. Responses of proximal tubular cells to injury in congenital renal disease: Fight or flight. *Pediatr. Nephrol.* **2013**, *29*, 537–541. [CrossRef]
44. Raggi, C.; Luciani, A.; Nevo, N.; Antignac, C.; Terryn, S.; Devuyst, O. Dedifferentiation and aberrations of the endolysosomal compartment characterize the early stage of nephropathic cystinosis. *Hum. Mol. Genet.* **2013**, *23*, 2266–2278. [CrossRef]
45. Greco, M.; Brugnara, M.; Zaffanello, M.; Taranta, A.; Pastore, A.; Emma, F. Long-term outcome of nephropathic cystinosis: A 20-year single-center experience. *Pediatr. Nephrol.* **2010**, *25*, 2459–2467. [CrossRef]
46. Brodin-Sartorius, A.; Tête, M.-J.; Niaudet, P.; Antignac, C.; Guest, G.; Ottolenghi, C.; Charbit, M.; Moyse, D.; Legendre, C.; Lesavre, P.; et al. Cysteamine therapy delays the progression of nephropathic cystinosis in late adolescents and adults. *Kidney Int.* **2012**, *81*, 179–189. [CrossRef]
47. Emma, F.; Hoff, W.V.; Hohenfellner, K.; Topaloglu, R.; Greco, M.; Ariceta, G.; Bettini, C.; Bockenhauer, D.; Veys, K.; Pape, L.; et al. An international cohort study spanning five decades assessed outcomes of nephropathic cystinosis. *Kidney Int.* **2021**, *100*, 1112–1123. [CrossRef]
48. Langman, C.B.; Barshop, B.A.; Deschenes, G.; Emma, F.; Goodyer, P.; Lipkin, G.; Midgley, J.P.; Ottolenghi, C.; Servais, A.; Soliman, N.A.; et al. Controversies and research agenda in nephropathic cystinosis: Conclusions from a "Kidney Disease: Improving Global Outcomes" (KDIGO) Controversies Conference. *Kidney Int.* **2016**, *89*, 1192–1203. [CrossRef] [PubMed]
49. Topaloglu, R.; Gulhan, B.; Inözü, M.; Canpolat, N.; Yilmaz, A.; Noyan, A.; Dursun, I.; Gökce, I.; Gürgöze, M.K.; Akinci, N.; et al. The Clinical and Mutational Spectrum of Turkish Patients with Cystinosis. *Clin. J. Am. Soc. Nephrol.* **2017**, *12*, 1634–1641. [CrossRef] [PubMed]
50. Broyer, M.; Tete, M.-J. Outcome of cystinosis after 20 years of age. A study of the Enfants-Malades series. In *Pediatric Nephrology*; Springer: New York, NY, USA, 2008; pp. 1910–1911.

51. Vaisbich, M.H.; Koch, V.H. Report of a Brazilian Multicenter Study on Nephropathic Cystinosis. *Nephron Clin. Pract.* **2010**, *114*, c12–c18. [CrossRef] [PubMed]
52. Bertholet-Thomas, A.; Berthiller, J.; Tasic, V.; Kassai, B.; Otukesh, H.; Greco, M.; Ehrich, J.; Bernardes, R.D.P.; Deschênes, G.; Hulton, S.-A.; et al. Worldwide view of nephropathic cystinosis: Results from a survey from 30 countries. *BMC Nephrol.* **2017**, *18*, 210. [CrossRef]
53. Ariceta, G.; Giordano, V.; Santos, F. Effects of long-term cysteamine treatment in patients with cystinosis. *Pediatr. Nephrol.* **2017**, *34*, 571–578. [CrossRef]
54. Viltz, L.; Trauner, D.A. Effect of Age at Treatment on Cognitive Performance in Patients with Cystinosis. *J. Pediatr.* **2013**, *163*, 489–492. [CrossRef]
55. Nesterova, G.; Gahl, W.A. Cystinosis: The evolution of a treatable disease. *Pediatr. Nephrol.* **2012**, *28*, 51–59. [CrossRef]
56. Cohen, C.; Charbit, M.; Chadefaux-Vekemans, B.; Giral, M.; Garrigue, V.; Kessler, M.; Antoine, C.; Snanoudj, R.; Niaudet, P.; Kreis, H.; et al. Excellent long-term outcome of renal transplantation in cystinosis patients. *Orphanet J. Rare Dis.* **2015**, *10*, 90. [CrossRef]
57. Spicer, R.A.; Clayton, P.A.; McTaggart, S.J.; Zhang, G.Y.; Alexander, S.I. Patient and Graft Survival Following Kidney Transplantation in Recipients With Cystinosis: A Cohort Study. *Am. J. Kidney Dis.* **2015**, *65*, 172–173. [CrossRef]
58. Markello, T.C.; Bernardini, I.M.; Gahl, W.A. Improved Renal Function in Children with Cystinosis Treated with Cysteamine. *N. Engl. J. Med.* **1993**, *328*, 1157–1162. [CrossRef]
59. Nesterova, G.; Gahl, W.A. Cystinosis, GeneReviews. Available online: https://www.ncbi.nlm.nih.gov/books/NBK1400/ (accessed on 13 February 2022).
60. Gahl, W.A.; Thoene, J.G.; Schneider, J.A. Cystinosis: A disorder of lysosomal membrane transport. *Metab. Mol. Bases Inherit. Dis.* **2001**, *4*, 5085–5108.
61. David, D.; Berlingerio, S.P.; Elmonem, M.A.; Arcolino, F.O.; Soliman, N.; Heuvel, B.V.D.; Gijsbers, R.; Levtchenko, E. Molecular Basis of Cystinosis: Geographic Distribution, Functional Consequences of Mutations in the CTNS Gene, and Potential for Repair. *Nephron Exp. Nephrol.* **2018**, *141*, 133–146. [CrossRef] [PubMed]
62. Forestier, L.; Jean, G.; Attard, M.; Cherqui, S.; Lewis, C.; Hoff, W.V.; Broyer, M.; Town, M.; Antignac, C. Molecular Characterization of CTNS Deletions in Nephropathic Cystinosis: Development of a PCR-Based Detection Assay. *Am. J. Hum. Genet.* **1999**, *65*, 353–359. [CrossRef] [PubMed]
63. Shotelersuk, V.; Larson, D.; Anikster, Y.; McDowell, G.; Lemons, R.; Bernardini, I.; Guo, J.; Thoene, J.; Gahl, W.A. CTNS Mutations in an American-Based Population of Cystinosis Patients. *Am. J. Hum. Genet.* **1998**, *63*, 1352–1362. [CrossRef] [PubMed]
64. Kiehntopf, M.; Schickel, J.; von der Gönne, B.; Koch, H.G.; Superti-Furga, A.; Steinmann, B.; Deufel, T.; Harms, E. Analysis of the CTNS gene in patients of German and Swiss origin with nephropathic cystinosis. *Hum. Mutat.* **2002**, *20*, 237. [CrossRef]
65. Alcántara-Ortigoza, M.; Belmont-Martínez, L.; Vela-Amieva, M.; Angel, A.G.-D. Analysis of the CTNS Gene in Nephropathic Cystinosis Mexican Patients: Report of Four Novel Mutations and Identification of a False Positive 57-kb Deletion Genotype with LDM-2/Exon 4 Multiplex PCR Assay. *Genet. Test.* **2008**, *12*, 409–414. [CrossRef]
66. Mason, S.; Pepe, G.; Dall'Amico, R.; Tartaglia, S.; Casciani, S.; Greco, M.; Bencivenga, P.; Murer, L.; Rizzoni, G.; Tenconi, R.; et al. Mutational spectrum of the CTNS gene in Italy. *Eur. J. Hum. Genet.* **2003**, *11*, 503–508. [CrossRef]
67. Soliman, N.A.; Elmonem, M.A.; Heuvel, L.V.D.; Hamid, R.H.A.; Gamal, M.; Bongaers, I.; Marie, S.; Levtchenko, E.; Zschocke, J.; Gibson, K.M. Mutational Spectrum of the CTNS Gene in Egyptian Patients with Nephropathic Cystinosis. *JIMD Rep.* **2014**, *14*, 87–97. [CrossRef]
68. Topaloglu, R.; Vilboux, T.; Coskun, T.; Ozaltin, F.; Tinloy, B.; Gunay-Aygun, M.; Bakkaloglu, A.; Besbas, N.; Heuvel, L.V.D.; Kleta, R.; et al. Genetic basis of cystinosis in Turkish patients: A single-center experience. *Pediatr. Nephrol.* **2011**, *27*, 115–121. [CrossRef]
69. Shahkarami, S.; Galehdari, H.; Ahmadzadeh, A.; Babaahmadi, M.; Pedram, M. The first Molecular genetics analysis of individuals suffering from nephropatic cystinosis in the Southwestern Iran. *Nefrología* **2013**, *33*, 308–315. [CrossRef]
70. Owen, E.P.; Nandhlal, J.; Leisegang, F.; Van Der Watt, G.; Nourse, P.; Gajjar, P. Common mutation causes cystinosis in the majority of black South African patients. *Pediatr. Nephrol.* **2014**, *30*, 595–601. [CrossRef] [PubMed]
71. Brasell, E.J.; Chu, L.; El Kares, R.; Seo, J.H.; Loesch, R.; Iglesias, D.M.; Goodyer, P. The aminoglycoside geneticin permits translational readthrough of the CTNS W138X nonsense mutation in fibroblasts from patients with nephropathic cystinosis. *Pediatr. Nephrol.* **2018**, *34*, 873–881. [CrossRef] [PubMed]
72. Kalatzis, V.; Nevo, N.; Cherqui, S.; Gasnier, B.; Antignac, C. Molecular pathogenesis of cystinosis: Effect of CTNS mutations on the transport activity and subcellular localization of cystinosin. *Hum. Mol. Genet.* **2004**, *13*, 1361–1371. [CrossRef] [PubMed]
73. Jinks, D.C.; Minter, M.; Tarver, D.A.; Vanderford, M.; Hejtmancik, J.F.; McCabe, E.R.B. Molecular genetic diagnosis of sickle cell disease using dried blood specimens on blotters used for newborn screening. *Qual. Life Res.* **1989**, *81*, 363–366. [CrossRef] [PubMed]
74. Friedman, J.M.; The Global Alliance for Genomics and Health Regulatory and Ethics Working Group Paediatric Task Team; Cornel, M.C.; Goldenberg, A.J.; Lister, K.J.; Sénécal, K.; Vears, D.F. Genomic newborn screening: Public health policy considerations and recommendations. *BMC Med. Genom.* **2017**, *10*, 9. [CrossRef]
75. Fleige, T.; Burggraf, S.; Czibere, L.; Häring, J.; Glück, B.; Keitel, L.M.; Landt, O.; Harms, E.; Hohenfellner, K.; Durner, J.; et al. Next generation sequencing as second-tier test in high-throughput newborn screening for nephropathic cystinosis. *Eur. J. Hum. Genet.* **2019**, *28*, 193–201. [CrossRef]

76. Czibere, L.; Burggraf, S.; Fleige, T.; Glück, B.; Keitel, L.M.; Landt, O.; Durner, J.; Röschinger, W.; Hohenfellner, K.; Wirth, B.; et al. High-throughput genetic newborn screening for spinal muscular atrophy by rapid nucleic acid extraction from dried blood spots and 384-well qPCR. *Eur. J. Hum. Genet.* **2019**, *28*, 23–30. [CrossRef]
77. Gemeinsamer Bundesauschuss. Beschluss Kinder-Richtlinie: Neugeborenen-Screening Auf 5q-Assoziierte Spinale Muskelatrophie. Available online: https://www.g-ba.de/beschluesse/4617/ (accessed on 13 February 2022).
78. Hohenfellner, K.; Bergmann, C.; Fleige, T.; Janzen, N.; Burggraf, S.; Olgemöller, B.; Gahl, W.A.; Czibere, L.; Froschauer, S.; Röschinger, W.; et al. Molecular based newborn screening in Germany: Follow-up for cystinosis. *Mol. Genet. Metab. Rep.* **2019**, *21*, 100514. [CrossRef]
79. Elmonem, M.A.; Veys, K.R.; Soliman, N.A.; Van Dyck, M.; Heuvel, L.P.V.D.; Levtchenko, E. Cystinosis: A review. *Orphanet J. Rare Dis.* **2016**, *11*, 47. [CrossRef]
80. Gahl, W.A.; Reed, G.F.; Thoene, J.G.; Schulman, J.D.; Rizzo, W.B.; Jonas, A.J.; Denman, D.W.; Schlesselman, J.J.; Corden, B.J.; Schneider, J.A. Cysteamine Therapy for Children with Nephropathic Cystinosis. *N. Engl. J. Med.* **1987**, *316*, 971–977. [CrossRef]
81. Lu, C.; Tzovaras, B.G.; Gough, J. A survey of direct-to-consumer genotype data, and quality control tool (GenomePrep) for research. *Comp. Struc. Biot. J.* **2021**, *19*, 3747–3754. [CrossRef] [PubMed]
82. DeCristo, D.M.; Milko, L.V.; O'Daniel, J.M.; Foreman, A.K.M.; Mollison, L.F.; Powell, B.C.; Powell, C.M.; Berg, J.S. Actionability of commercial laboratory sequencing panels for newborn screening and the importance of transparency for parental decision-making. *Genome Med.* **2021**, *13*, 50. [CrossRef] [PubMed]

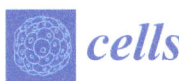

Review

Biomarkers in Nephropathic Cystinosis: Current and Future Perspectives

Francesco Emma [1], Giovanni Montini [2,3], Marco Pennesi [4], Licia Peruzzi [5], Enrico Verrina [6], Bianca Maria Goffredo [7], Fabrizio Canalini [8], David Cassiman [9], Silvia Rossi [8] and Elena Levtchenko [10,*]

1. Department of Pediatric Subspecialties, Division of Nephrology, Bambino Gesù Children's Hospital-IRCCS, 00165 Rome, Italy; francesco.emma@opbg.net
2. Pediatric Nephrology, Dialysis and Transplant Unit, Fondazione Ca' Grande IRRCS Ospedale Maggiore Policlinico, 20122 Milan, Italy; giovanni.montini@unimi.it
3. Department of Clinical Sciences and Community Health, University of Milan, 20122 Milan, Italy
4. Institute for Maternal and Child Health, IRCCS Burlo Garofolo, 34137 Trieste, Italy; pennesi@burlo.trieste.it
5. Pediatric Nephrology Unit, Regina Margherita Children's Hospital, AOU Città della Salute e della Scienza di Torino, 10126 Turin, Italy; licia.peruzzi@unito.it
6. Dialysis Unit, Department of Pediatrics, IRCCS Istituto Giannina Gaslini, 16147 Genoa, Italy; enricoverrina@ospedale-gaslini.ge.it
7. Department of Pediatric Subspecialties, Division of Metabolic Diseases, Bambino Gesù Children's Hospital-IRCCS, 00165 Rome, Italy; biancamaria.goffredo@opbg.net
8. Medical Department, Chiesi Pharmaceutics, 43100 Parma, Italy; f.canalini@chiesi.com (F.C.); si.rossi@chiesi.com (S.R.)
9. Department of Metabolic Diseases, University Hospitals Leuven, 3000 Leuven, Belgium; david.cassiman@uzleuven.be
10. Department of Pediatric Nephrology and Development and Regeneration, University Hospitals Leuven, University of Leuven, 3000 Leuven, Belgium
* Correspondence: elena.levtchenko@uzleuven.be

Abstract: Early diagnosis and effective therapy are essential for improving the overall prognosis and quality of life of patients with nephropathic cystinosis. The severity of kidney dysfunction and the multi-organ involvement as a consequence of the increased intracellular concentration of cystine highlight the necessity of accurate monitoring of intracellular cystine to guarantee effective treatment of the disease. Cystine depletion is the only available treatment, which should begin immediately after diagnosis, and not discontinued, to significantly slow progression of renal and extra-renal organ damage. This review aims to discuss the importance of the close monitoring of intracellular cystine concentration to optimize cystine depletion therapy. In addition, the role of new biomarkers in the management of the disease, from timely diagnosis to implementing treatment during follow-up, is overviewed.

Keywords: nephropathic cystinosis; biomarkers; cystine; cysteamine; kidney; therapeutic monitoring

Citation: Emma, F.; Montini, G.; Pennesi, M.; Peruzzi, L.; Verrina, E.; Goffredo, B.M.; Canalini, F.; Cassiman, D.; Rossi, S.; Levtchenko, E. Biomarkers in Nephropathic Cystinosis: Current and Future Perspectives. *Cells* **2022**, *11*, 1839. https://doi.org/10.3390/cells11111839

Academic Editors: Cord Brakebusch and Alfonso Eirin

Received: 23 March 2022
Accepted: 2 June 2022
Published: 4 June 2022

Publisher's Note: MDPI stays neutral with regard to jurisdictional claims in published maps and institutional affiliations.

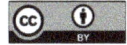

Copyright: © 2022 by the authors. Licensee MDPI, Basel, Switzerland. This article is an open access article distributed under the terms and conditions of the Creative Commons Attribution (CC BY) license (https://creativecommons.org/licenses/by/4.0/).

1. Introduction

Cystinosis is a rare lysosomal storage disorder caused by autosomal recessive mutations in the *CTNS* gene that encodes the cystine transporter cystinosin, a ubiquitously expressed lysosomal cystine–proton co-transporter, which is expressed at the lysosomal membrane and mediates the efflux of cystine from the lysosome [1–3]. *CTNS* gene mutations lead to a deficiency or absence of cystinosin, with consequent accumulation of free cystine in lysosomes and buildup of toxic crystals that ultimately lead to tissue and organ damage. Cystinosis is a systemic metabolic disorder that initially affects the kidneys, as well as the eyes with accumulation of corneal cystine crystals, and, subsequently, endocrine and reproductive organs, muscles, bones, lungs, skin, and the central nervous system [4].

Based on the severity of presentation and age of onset, three clinical forms of the disease can be defined: infantile or early-onset nephropathic [5], juvenile or late-onset nephropathic [6], and the adult or ocular non-nephropathic form [7,8]. At present, more than 140 mutations have been reported [9,10], with the infantile form of cystinosis being associated with severe *CTNS* mutations on both alleles, and the juvenile and ocular forms mostly being associated with milder mutations in at least one allele [8,10].

The estimated incidence of cystinosis is 1 in 100,000–200,000 live births [7,8]. Infantile nephropathic cystinosis is the most common (95% of total cases) and severe clinical form of the disease, and is associated with high morbidity and mortality. The infantile form phenotypically manifests as renal Fanconi syndrome by 6–12 months of age [8]. With time, chronic kidney disease (CKD) develops [11]. Additional clinical characteristics include poor growth and failure to thrive, severe polyuria, polydipsia and dehydration, vomiting and feeding difficulties, and vitamin D-resistant hypophosphatemic rickets in children and osteomalacia in adults. During the first months of life, patients are usually asymptomatic. However, they already demonstrate elevated amounts of amino acids, low molecular weight proteins, and glucose in their urines. These represent early, although not necessarily specific, biomarkers [12]. If untreated, nephropathic cystinosis can lead to end-stage kidney disease (ESKD) by 10–12 years of age and systemic disease with multi-organ involvement, requiring treatment with dialysis and kidney transplantation [13–16]. Delayed diagnosis may occur because of the rarity of the disease and its incomplete clinical presentation at an early age. Patients with juvenile cystinosis can mimic other proteinuric conditions or might present with impaired kidney function of unknown etiology or bone complaints, as renal Fanconi syndrome is mild compared with patients having infantile cystinosis. Nevertheless, a careful examination of those patients reveals signs of proximal tubular dysfunction (aminoaciduria, low molecular weight proteinuria, glucosuria, and phosphaturia) suggesting the possibility of cystinosis [17]. Patients with all three clinical forms (infantile, juvenile, ocular) demonstrate the pathognomonic cornea cystine crystals, allowing the immediate diagnosis of cystinosis prior to confirmation by while blood cells cystine measurements and genetic testing [5–8].

Cystine-depletion therapy with cysteamine allows significant improvement in life expectancy [14,18], but cannot prevent the development of CKD and other systemic complications, and needs to be continued after kidney transplantation [7]. Recent data have demonstrated that lysosomal cystine accumulation is not the only pathological event related to the absence of functional cystinosin [19], which might explain why treatment with cysteamine is not curative. It is, however, the only available treatment for these patients. Adequate depletion is therefore needed and since the efficacy of cystine-depletion may be different due to inter-individual variability [20], precise evaluation of patient's cystine levels needs to be monitored in clinical practice to tailor the individual cysteamine dose adjustment. Therefore, there is an urgent need to identify novel biomarkers not only for monitoring the progression of the disease, but also its prognosis in light of understanding the role of mechanisms other than cystine accumulation in the onset of pathological events. In this review, we focus on biomarkers of cystine accumulation, which remains the key feature of cystinosis and a target of cysteamine therapy.

2. Methods for Measuring Intracellular Leucocyte Cystine

The quantification of intracellular cystine is important for both diagnosis and monitoring of cystinosis therapy. Different methods have been developed to measure cystine content in leucocytes, which are the best cells for these analyses because they are easily and repeatedly accessible; in these cells, the cystine concentration is increased up to 80-fold compared with normal individuals [21,22]. Historically, quantification of intracellular leucocyte cystine (ILC) was performed using cystine-binding protein derived from *E. coli* [23,24]. This method was later abandoned given its high cost and use of radioactivity. Ion exchange chromatography, HPLC, and tandem mass spectrometry (MS) [25–27] are currently used by different laboratories, with tandem MS being the most sensitive method.

2.1. Cell Isolation

One of the most critical steps in ILC determination is the isolation of cells from whole blood. Intracellular cystine mainly accumulates in phagocytic cells—polymorphonuclear (PMN) leukocytes and monocytes—and not in lymphocytes [21]. Initially, cystine was measured on mixed leukocyte samples [28]. The results, however, are less reliable because they depend on the composition of white blood cells. For example, since lymphocytes usually predominate in young children, their mixed leukocyte ILC content is usually lower and in some cases can even delay diagnosis [29].

The type of anticoagulant used in blood collection is also important, with acid citrate dextrose or heparin being preferred over EDTA [30]. Two methods have been used for PMN isolation, namely Ficoll gradient centrifugation [31], and more recently, immunomagnetic granulocyte purification [32].

After isolation, sulfhydryl exchange needs to be blocked with reagents such as N-ethylmaleimide that prevent oxidation of cysteine into cystine. After this stage, samples can be stored at $-80\ °C$ if cystine measurements will be delayed or in samples that need to be shipped. The shipping of blood samples also allows for the frequent monitoring of patients who are far from the analytical laboratory, thus improving disease control. Before measuring cystine, samples are sonicated to disrupt the lysosomal membrane and acidified with sulfosalicylic acid [26]. According to local protocols, samples that need to be shipped are pre-treated or are shipped as fresh samples and immediately processed upon arrival. In this latter case, samples should arrive at the laboratory no later than 24 h after collection.

2.2. Cystine and Protein Determination

The first method to quantify cystine used a cystine-binding protein assay, which allowed the detection of nanomolar concentrations of cystine by isotopic dilution [23,24]. Alternatively, ion exchange chromatography has been used. This technique, however, is less sensitive and sometimes generated false results when samples were too small [8].

Current techniques for the assessment of ILC levels include high-performance liquid chromatography (HPLC) and liquid chromatography-tandem mass spectrometry (LC-MS/MS) [25–27]. Both techniques require specialized personnel and specific equipment. For these reasons, they are only performed in a few specialized centers. Compared to HPLC, LC-MS/MS allows measuring ILC on smaller amounts of blood, and for this reason is increasingly used. Before measuring cystine, the protein fraction is precipitated, internal standards are added, and the final solution is extracted with acetonitrile. Centrifuged samples can be analyzed at a later time. The pellet is re-suspended to measure protein content.

ILC is expressed as nanomoles of half-cystine (each molecule of cystine is composed of 2 cysteine moieties linked by a disulfide bond) normalized per milligram of protein. Often, proteins are evaluated by the classic Lowry method [33]. The best method for determination of protein is a matter of debate. There may be some preference for the use of the bicinchoninic acid method over the Lowry method [34]. The method for protein determination is important because it affects the denominator of the ILC value and the reference range for a given laboratory. For mixed-leukocyte preparations, a correction factor of 0.65 has been proposed to compare values of ILC obtained using the bicinchoninic acid vs. the Lowry assay [35]. Each laboratory needs to establish its own reference intervals for control subjects, healthy heterozygotes, and patients at diagnosis, also considering differences in age and gender [36].

3. Prenatal and Neonatal Diagnosis

Diagnosis of cystinosis should always be confirmed with genetic testing. Early diagnosis is crucial as it allows the early initiation of therapy. This is important for better prognosis of long-term kidney function [37].

3.1. Prenatal Diagnosis

Prenatal diagnosis of cystinosis can be performed in at-risk pregnancies by molecular analysis of the *CTNS* gene in chorionic villi or circulating fetal cells. Traditionally, the quantification of cystine was performed in chorionic villi or cultured amniocytes using [^{14}C]-cystine [38]. This method is no longer used and has been replaced by genetic testing, a safer, faster, and cost-effective test.

3.2. Neonatal Diagnosis in at Risk Siblings

When prenatal evaluation in at-risk pregnancies is not feasible, DNA testing can be performed immediately after birth. Early diagnosis before four weeks of age, followed by prompt treatment with cysteamine from the age of five weeks, can protect tubular and glomerular function, at least during the first years of life [39]. Cystine content can be measured in peripheral leucocytes in samples obtained from placenta or in fibroblasts [40]. Since cystine crystals develop more rapidly in bone morrow compared to the cornea, detection of crystals in bone marrow was used in the past for diagnosis of cystinosis [41]. While this method is rapid and can allow the identification of cystine crystals during early life before they can be detected in the cornea, the aspiration of bone marrow is highly invasive and is not recommended in routine clinical practice.

3.3. Newborn Screening in Unaffected Population

Cystinosis is a treatable disease. Early treatment significantly impacts long-term kidney function [37]. Several groups have investigated strategies for newborn screening. Measuring cystine concentrations in dry blood spots is not reliable due to oxidation of intracellular cysteine (authors' unpublished observation). The quantification of the seven-carbon sugar sedoheptulose in dried blood spots has been proposed as a quick pre-symptomatic method for detection of homozygosity for the most common *CTNS* 57-kb deletion. However, this method detects patients with a mutation that is prevalent only in Northern Europe [42].

Currently, detection of *CTNS* gene pathogenic variants by next-generation sequencing (NGS) is being investigated in several laboratories. A proof-of-principle demonstration of the validity of this approach has been recently produced in Germany by combining quantitative polymerase chain reaction (qPCR) and NGS [43]. In this study, one child was diagnosed in the neonatal period and was treated immediately with cysteamine; at 16 months of age, this patient had no signs of renal Fanconi syndrome [44].

4. Treatment Monitoring: Importance of Target Cystine Values

Maintenance of low ILC is currently the only way to monitor cysteamine treatment (Figure 1A,B).

Available preparations of cysteamine include immediate- and delayed-release formulations (IR-CYS and DR-CYS, respectively). The therapy is also complemented by the use of cysteamine eye drops to dissolve corneal cystine crystals, and by symptomatic treatments aiming at supplementing losses due to renal Fanconi syndrome and correcting the consequences of extra-renal intracellular cystine accumulation.

Early treatment initiation and constant monitoring of the effective cystine depletion in each patient has an impact on disease progression by protecting from cellular and tissue damage in both renal and extra-renal tissues. Oral cysteamine therapy should begin as soon as the diagnosis is made, should not be discontinued, and should be monitored for efficacy [14,45]. Early, continuous, and effective depletion therapy is able to modify the course of the disease, postponing ESKD and also reducing the incidence and severity of pathologies that are consequences of the systemic deposition of cystine, such as hypothyroidism, diabetes mellitus, neuromuscular dysfunction, and cerebral atrophy, with a general improvement in the both the quality of life and life expectancy [8,16,46–49].

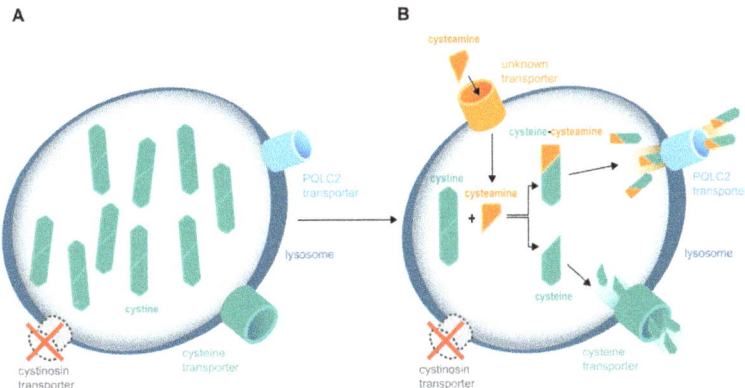

Figure 1. Cysteamine depletes lysosomal cystine accumulation in cystinosis. (**A**) The absence or the lack of function of the cystinosin transporter causes intracellular accumulation of cystine. (**B**) The administration of cysteamine allows the depletion of excess cystine from lysosomes in cells.

Continuous cysteamine therapy shows remarkable long-term benefits as long as the treatment is adequate. The appropriateness of therapy is defined by its ability to maintain an optimal low intracellular concentration of cystine [16]. In order to delay or avoid the progression of multi-organ dysfunction and comorbidities, and to decrease mortality [50], therapeutic monitoring needs to be consistent, and dose adjustments of cysteamine should be made on the basis of ILC levels. The cystine concentration within cells of healthy individuals is below 0.2 nmol half-cystine/mg protein and below 1 nmol half-cystine/mg protein in heterozygous subjects who present the gene mutation/deletion in one allele and no clinical symptoms [51]. Homozygous patients who are not subjected to therapy have intracellular cystine levels that are >2 nmol half-cystine/mg of protein.

The optimal cut-off value for appropriate therapy is defined by most laboratories as 1 nmol half-cystine/mg of protein in mixed WBC preparations, i.e., the level seen in heterozygous individuals without clinical symptoms [52]. Cystine levels between 1 and 2 nmol half-cystine/mg of protein, although not optimal, are considered acceptable. Indeed, in some patients the optimal value cannot be reached as high cysteamine dosages are not tolerated. For concentrations > 2 nmol half-cystine/mg of protein, important clinical consequences become evident: for instance, every year of sub-optimal treatment has been shown to correspond to a loss of 0.9 years of renal glomerular function [45] (Table 1).

Of note, cystine levels in PMN leukocytes are usually higher than those in mixed leukocyte preparations, and laboratories measuring cystine in these cells might have slightly higher target values. Hence, the use of granulocyte cystine levels as a diagnostic tool or for therapeutic monitoring requires additional validation to determine what levels depict global cystine burden and proper therapeutic adherence [36]. Until consensus is reached on the use of granulocytes, it is fundamental that laboratories assessing elevated cystine levels in different leucocyte populations and with different methods provide their own reference values for diagnosis and therapeutic monitoring [47].

Table 1. Clinical consequences of inadequate cystine depletion therapy.

Study	Kidney Outcome	Extra-Renal Outcome	Reference
US study; children treated with cysteamine up to 73 months (n = 93)	Mean creatinine clearance reduced in patients not adequately depleted (< 1 vs. > 3 nmol half-cystine/mg protein: 50.5 vs. 29.7 mL per min per 1.73 m^2)		[53]
US single center study; patients analyzed between 1960 and 1992 (n = 76)	Non-adequate treatment as shown by leucocyte cystine levels > 2 nmol half-cystine/mg protein. Treatment started at > 2 y with reduced creatinine clearance and early onset of renal impairment (mean creatinine clearance predicted = 0 ml at the age of 20 vs. 74 y for children receiving adequate treatment compared to those with only partial treatment)		[52]
US database; age 18–45 y analyzed between January 1985 and May 2006 (n = 100)	Non-adequate treatment, highlighted by leucocyte cystine levels above the cut-off, need for kidney transplantation at least 3.8 y earlier	Non-adequate treatment associated with an increased incidence of hypothyroidism (87% vs. 56%) and death (49% vs. 8%)	[16]
French study; age $\geq$ 15 y, diagnosis time: 1961–1995, mean follow-up 24.6 y (n = 86)	Patients with leucocyte cystine levels > 3 nmol half-cystine/mg protein show early onset ESRD compared to adequately depleted patients (p < 0.0001)		[14]
Turkish study; single center retrospective study, age 0.5–29 y, median follow-up 8 y (n = 21)		Non-adequate treatment associated with an increased incidence of complications; < 2 vs. $\geq$2 nmol half-cystine/mg protein with deficit of growth (66.6% vs. 90.9%), pubertal delay (0% vs 66.6%), hypothyroidism (33.3% vs. 54.5%), and diabetes (0% vs 18.1%)	[6]
US database; age 11–48 y analyzed between 1975 and 2005 (n = 147)	Adequate treatment associated with delayed onset ESRD (R^2 = 0.997) Every year of sub-optimal treatment corresponded to a loss of 0.9 y of renal glomerular function 21 patients (born in the 1960s and 1970s) reached ESKD in the first 8 years of life	Mean leucocyte cystine levels (p = 0.01), and earlier initiation of cysteamine therapy (p = 0.03) significantly associated with improved growth Children reaching CKD stage 5 before 15 years of age grew on average 0.55 height standard deviation scores worse than children that reached dialysis after their 15th birthday (95% CI: 0.09–1.01; p = 0.03)	[45]
International European cohort of patients born between 1964 and 2016 (n = 453)	Earlier age at start of cysteamine and lower mean leucocyte cystine levels are associated with delayed development of CKD stage 5		[37]

5. Limitations of Current Monitoring

While ILC is currently accepted as a gold standard for therapeutic monitoring of cystinosis, the method has several limitations related to technical and economic issues of sample measurement and storage. For instance, for reliable results, leucocytes should be isolated as soon as possible after blood collection to guarantee integrity, potentially becoming an issue for centers distantly located from the analytical laboratory. In addition, biochemical and instrumental analyses are time-consuming, and keeping analytical techniques such as LC-MS/MS routinely active may be expensive for some small centers and low-income countries, both in terms of equipment needed and personnel expertise. As previously mentioned, proper therapeutic monitoring is mandatory for follow-up given the large variability in the pharmacokinetics of cysteamine, which shows a somewhat poor correlation between the cysteamine dose and ILC levels [20,49]. Therefore, it is always necessary to quantify the actual cystine depletion to ensure that it is maintained below the validated cut-off value, and not simply rely on patient adherence to cysteamine therapy.

Moreover, because of the short lifespan of leucocytes, ILC levels may not sufficiently reflect renal and extra-renal tissue levels of cystine. Finally, with the exception of cystine in the cornea [54], there is no direct evidence that detection of cystine in other organs, such as the skin [55], can offer a reliable tool for therapeutic monitoring.

6. Novel Biomarkers

6.1. Biochemical Biomarkers

6.1.1. Chitotriosidase

In order to obtain a better picture of the burden of cystine on the entire body, macrophage activation biomarkers have recently been proposed as additional therapeutic monitoring tools for cystinosis [4,56–58]. Macrophages are long-living cells, and their activation is an important pathogenic mechanism present in cystinosis [56,57,59]. Indeed, cystine crystals containing macrophages have been identified in several tissues, including kidney, liver, and the skin [60–64]. Upon activation, macrophages release high levels of inflammatory biomarkers.

A recent study established the validity of plasma chitotriosidase, an enzyme produced by activated macrophages, as a reliable biomarker for long-term therapeutic monitoring of nephropathic cystinosis [58]. In a cohort of 57 patients, this prospective international, multi-center study collected and compared the levels of ILC with four biomarkers of macrophage activation over a period of two years: interleukin (IL)-1β, IL-6, IL-18, and plasma chitotriosidase. Of these, plasma chitotriosidase levels were found to be significantly correlated with ILC levels. Specifically, a cut-off value for chitotriosidase activity of 150 nmol/ml plasma per hour was demonstrated to be both reliable and specific in distinguishing good versus poor therapeutic control compared to ILC reference values (<2 versus ≥2 nmol half-cystine/mg protein). Moreover, chitotriosidase activity was also significantly correlated with the number of extrarenal complications burdening patients. In this case, a cut-off value for chitotriosidase of 250 nmol/mL plasma per hour was found to have a specificity of 93% in identifying patients suffering from multiple extrarenal complications, thus acting as a predictor of disease severity. From a technical point of view, the use of chitotriosidase as a biomarker presents several benefits, such as the stability of chitotriosidase in plasma for longer periods of time compared to leucocytes, i.e., over 1 month at room temperature, and over 4 months when stored at +4 °C, compared to less than 24 h for leucocytes [65,66]. It is also simpler, faster, and less expensive, as well as being an easily accessible fluorometric assay compared to LC-MS/MS. The drawback of this biomarker is that about 5% of the population carry a mutation in the chitotriosidase gene, which precludes its use.

6.1.2. Alpha-Ketoglutarate

Metabolomic analysis of $CTNS^{-/-}$ proximal tubule cell lines revealed altered metabolic pathways (glycolysis, TCA cycle, DNA replication, and DNA repair) and a reduction of lysosomal catalytic proteins expression. One of the differentially expressed metabolites is alpha-ketoglutarate (AKG), which is significantly increased in proximal tubular cells and plasma in patients with cystinosis. AKG is a key molecule in the Krebs cycle, acting as a nitrogen scavenger and a source of glutamate and glutamine that stimulates protein synthesis and inhibits protein degradation. AKG plays a pivotal role in the regulation of autophagy and apoptosis, potentially bridging the latter to the loss of cystinosin and kidney proximal tubule impairment in cystinosis. [67]. Alpha-ketoglutarate might therefore be considered a new biochemical biomarker of cystinosis.

Bicalutamide, a drug used in the treatment of prostate cancer, was able to re-establish metabolic homeostasis and reduce alpha-ketoglutarate levels in an organoid model (patient-derived tubuloids), and in cystinotic zebrafish. Although an anti-androgenic effect of bicalutamide should be taken into account, combined treatment with cysteamine might be a promising therapy that can potentially act on improving proximal tubule cell function while reducing cystine levels [67].

6.2. Quantification of Cystine Crystals

6.2.1. Intestinal Cystine Crystals

Besides the determination in the cornea [27], cystine crystals can be detected, upon biopsy, in intestinal mucosa, where they tend to diminish following adequate cysteamine therapy. However, they are still present even when levels of cystine in white blood cells are low, thus suggesting that cysteamine treatment may not be completely effective within tissues [62]. As in other organs, cystine crystals in gastric and intestinal mucosa preferentially accumulate within interstitial macrophages [68]. Obviously, routinely performing gastric or intestinal biopsies is not suitable for therapeutic disease monitoring due to the invasiveness of the procedure and low reproducibility.

6.2.2. Intradermal Cystine Crystal Determination and Skin Aging

Accelerated skin aging is characteristic of cystinosis patients [63], where cystine crystals accumulate in dermal macrophages and fibroblasts. Crystals in skin can be determined in vivo by advanced non-invasive methods, such as high-definition optical coherence tomography [69] and reflectance confocal microscopy [55]. High-definition optical coherence tomography in skin from patients with cystinosis reveals a significant reduction in epidermal and papillary dermis thickness with respect to healthy controls. Moreover, the reduced thickness of epidermis in subjects characterized by *CTNS* mutations was found to be predictive of extrarenal manifestations such as retinopathy and primary hypothyroidism [69].

Reflectance confocal microscopy allows differentiation of the density, within skin, of crystal-containing particles that are present in higher quantities in older patients and in those who started cysteamine treatment later [55]. This method, coupled with an automated and unbiased imaging tool for the quantification of crystal area and volume, makes cystine crystals in skin a novel biomarker that can facilitate long-term monitoring of cystinosis patients in clinical practice [70]. The study by Bengali et al. [70] expanded the observation of Chiaverini et al. [55], monitoring 70 cystinosis patients for over two years through analysis of punch skin biopsy and the quantification of images of 2D area and 3D volume of crystals in dermis, compared to 27 healthy controls. Images were automatically processed and showed significantly different mean values in cystinosis patients vs. controls. Moreover, the normalized confocal crystal volume increased with age and was also associated with the stage of CKD and diagnosis of hypothyroidism, thus showing its potential as a biomarker of disease severity over time [70].

Novel biomarkers for cystine are summarized in Table 2.

Table 2. Novel biomarkers for determination of cystine content in cells and tissues.

Biomarker	Cell/Tissue	Reference
Chitotriosidase	Macrophages	[58]
Alpha-ketoglutarate	Plasma	[67]
Cystine crystals	Skin	[55,69,70]

7. Conclusions

Prognosis of nephropathic cystinosis has dramatically improved due to the introduction of cystine-depleting therapy and renal replacement therapy. Patients receiving early diagnosis and early treatment have an increased life expectancy and better quality of life. Early, continuous, and appropriate cysteamine depletion therapy allows the maintenance of intracellular cystine within optimal cut-off values. Despite the limitations, leucocyte cystine measurements is the only validated tool for disease monitoring, and its use for optimization of depleting treatment is crucial. Nevertheless, it is pivotal to develop alternative strategies for therapeutic monitoring to overcome the limitations of this marker. Further research is required to validate and integrate different novel biomarkers to be used as a single tool which will allow accurate estimation of the efficiency of treatment and long-term prognosis of patients with cystinosis.

Author Contributions: F.E., G.M., M.P., L.P., E.V., B.M.G., F.C., D.C., S.R. and E.L. conceptualized and searched the literature. F.E. and E.L. wrote the manuscript. F.E., G.M., M.P., L.P., E.V., B.M.G., F.C., D.C., S.R. and E.L. reviewed and edited the manuscript. All authors have read and agreed to the published version of the manuscript.

Funding: This research received no external funding.

Data Availability Statement: Not applicable.

Acknowledgments: Editorial assistance was provided by Irene Sebastianutto, and Barbara Bartolini, on behalf of Health Publishing and Services srl. Medical writing and editorial assistance were funded by Chiesi Italia S.p.A. The Special Issue of Cells is financially supported by Cystinosis Research Ireland, Cystinosis Foundation UK, Cystinosis Research Network and Cystinosis Network Europe. E.L. is supported by the Fund Scientific Research Flanders (F.W.O Vlaanderen), grant 1801110N, the Cystinosis Research Network and Cystinosis Ireland. F.E. is supported by the Cystinosis Research Foundation. F.E., E.L., G.M., L.P., E.V. acknowledge European Reference Kidney Network (ERKNet).

Conflicts of Interest: F.E. received fees and honoraria in the past 24 months from Chiesi Farmaceutica Spa, Recordati Rare Diseases, Kyowa Kirin, Avrobio, Otsuka Pharmaceuticals. S.R. and F.C. are employees of Chiesi Italia S.p.A, Parma, Italy. D.C. declares to be involved in multiple industry-driven trial protocols, as P.I. and sub-P.I. since 2005. He occasionally consults for regulatory agencies (RIZIV-INAMI, CTG, EMA), health care consultants and many large and small pharma and biotech companies. He has received speaker fees and advisory board compensations from companies active in the field of Inborn Errors of Metabolism, e.g., Alexion, Alnylam, Sanofi-Genzyme, Orphalan, Takeda. The University of Leuven (Leuven Research and Development, LRD) and University Hospitals Leuven have— on his behalf—received research grants, travel and conference bursaries, and speaker fees and advisory board compensations from a.o. Sanofi-Genzyme, Takeda-Shire, Alexion, Alnylam, Amicus, Actelion, Bayer, Biomarin, BMS, Chiesi, Orpha Labs, Orphalan, Roche, Schering-Plough, Sobi, Synageva. E.L. received consultancy fees and is a member of advisory board of Recordati and Chiesi. G.M., M.P., L.P., E.V., B.M.G. declare no conflict of interest.

References

1. Thoene, J.; Lemons, R.; Anikster, Y.; Mullet, J.; Paelicke, K.; Lucero, C.; Gahl, W.; Schneider, J.; Shu, S.G.; Campbell, H.T. Mutations of CTNS causing intermediate cystinosis. *Mol. Genet. Metab.* **1999**, *67*, 283–293. [CrossRef] [PubMed]
2. Town, M.; Jean, G.; Cherqui, S.; Attard, M.; Forestier, L.; Whitmore, S.A.; Callen, D.F.; Gribouval, O.; Broyer, M.; Bates, G.P.; et al. A novel gene encoding an integral membrane protein is mutated in nephropathic cystinosis. *Nat. Genet.* **1998**, *18*, 319–324. [CrossRef] [PubMed]
3. The Cystinosis Collaborative Research Group. Linkage of the gene for cystinosis to markers on the short arm of chromosome 17. *Nat. Genet.* **1995**, *10*, 246–248. [CrossRef] [PubMed]
4. Veys, K.R.; Elmonem, M.A.; Arcolino, F.O.; van den Heuvel, L.; Levtchenko, E. Nephropathic cystinosis: An update. *Curr. Opin. Pediatr.* **2017**, *29*, 168–178. [CrossRef]
5. Besouw, M.T.; Van Dyck, M.; Cassiman, D.; Claes, K.J.; Levtchenko, E.N. Management dilemmas in pediatric nephrology: Cystinosis. *Pediatr. Nephrol.* **2015**, *30*, 1349–1360. [CrossRef]
6. Gultekingil Keser, A.; Topaloglu, R.; Bilginer, Y.; Besbas, N. Long-term endocrinologic complications of cystinosis. *Minerva. Pediatr.* **2014**, *66*, 123–130.
7. Emma, F.; Nesterova, G.; Langman, C.; Labbe, A.; Cherqui, S.; Goodyer, P.; Janssen, M.C.; Greco, M.; Topaloglu, R.; Elenberg, E.; et al. Nephropathic cystinosis: An international consensus document. *Nephrol. Dial. Transpl.* **2014**, *29* (Suppl. 4), iv87–iv94. [CrossRef]
8. Gahl, W.A.; Thoene, J.G.; Schneider, J.A. Cystinosis. *N. Engl. J. Med.* **2002**, *347*, 111–121. [CrossRef]
9. Topaloglu, R. Nephropathic cystinosis: An update on genetic conditioning. *Pediatr. Nephrol.* **2021**, *36*, 1347–1352. [CrossRef]
10. David, D.; Princiero Berlingerio, S.; Elmonem, M.A.; Oliveira Arcolino, F.; Soliman, N.; van den Heuvel, B.; Gijsbers, R.; Levtchenko, E. Molecular Basis of Cystinosis: Geographic Distribution, Functional Consequences of Mutations in the CTNS Gene, and Potential for Repair. *Nephron.* **2019**, *141*, 133–146. [CrossRef]

11. Ivanova, E.A.; Arcolino, F.O.; Elmonem, M.A.; Rastaldi, M.P.; Giardino, L.; Cornelissen, E.M.; van den Heuvel, L.P.; Levtchenko, E.N. Cystinosin deficiency causes podocyte damage and loss associated with increased cell motility. *Kidney Int.* **2016**, *89*, 1037–1048. [CrossRef] [PubMed]
12. Levtchenko, E.; Monnens, L. Development of Fanconi syndrome during infancy in a patient with cystinosis. *Acta. Paediatr.* **2006**, *95*, 379–380. [CrossRef] [PubMed]
13. Long, W.S.; Seashore, M.R.; Siegel, N.J.; Bia, M.J. Idiopathic Fanconi syndrome with progressive renal failure: A case report and discussion. *Yale. J. Biol. Med.* **1990**, *63*, 15–28. [PubMed]
14. Brodin-Sartorius, A.; Tete, M.J.; Niaudet, P.; Antignac, C.; Guest, G.; Ottolenghi, C.; Charbit, M.; Moyse, D.; Legendre, C.; Lesavre, P.; et al. Cysteamine therapy delays the progression of nephropathic cystinosis in late adolescents and adults. *Kidney Int.* **2012**, *81*, 179–189. [CrossRef]
15. Nesterova, G.; Gahl, W.A. Cystinosis: Tthe evolution of a treatable disease. *Pediatr. Nephrol.* **2013**, *28*, 51–59. [CrossRef]
16. Gahl, W.A.; Balog, J.Z.; Kleta, R. Nephropathic cystinosis in adults: Natural history and effects of oral cysteamine therapy. *Ann. Intern. Med.* **2007**, *147*, 242–250. [CrossRef]
17. Schiefer, J.; Zenker, M.; Grone, H.J.; Chatzikyrkou, C.; Mertens, P.R.; Liakopoulos, V. Unrecognized juvenile nephropathic cystinosis. *Kidney. Int.* **2018**, *94*, 1027. [CrossRef]
18. Manz, F.; Gretz, N. Cystinosis in the Federal Republic of Germany. Coordination and analysis of the data. *J. Inherit. Metab. Dis.* **1985**, *8*, 2–4. [CrossRef]
19. Cherqui, S.; Courtoy, P.J. The renal Fanconi syndrome in cystinosis: Pathogenic insights and therapeutic perspectives. *Nat. Rev. Nephrol.* **2017**, *13*, 115–131. [CrossRef]
20. Greco, M.; Brugnara, M.; Zaffanello, M.; Taranta, A.; Pastore, A.; Emma, F. Long-term outcome of nephropathic cystinosis: A 20-year single-center experience. *Pediatr. Nephrol.* **2010**, *25*, 2459–2467. [CrossRef]
21. Schulman, J.D.; Wong, V.G.; Kuwabara, T.; Bradley, K.H.; Seegmiller, J.E. Intracellular cystine content of leukocyte populations in cystinosis. *Arch. Intern. Med.* **1970**, *125*, 660–664. [CrossRef] [PubMed]
22. Schneider, J.A.; Bradley, K.; Seegmiller, J.E. Increased cystine in leukocytes from individuals homozygous and heterozygous for cystinosis. *Science* **1967**, *157*, 1321–1322. [CrossRef]
23. Oshima, R.G.; Willis, R.C.; Furlong, C.E.; Schneider, J.A. Binding assays for amino acids. The utilization of a cystine binding protein from Escherichia coli for the determination of acid-soluble cystine in small physiological samples. *J. Biol. Chem.* **1974**, *249*, 6033–6039. [CrossRef]
24. Smith, F.; Furlong, C.E.; Greene, A.A.; Schneider, J.A. Cystine: Binding protein assay. *Methods Enzymol.* **1987**, *143*, 144–148. [CrossRef] [PubMed]
25. Chabli, A.; Aupetit, J.; Raehm, M.; Ricquier, D.; Chadefaux-Vekemans, B. Measurement of cystine in granulocytes using liquid chromatography-tandem mass spectrometry. *Clin. Biochem.* **2007**, *40*, 692–698. [CrossRef]
26. de Graaf-Hess, A.; Trijbels, F.; Blom, H. New method for determining cystine in leukocytes and fibroblasts. *Clin. Chem.* **1999**, *45*, 2224–2228. [CrossRef]
27. Elmonem, M.A.; Veys, K.R.; Soliman, N.A.; van Dyck, M.; van den Heuvel, L.P.; Levtchenko, E. Cystinosis: A review. *Orphanet. J. Rare. Dis.* **2016**, *11*, 47. [CrossRef]
28. Smolin, L.A.; Clark, K.F.; Schneider, J.A. An improved method for heterozygote detection of cystinosis, using polymorphonuclear leukocytes. *Am. J. Hum. Genet.* **1987**, *41*, 266–275.
29. Levtchenko, E.; de Graaf-Hess, A.; Wilmer, M.; van den Heuvel, L.; Monnens, L.; Blom, H. Comparison of cystine determination in mixed leukocytes vs polymorphonuclear leukocytes for diagnosis of cystinosis and monitoring of cysteamine therapy. *Clin. Chem.* **2004**, *50*, 1686–1688. [CrossRef]
30. Fowler, B.; Bielsky, M.C.; Farrington, Z. *White Cell Cystine Group*; BIMDG Bulletin Spring 2001, WCYS Compiled.doc.; BIMDG: Cambridge, UK, 2001.
31. Chadefaux-Vekemans, B. *White Cell Cystine Group: Guideline no. 2. Polymorphonuclear Leucocyte Preparation*; BIMDG Bulletin Spring 2001; BIMDG: Cambridge, UK, 2001.
32. Gertsman, I.; Johnson, W.S.; Nishikawa, C.; Gangoiti, J.A.; Holmes, B.; Barshop, B.A. Diagnosis and Monitoring of Cystinosis Using Immunomagnetically Purified Granulocytes. *Clin. Chem.* **2016**, *62*, 766–772. [CrossRef]
33. Lowry, O.H.; Rosebrough, N.J.; Farr, A.L.; Randall, R.J. Protein measurement with the Folin phenol reagent. *J. Biol. Chem.* **1951**, *193*, 265–275. [CrossRef]
34. Smith, P.K.; Krohn, R.I.; Hermanson, G.T.; Mallia, A.K.; Gartner, F.H.; Provenzano, M.D.; Fujimoto, E.K.; Goeke, N.M.; Olson, B.J.; Klenk, D.C. Measurement of protein using bicinchoninic acid. *Anal. Biochem.* **1985**, *150*, 76–85. [CrossRef]
35. Powell, K.L.; Langman, C.B. An unexpected problem in the clinical assessment of cystinosis. *Pediatr. Nephrol.* **2012**, *27*, 687–688. [CrossRef]
36. Langman, C.B.; Barshop, B.A.; Deschenes, G.; Emma, F.; Goodyer, P.; Lipkin, G.; Midgley, J.P.; Ottolenghi, C.; Servais, A.; Soliman, N.A.; et al. Controversies and research agenda in nephropathic cystinosis: Conclusions from a "Kidney Disease: Improving Global Outcomes" (KDIGO) Controversies Conference. *Kidney. Int.* **2016**, *89*, 1192–1203. [CrossRef]
37. Emma, F.; Hoff, W.V.; Hohenfellner, K.; Topaloglu, R.; Greco, M.; Ariceta, G.; Bettini, C.; Bockenhauer, D.; Veys, K.; Pape, L.; et al. An international cohort study spanning five decades assessed outcomes of nephropathic cystinosis. *Kidney. Int.* **2021**, *100*, 1112–1123. [CrossRef]

38. Jackson, M.; Young, E. Prenatal diagnosis of cystinosis by quantitative measurement of cystine in chorionic villi and cultured cells. *Prenat. Diagn.* **2005**, *25*, 1045–1047. [CrossRef]
39. da Silva, V.A.; Zurbrugg, R.P.; Lavanchy, P.; Blumberg, A.; Suter, H.; Wyss, S.R.; Luthy, C.M.; Oetliker, O.H. Long-term treatment of infantile nephropathic cystinosis with cysteamine. *N. Engl. J. Med.* **1985**, *313*, 1460–1463. [CrossRef]
40. Gahl, W.A.; Thoene, J.G. Cystinosis: A disorder of lysosomal membrane transport. In *The Metabolic and Molecular Bases of Inherited Disease*; Scriver, C.R., Sly, W.S., Childs, B., Beaudet, A.L., Valle, D., Kinzler, K.W., Vogelstein, B., Eds.; McGraw-Hill: New York, NY, USA, 2001; pp. 5085–5108.
41. Surmeli Doven, S.; Delibas, A.; Kayacan, U.R.; Unal, S. Short-cut diagnostic tool in cystinosis: Bone marrow aspiration. *Pediatr. Int.* **2017**, *59*, 1178–1182. [CrossRef]
42. Wamelink, M.M.; Struys, E.A.; Jansen, E.E.; Blom, H.J.; Vilboux, T.; Gahl, W.A.; Komhoff, M.; Jakobs, C.; Levtchenko, E.N. Elevated concentrations of sedoheptulose in bloodspots of patients with cystinosis caused by the 57-kb deletion: Implications for diagnostics and neonatal screening. *Mol. Genet. Metab.* **2011**, *102*, 339–342. [CrossRef]
43. Fleige, T.; Burggraf, S.; Czibere, L.; Haring, J.; Gluck, B.; Keitel, L.M.; Landt, O.; Harms, E.; Hohenfellner, K.; Durner, J.; et al. Next generation sequencing as second-tier test in high-throughput newborn screening for nephropathic cystinosis. *Eur. J. Hum. Genet.* **2020**, *28*, 193–201. [CrossRef]
44. Hohenfellner, K.; Bergmann, C.; Fleige, T.; Janzen, N.; Burggraf, S.; Olgemoller, B.; Gahl, W.A.; Czibere, L.; Froschauer, S.; Roschinger, W.; et al. Molecular based newborn screening in Germany: Follow-up for cystinosis. *Mol. Genet. Metab. Rep.* **2019**, *21*, 100514. [CrossRef] [PubMed]
45. Nesterova, G.; Williams, C.; Bernardini, I.; Gahl, W.A. Cystinosis: Renal glomerular and renal tubular function in relation to compliance with cystine-depleting therapy. *Pediatr. Nephrol.* **2015**, *30*, 945–951. [CrossRef] [PubMed]
46. Servais, A.; Saitovitch, A.; Hummel, A.; Boisgontier, J.; Scemla, A.; Sberro-Soussan, R.; Snanoudj, R.; Lemaitre, H.; Legendre, C.; Pontoizeau, C.; et al. Central nervous system complications in adult cystinosis patients. *J. Inherit. Metab. Dis.* **2020**, *43*, 348–356. [CrossRef] [PubMed]
47. Wilmer, M.J.; Schoeber, J.P.; van den Heuvel, L.P.; Levtchenko, E.N. Cystinosis: Practical tools for diagnosis and treatment. *Pediatr. Nephrol.* **2011**, *26*, 205–215. [CrossRef]
48. Levtchenko, E.N.; van Dael, C.M.; de Graaf-Hess, A.C.; Wilmer, M.J.; van den Heuvel, L.P.; Monnens, L.A.; Blom, H.J. Strict cysteamine dose regimen is required to prevent nocturnal cystine accumulation in cystinosis. *Pediatr. Nephrol.* **2006**, *21*, 110–113. [CrossRef]
49. Linden, S.; Klank, S.; Harms, E.; Gruneberg, M.; Park, J.H.; Marquardt, T. Cystinosis: Therapy adherence and metabolic monitoring in patients treated with immediate-release cysteamine. *Mol. Genet. Metab. Rep.* **2020**, *24*, 100620. [CrossRef]
50. Ariceta, G.; Giordano, V.; Santos, F. Effects of long-term cysteamine treatment in patients with cystinosis. *Pediatr. Nephrol.* **2019**, *34*, 571–578. [CrossRef]
51. Kleta, R.; Kaskel, F.; Dohil, R.; Goodyer, P.; Guay-Woodford, L.M.; Harms, E.; Ingelfinger, J.R.; Koch, V.H.; Langman, C.B.; Leonard, M.B.; et al. Diseases, N.I.H.O.o.R. First NIH/Office of Rare Diseases Conference on Cystinosis: Past, present, and future. *Pediatr. Nephrol.* **2005**, *20*, 452–454. [CrossRef]
52. Markello, T.C.; Bernardini, I.M.; Gahl, W.A. Improved renal function in children with cystinosis treated with cysteamine. *N. Engl. J. Med.* **1993**, *328*, 1157–1162. [CrossRef]
53. Gahl, W.A.; Reed, G.F.; Thoene, J.G.; Schulman, J.D.; Rizzo, W.B.; Jonas, A.J.; Denman, D.W.; Schlesselman, J.J.; Corden, B.J.; Schneider, J.A. Cysteamine therapy for children with nephropathic cystinosis. *N. Engl. J. Med.* **1987**, *316*, 971–977. [CrossRef]
54. Labbe, A.; Niaudet, P.; Loirat, C.; Charbit, M.; Guest, G.; Baudouin, C. In vivo confocal microscopy and anterior segment optical coherence tomography analysis of the cornea in nephropathic cystinosis. *Ophthalmology* **2009**, *116*, 870–876. [CrossRef] [PubMed]
55. Chiaverini, C.; Kang, H.Y.; Sillard, L.; Berard, E.; Niaudet, P.; Guest, G.; Cailliez, M.; Bahadoran, P.; Lacour, J.P.; Ballotti, R.; et al. In vivo reflectance confocal microscopy of the skin: A noninvasive means of assessing body cystine accumulation in infantile cystinosis. *J. Am. Acad. Dermatol.* **2013**, *68*, e111–e116. [CrossRef] [PubMed]
56. Elmonem, M.A.; Makar, S.H.; van den Heuvel, L.; Abdelaziz, H.; Abdelrahman, S.M.; Bossuyt, X.; Janssen, M.C.; Cornelissen, E.A.; Lefeber, D.J.; Joosten, L.A.; et al. Clinical utility of chitotriosidase enzyme activity in nephropathic cystinosis. *Orphanet. J. Rare. Dis.* **2014**, *9*, 155. [CrossRef]
57. Prencipe, G.; Caiello, I.; Cherqui, S.; Whisenant, T.; Petrini, S.; Emma, F.; De Benedetti, F. Inflammasome activation by cystine crystals: Implications for the pathogenesis of cystinosis. *J. Am. Soc. Nephrol.* **2014**, *25*, 1163–1169. [CrossRef]
58. Veys, K.R.P.; Elmonem, M.A.; Van Dyck, M.; Janssen, M.C.; Cornelissen, E.A.M.; Hohenfellner, K.; Prencipe, G.; van den Heuvel, L.P.; Levtchenko, E. Chitotriosidase as a Novel Biomarker for Therapeutic Monitoring of Nephropathic Cystinosis. *J. Am. Soc. Nephrol.* **2020**, *31*, 1092–1106. [CrossRef]
59. Lobry, T.; Miller, R.; Nevo, N.; Rocca, C.J.; Zhang, J.; Catz, S.D.; Moore, F.; Thomas, L.; Pouly, D.; Bailleux, A.; et al. Interaction between galectin-3 and cystinosin uncovers a pathogenic role of inflammation in kidney involvement of cystinosis. *Kidney Int.* **2019**, *96*, 350–362. [CrossRef] [PubMed]
60. Brown, R.J. A clinico-pathological study of cystinosis in two siblings. *Arch. Dis. Child.* **1952**, *27*, 428–433. [CrossRef]
61. DiDomenico, P.; Berry, G.; Bass, D.; Fridge, J.; Sarwal, M. Noncirrhotic portal hypertension in association with juvenile nephropathic cystinosis: Case presentation and review of the literature. *J. Inherit. Metab. Dis.* **2004**, *27*, 693–699. [CrossRef]

62. Dohil, R.; Carrigg, A.; Newbury, R. A potential new method to estimate tissue cystine content in nephropathic cystinosis. *J. Pediatr.* **2012**, *161*, 531–535.e1. [CrossRef]
63. Guillet, G.; Sassolas, B.; Fromentoux, S.; Gobin, E.; Leroy, J.P. Skin storage of cystine and premature skin ageing in cystinosis. *Lancet* **1998**, *352*, 1444–1445. [CrossRef]
64. Monier, L.; Mauvieux, L. Cystine crystals in bone marrow aspirate. *Blood* **2015**, *126*, 1515. [CrossRef] [PubMed]
65. Elmonem, M.A.; Ramadan, D.I.; Issac, M.S.; Selim, L.A.; Elkateb, S.M. Blood spot versus plasma chitotriosidase: A systematic clinical comparison. *Clin. Biochem.* **2014**, *47*, 38–43. [CrossRef]
66. Guo, Y.; He, W.; Boer, A.M.; Wevers, R.A.; de Bruijn, A.M.; Groener, J.E.; Hollak, C.E.; Aerts, J.M.; Galjaard, H.; van Diggelen, O.P. Elevated plasma chitotriosidase activity in various lysosomal storage disorders. *J. Inherit. Metab. Dis.* **1995**, *18*, 717–722. [CrossRef] [PubMed]
67. Jamalpoor, A.; van Gelder, C.A.; Yousef Yengej, F.A.; Zaal, E.A.; Berlingerio, S.P.; Veys, K.R.; Pou Casellas, C.; Voskuil, K.; Essa, K.; Ammerlaan, C.M.; et al. Cysteamine-bicalutamide combination therapy corrects proximal tubule phenotype in cystinosis. *EMBO Mol. Med.* **2021**, *13*, e13067. [CrossRef] [PubMed]
68. Elmonem, M.A.; Veys, K.; Oliveira Arcolino, F.; Van Dyck, M.; Benedetti, M.C.; Diomedi-Camassei, F.; De Hertogh, G.; van den Heuvel, L.P.; Renard, M.; Levtchenko, E. Allogeneic HSCT transfers wild-type cystinosin to nonhematological epithelial cells in cystinosis: First human report. *Am. J. Transplant.* **2018**, *18*, 2823–2828. [CrossRef]
69. Veys, K.R.P.; Elmonem, M.A.; Dhaenens, F.; Van Dyck, M.; Janssen, M.; Cornelissen, E.A.M.; Hohenfellner, K.; Reda, A.; Quatresooz, P.; van den Heuvel, B.; et al. Enhanced Intrinsic Skin Aging in Nephropathic Cystinosis Assessed by High-Definition Optical Coherence Tomography. *J. Investig. Dermatol.* **2019**, *139*, 2242–2245. [CrossRef]
70. Bengali, M.; Goodman, S.; Sun, X.; Dohil, M.A.; Dohil, R.; Newbury, R.; Lobry, T.; Hernandez, L.; Antignac, C.; Jain, S.; et al. Non-invasive intradermal imaging of cystine crystals in cystinosis. *PLoS ONE* **2021**, *16*, e0247846. [CrossRef]

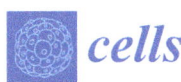

Review

Muscle and Bone Impairment in Infantile Nephropathic Cystinosis: New Concepts

Dieter Haffner [1,2,*], Maren Leifheit-Nestler [1,2], Candide Alioli [3] and Justine Bacchetta [3,4]

1. Department of Pediatric Kidney, Liver and Metabolic Diseases, Hannover Medical School, Carl-Neuberg-Str. 1, 30625 Hannover, Germany; Leifheit-Nestler.Maren@mh-hannover.de
2. Pediatric Research Center, Hannover Medical School, Carl-Neuberg-Str. 1, 30625 Hannover, Germany
3. INSERM Research Unit 1033, Pathophysiology of Bone Disease, Faculté de Médecine Lyon Est, Université de Lyon, Rue Guillaume Paradin, 69008 Lyon, France; candide.alioli@inserm.fr (C.A.); justine.bacchetta@chu-lyon.fr (J.B.)
4. Reference Center for Rare Renal Diseases, Reference Center for Rare Diseases of Calcium and Phosphate Metabolism, Pediatric Nephrology, Rheumatology and Dermatology Unit, Hôpital Femme Mère Enfant, Boulevard Pinel, 69500 Bron, France
* Correspondence: haffner.dieter@mh-hannover.de

Abstract: Cystinosis Metabolic Bone Disease (CMBD) has emerged during the last decade as a well-recognized, long-term complication in patients suffering from infantile nephropathic cystinosis (INC), resulting in significant morbidity and impaired quality of life in teenagers and adults with INC. Its underlying pathophysiology is complex and multifactorial, associating complementary, albeit distinct entities, in addition to ordinary mineral and bone disorders observed in other types of chronic kidney disease. Amongst these long-term consequences are renal Fanconi syndrome, hypophosphatemic rickets, malnutrition, hormonal abnormalities, muscular impairment, and intrinsic cellular bone defects in bone cells, due to *CTNS* mutations. Recent research data in the field have demonstrated abnormal mineral regulation, intrinsic bone defects, cysteamine toxicity, muscle wasting and, likely interleukin-1-driven inflammation in the setting of CMBD. Here we summarize these new pathophysiological deregulations and discuss the crucial interplay between bone and muscle in INC. In future, vitamin D and/or biotherapies targeting the IL1β pathway may improve muscle wasting and subsequently CMBD, but this remains to be proven.

Keywords: infantile nephropathic cystinosis; bone-muscle wasting; fibroblast growth factor 23; osteoclasts; sclerostin; leptin; fractures; cysteamine

1. Introduction

Infantile nephropathic cystinosis (INC) is a rare autosomal recessive storage disease, due to mutations in the *CTNS* gene encoding for the lysosomal cystine transporter cystinosin [1]. CTNS malfunction results in an accumulation of cystine in all organs, primarily the kidneys, leading to Fanconi syndrome, a global defect of the proximal renal tubules, and progressive chronic kidney disease (CKD), which can be ameliorated by early treatment with the cystine-depleting agent cysteamine [2,3]. Severe bone and muscle impairment are other important complications of INC, which often persist or are even aggravated, despite measures for Fanconi syndrome, cysteamine therapy, and kidney replacement therapy (dialysis or kidney transplantation) [4–7]. Initial studies suggest that bone and muscle impairment in INC are the primary consequences of Fanconi syndrome, and later, of mineral and bone disorder associated with CKD (CKD-MBD) [8,9]. The former results in impairment of calcium and phosphate homeostasis, with the clinical consequences of hypophosphatemic rickets and muscle weakness, whereas the latter describes the complexity of renal osteodystrophy, alterations in mineral and vitamin D metabolism, and cardiovascular complications, as seen in CKD patients with other underlying causes of

Citation: Haffner, D.; Leifheit-Nestler, M.; Alioli, C.; Bacchetta, J. Muscle and Bone Impairment in Infantile Nephropathic Cystinosis: New Concepts. *Cells* **2022**, *11*, 170. https://doi.org/10.3390/cells11010170

Academic Editor: Alexander E. Kalyuzhny

Received: 11 November 2021
Accepted: 1 January 2022
Published: 5 January 2022

Publisher's Note: MDPI stays neutral with regard to jurisdictional claims in published maps and institutional affiliations.

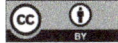

Copyright: © 2022 by the authors. Licensee MDPI, Basel, Switzerland. This article is an open access article distributed under the terms and conditions of the Creative Commons Attribution (CC BY) license (https://creativecommons.org/licenses/by/4.0/).

CKD [2,10]. Recent clinical and experimental studies provide increasing evidence that bone and muscle impairment in INC is much more complex and, at least partly, due to an intrinsic bone defect and elevated leptin signaling, promoting muscle wasting [11–17]. The term cystinosis metabolic bone disease (CMBD) was coined by an international guideline initiative to describe this complex bone phenotype in INC patients (Figure 1) [18]. This review highlights the recent insights in the pathophysiology of muscle and bone impairment and their interplay in INC.

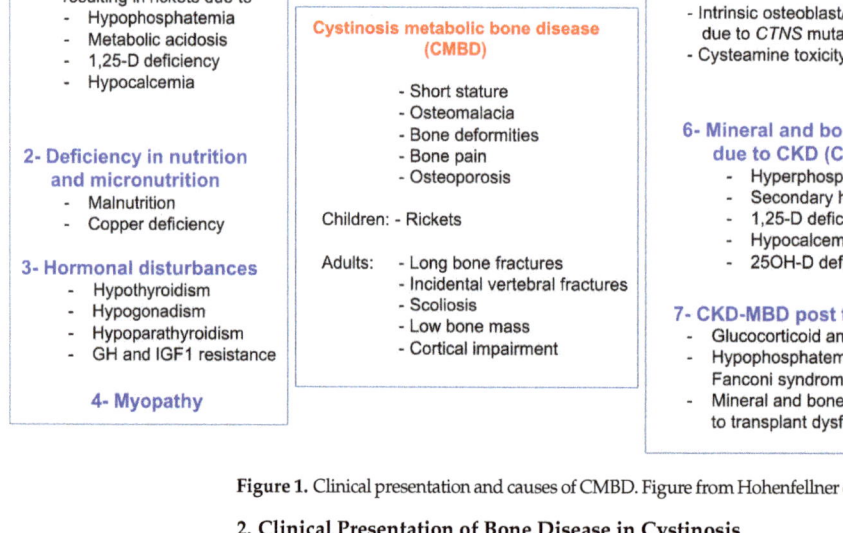

Figure 1. Clinical presentation and causes of CMBD. Figure from Hohenfellner et al., with permission [18].

2. Clinical Presentation of Bone Disease in Cystinosis

The early use (<2 years) of cysteamine treatment has postponed end-stage kidney disease and extra-renal complications beyond the second decade of life [19]. However, as patient survival improves [20], bone impairment was recently described as a "novel" complication of cystinosis resulting in substantial comorbidity during puberty or early adulthood [5–8,21]. This complication may dramatically alter the quality of life of patients: "As patients with cystinosis now routinely survive well into adulthood, additional challenges to lifelong bone health have emerged" [8]. In 2016, we reported on three teenagers with INC, displaying a severe bone phenotype that was characterized by unusual resorption areas on bone biopsy [5]. Later, a French observational study was carried out on 10 INC patients (median age 23 years, range 10–35) using biomarkers and High Resolution peripheral Quantitative Computed Tomography (HR-pQCT) at the ultra-distal tibia [6]. Seven patients (70%) complained of at least one bone symptom, namely, bone pain and/or deformation and/or history of fractures. Significant alterations in cortical parameters and, notably, cortical thickness were noted in INC patients compared to healthy subjects, similar to what was observed in $CTNS^{-/-}$ knockout mice (vide infra). Circulating and urinary calcium, as well as alkaline phosphatase (ALP) levels, were normal. However, there was a tendency towards low parathyroid hormone (PTH) and low fibroblast growth factor 23 (FGF23) levels, likely reflecting the consequences of chronic tubular phosphate wasting, although Fanconi syndrome appeared to be well controlled in these patients. These results were further confirmed in 2020, both in a German and an American study, clearly showing decreased FGF23 levels in INC patients when corrected for the stage of CKD [13,14].

A North American team also performed bone and mineral evaluations in 30 INC patients with a mean age of 20 years (range 5–44 y) [7]. Bone mineral density was reduced at all sites; low bone mass in at least one evaluation zone was present in 46% of patients. A large proportion of patients displayed bone symptoms: one or more fractures of the long bones (27%), incidental vertebral fractures (32%), limb deformities (34%), and scoliosis (50%).

An international guideline on the diagnosis and management of CMBD was published in 2019 [18]. Briefly, assessment of CMBD involves; regular monitoring of longitudinal growth, blood levels of phosphate, calcium, ALP, and bicarbonate, and, depending on the clinical and biochemical findings, bone radiography, and assessment of hormone levels and vitamins, such as thyroid hormone, PTH, 25 OH vitamin D, and testosterone in males, and surveillance for non-renal complications of INC including myopathy. Patients require a multi-disciplinary and comprehensive management of CMBD. Urinary loss due to Fanconi syndrome should be replaced, including phosphate and bicarbonate). Patients require adequate cystine-depleting treatment with cysteamine, adequate caloric and protein intake, supplementation with native vitamin D, in cases of vitamin D deficiency, treatment with active vitamin D to support the treatment of rickets, and eventually hormone replacement/therapy (thyroid hormone, testosterone in males, and recombinant growth hormone in cases of persistent short stature) [22], physical therapy, and orthopedic surgery in cases of persistent, significant limb deformities despite adequate treatment for Fanconi syndrome [18].

3. Cystinosis Metabolic Bone Disease

The pathophysiology of the bone phenotype in INC is complex. At least eight distinct factors contribute to CMBD (see Figure 1), which are outlined in the following section [18].

3.1. Fanconi Syndrome

Fanconi syndrome, due to cystine accumulation in renal proximal tubules, emerges around the age of 6 months, resulting in renal phosphate wasting and consecutive hypophosphatemia, metabolic acidosis, 1,25-vitamin D deficiency, and hypocalcemia. All of these factors promote the development of hypophosphatemic rickets [2,13,18]. However, hypophosphatemia is thought to be the most crucial factor, as it was shown to impair apoptosis of hypertrophic chondrocytes in the growth plate, the decisive cellular defect in all forms of rickets [23]. In addition, metabolic acidosis was shown to impair both, bone mineralization and linear growth in children [24,25].

3.2. Deficiency in Nutrition and Micronutrition

Children with INC often present with impaired appetite and frequent vomiting, due to excessive fluid intake demands due to Fanconi syndrome-associated polyuria, resulting in caloric and protein malnutrition and eventually copper deficiency, which all contribute to impaired bone growth [26,27].

3.3. Hormonal Disturbances

Hormonal disturbances due to cystine accumulation in endocrine organs may result in hypothyroidism, hypogonadism, and hypoparathyroidism, all of which are known inhibitors of longitudinal bone growth [28,29]. Gonadal dysfunction affecting males is characterized by hypergonadotropic hypogonadism, i.e., high luteinizing hormone (LH) and follicle-stimulating hormone (FSH), in association with low testosterone [30]. This is due to the lysosomal overload of Sertoli and Leydig cells in the testes, which can be ameliorated by cysteamine therapy [31]. In addition, INC patients develop an insensitivity to the actions of growth hormone (GH) and insulin-like growth factor 1 (IGF1), as noted in other patients suffering from advanced CKD, which further hinders growth and can be overcome by treatment with recombinant human GH [22,32,33].

3.4. Myopathy

Distal myopathy presents around the second decade of life in children with INC and primarily involves the hand muscles [28,34]. It may even be detected in patients with no overt muscle weakness. Later, patients may develop dysphagia and restrictive lung disease [35–37]. Myopathy is mainly due to cystine accumulation in striated muscles, which may be aggravated by concomitant hypophosphatemia and hypocalcemia due to Fanconi syndrome. Biopsy studies of affected muscles show marked fiber-size variability, vacuoles, and impaired grouping of fiber type [38]. Interestingly, cysteine crystals were found in perimysial cells, whereas no crystals could be detected in cell vacuoles. Electrophysiological studies of affected muscles show diminished amplitude and duration. Muscle weakness may initially be mild, primarily involving intrinsic hand muscles. Later, patients show pronounced distal weakness, more so than proximal weakness and contractures [35]. A recent study in 76 pediatric and adult INC patients showed a mean grip strength SD-score of -2.1, which was significantly lower compared to CKD patients with other underlying kidney diseases [39]. Reduced grip strength was associated with the male gender, delayed cysteamine therapy, and low levels of physical activity. Impaired muscle function leads to impaired bone health through reduced mechanical loads on bone. This is supported by the findings that the strength of load-bearing bones largely depends on growing muscle strength [40].

3.5. Mineral and Bone Disorders Due to CKD (CKD-MBD)

CKD-MBD, due to a progressive decline in glomerular function, leads to impaired bone health, well known from CKD patients suffering from other kidney diseases [10]. The term CKD-MBD has replaced the old term renal osteodystrophy, which suggests that bone changes in CKD patients are primarily due to secondary hyperparathyroidism and vitamin D deficiency [41]. The first detectable bone abnormality in mild CKD not associated with renal Fanconi syndrome is an increased expression in the number of sclerostin and FGF23-expressing osteocytes, causing progressive elevations in the plasma concentrations of these bone-derived factors [41–43]. FGF23 acts, as PTH, as a phosphaturic hormone by inhibiting sodium (Na)-dependent phosphate (Pi) reabsorption via NaPi2a/2c after binding to the FGF receptor 1 and its cofactor Klotho [44]. This allows for normal phosphate homeostasis in the early stages of CKD, despite impaired renal excretory capacity. Elevated FGF23 levels also impair synthesis and increase degradation of calcitriol ($1,25(OH)_2D$), thereby promoting vitamin D deficiency [45]. Sclerostin was shown to directly inhibit the Wnt/Beta-catenin pathway in osteocytes. Its synthesis is already increased in patients with CKD stage 2, resulting in reduced bone remodeling [46]. Therefore, the current concept of CKD-MBD is that both increased FGF23 and sclerostin causes early bone loss in the early stages of CKD. It was thought that this is also the case in patients with INC. Recent studies show that INC is characterized by distinct CKD stage-dependent abnormalities in bone metabolism, including sclerostin and FGF23, which differs markedly to that observed in patients with other underlying causes of CKD as outlined below [13,14].

3.6. CKD-MBD Post Kidney Transplantation

Persistent elevation of both FGF23 and PTH levels are often noted in patients who received a kidney transplant, despite excellent transplant function, which may promote bone disease in these patients [47]. In addition, post-transplant growth can be markedly diminished due to glucocorticoid treatment which may also promote osteoporosis and increased risk of fractures in these patients, irrespective of the underlying renal disease [48].

3.7. Intrinsic Bone Defect

Cystinosin is expressed in bone cells, including osteoblasts and osteoclasts. $CTNS^{-/-}$ knockout mice do not develop overt Fanconi syndrome for, so far, unknown reasons [12]. Despite this, they display a clear bone phenotype, characterized by reduced trabecular bone, cortical thickness, and bone mineral density compared to healthy animals [12]. In addition, reduced osteoblast and osteoclast parameters were noted on tibiae histomorphometry of

$CTNS^{-/-}$ knockout mice compared to controls. In vitro experiments using osteoblasts from $CTNS^{-/-}$ knockout mice demonstrated elevated cystine content, reduced numbers of ALP-positive cells, diminished expression of differentiation and activity markers, and impaired mineralization, compared to cells taken from wild-type mice. Conforti et al. also reported that mesenchymal stem cells derived from an INC patient show a diminished ability to differentiate into osteoclasts [49]. Taken together, these observations suggest an intrinsic osteoblast and osteoclast defect in cystinosis.

This was further evaluated in studies using peripheral blood mononuclear cells (PBMCs) derived from INC patients. Claramunt-Taberner et al., demonstrated that CTNS was clearly expressed in human PBMCs derived from healthy subjects [11]. In addition, PBMCs derived from INC patients showed an increased number of tartrate-resistant acid phosphatase 5b (TRAP5b)-positive cells compared to healthy subjects, suggesting that cystinosis favors osteoclastogenesis [11]. The same group performed a subsequent study using PBMCs from patients with *CTNS* variants and residual cystine efflux activity, with inactive *CTNS* variants and with *CTNS* variants not allowing proper protein translation and presentation at the lysosomal membrane [15]. Interestingly, PBMCs with residual CTNS activity generated less osteoclasts compared to those with inactive or absent CTNS, indicating that CTNS may act as a negative regulator of osteoclast formation. In other words, loss of CTNS function may cause increased osteoclast activity. This is also supported by clinical studies in INC patients, using serum TRAP5b levels as a measure of osteoclast function [13]. Lysosomal dysfunction and defective autophagic mitochondria clearance have recently been showed in epithelial tubular cells [50], inducing increased oxidative cells. Since osteoclasts are giant multinucleated cells with a very high mitochondrial density, it is tempting to hypothesize a mitochondrial defect in cystinotic bone, but this remains to be proved [4].

3.8. Cysteamine Toxicity

There is increasing evidence that cysteamine treatment affects osteoblast and osteoclast function. In vitro studies using PBMCs from healthy donors and INC patients showed that cysteamine does not modify osteoclastogenesis [11]. However, high doses of cysteamine resulted in a clear reduction in bone resorption by PBMCs derived from INC patients, whereas low cysteamine doses stimulated osteoblastic differentiation and mineralization. This was later confirmed in a second study by the same group, showing that high dose cysteamine treatment exerts an inhibitory effect on osteoclastic differentiation in PBMCs derived from INC patients, irrespective of the severity of *CTNS* mutation, i.e., residual CTNS activity versus inactive or absent CTNS [15]. Thus, cysteamine, if given at high doses, may also impair bone health in INC patients.

4. Bone and Mineral Metabolism in INC Patients

Recently, the circulating parameters of bone and mineral metabolism were investigated in a cohort of 49 European children and adolescents with INC compared to 80 patients with other CKD entities [13]. The main parameters included; FGF23, soluble Klotho (sKlotho), sclerostin, bone alkaline phosphatase (BAP)—as a marker of bone formation, TRAP5b as an osteoclast marker and the receptor activator for the nuclear factor kappa-B ligand (RANKL)/osteoprotegerin (OPG) system, which is a strong regulator of osteoclast formation and activity. As expected, normalized serum phosphate levels were clearly decreased in INC patients with mild–moderate CKD compared to healthy children and CKD-controls, despite oral treatment with phosphate salts due to persistent renal phosphate wasting (Figure 2). INC patients showed a high frequency of reduced levels of phosphate, calcium PTH, and bicarbonate, and elevated BAP concentrations, which was associated with an 11-fold increased risk of skeletal comorbidity (reduced standardized height, limb deformities, and/or requirement for orthopedic surgery of the lower extremities) compared to CKD controls [13]. The markedly elevated BAP levels in INC patients across all CKD stages suggest persistent mineralization defects in INC patients despite measures for Fanconi syndrome. INC patients showed a specific CKD stage-dependent pattern of bone markers (Figure 3). As expected in CKD controls, FGF23 and sclerostin levels started to increase as early as in CKD stage 2 (eGFR < 90 mL/min/1.73 m^2). By contrast, INC patients demonstrated a delayed increase or lacked an increase in FGF23 and sclerostin serum levels in mild and moderate CKD [13]. FGF23 levels were independently associated with plasma phosphate, calcium and eGFR, suggesting that the delayed increase in FGF23 levels observed in INC patients compared to CKD controls was most likely due to concomitant hypophosphatemia and hypocalcemia. Both, eGFR and dosage of phosphate salts in INC patients correlated with sclerostin levels in the whole study cohort, suggesting that hypophosphatemia may prevent an increase in sclerostin levels in INC patients. Alternatively, the lack of increase in sclerostin levels may reflect a mechanism to compensate osteoblast malfunction due to *CNTS* mutations (vide supra). TRAP5b serum concentrations were elevated by approx. 1.7 SD score in INC patients compared to CKD controls, irrespective of eGFR. The diagnosis of INC was the only factor showing a significant association with sclerostin levels. TRAP5b is synthesized in osteoclasts and its serum levels were shown to correlate with osteoclast activity as well as numbers of osteoclasts. Therefore, elevated TRAP5b levels indicate that either the number of osteoclasts is increased or osteoblast activity is increased in INC patients, compared to other CKD patients of the same age and eGFR.

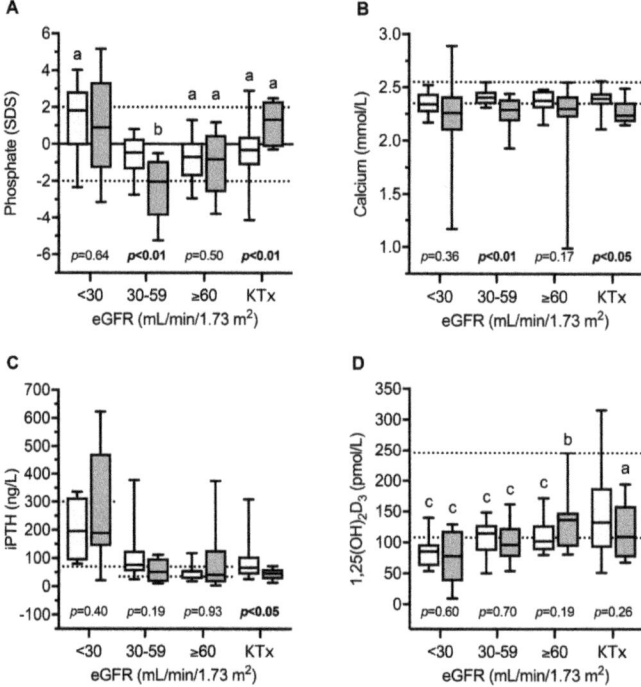

Figure 2. Serum levels of phosphate (**A**), calcium (**B**), intact parathyroid hormone (iPTH, (**C**)), and 1,25(OH)$_2$D$_3$ (**D**) in children with infantile nephropathic cystinosis (INC) and CKD controls as estimated glomerular filtration rate (eGFR) and after kidney transplantation (KTX). Gray box plots indicate INC patients; white box plots indicate CKD controls. Horizontal continuous and broken lines in (**A**) indicate the mean and upper and lower normal range; horizontal broken lines in (**B**,**C**) indicate the upper and lower normal range; horizontal broken lines in (**D**) indicate the PTH target range recommended by KDOQI; a, b, and c indicate $p < 0.05$, $p < 0.01$ and $p < 0.001$ versus healthy children, respectively. SDS, standard deviation score. Figure from Ewert et al., with permission [13].

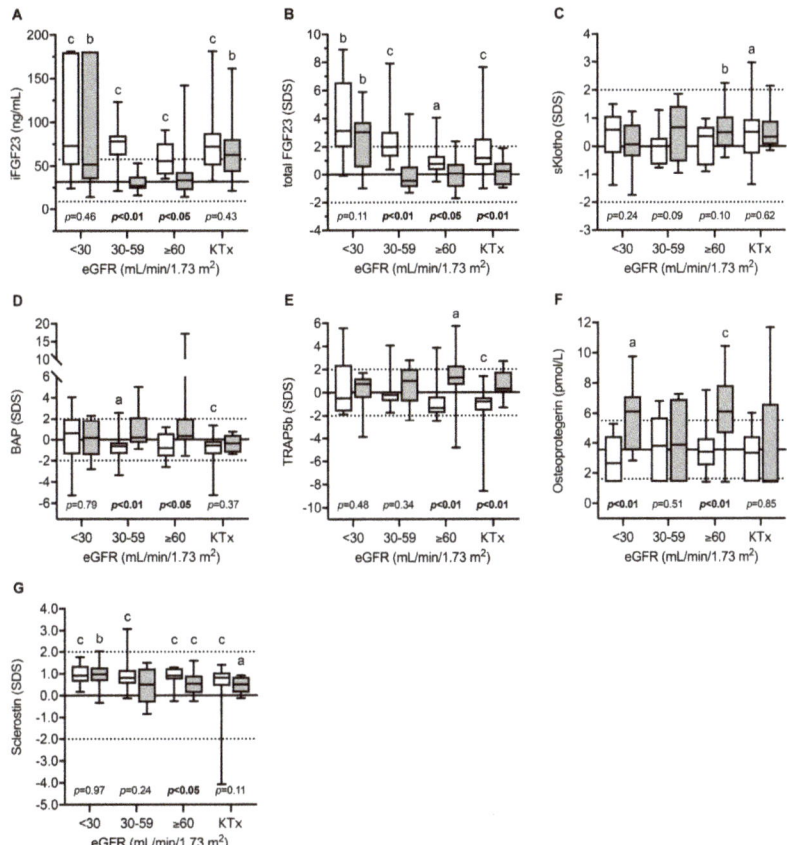

Figure 3. Circulating levels of intact (**A**) and total (**B**) fibroblast growth factor 23, soluble Klotho (**C**), bone alkaline phosphatase (**D**), tartrate-resistant acid phosphatase 5b (**E**), osteoprotegerin (**F**) and sclerostin (**G**) in children with infantile nephropathic cystinosis (INC), and CKD controls at various stages of CKD and after kidney transplantation (KTX): Gray box plots indicate INC patients while white box plots indicate CKD controls. Horizontal continuous and broken lines indicate the mean, upper, and lower normal range; a, b, and c indicate $p < 0.05$, $p < 0.01$, and $p < 0.001$ versus healthy children, respectively. eGFR, estimated glomerular filtration rate (eGFR); SDS, standard deviation score; iFGF23, intact fibroblast growth factor 23; BAP, bone alkaline phosphatase; TRAP5b, tartrate-resistant acid phosphatase 5b; OPG, osteoprotegerin; sKlotho, soluble Klotho. Figure from Ewert et al. with permission [13].

This confirms the results from the above-mentioned ex vivo studies, using PBMCs derived from INC patients, that *CTNS* malfunction results in increased osteoclastogenesis promoting increased bone resorption and reduced bone mass in INC patients. By contrast, no differences were observed with respect to OPG levels between INC patients and CKD controls [13].

Taken together, this study suggests that bone mineralization is markedly impaired in INC patients, despite treatment of Fanconi syndrome, which can only be partly normalized by kidney transplantation, and that CMBD is not only the consequence of Fanconi syndrome and progressive CKD resulting in CKD-MBD, but also an intrinsic osteoblast and osteoclast defect.

The distinct alterations in phosphate hemostasis and FGF23 levels in INC patients were later confirmed by Florenzano et al. [14]. They compared phosphate homeostasis and FGF23 levels in a cohort of 50 INC patients, with that of 97 CKD patients, matched for age and degree of renal insufficiency, with other underlying kidney diseases. INC patients displayed significantly lower circulating phosphate levels due to impaired tubular phosphate reabsorption and lower FGF23 concentrations compared to CKD controls, independent of eGFR. A multivariable analysis revealed that diagnosis of INC was independently associated with lower FGF23 levels after adjustment for age and eGFR. This study further supports the concept that phosphate is an important stimulator of FGF23 synthesis in bone and that the pathophysiology of bone disease in INC differs markedly from that in other CKD patients.

5. Towards an Interplay between Bone, Adipocytes, and Muscles

Osteoblasts, myocytes, and adipocytes both derive from mesenchymal stem cells (MSCs). As discussed above, myopathy is part of the complexity of CMBD, and the strength of load-bearing bones largely depends on growing muscle strength [40]. This is why the interplay between bone, adipocytes, and muscle is particularly relevant in patients with INC. We recently described the intrinsic cellular defects observed in bone cells from INC patients and animal models [11,12,49].

In 2016, Cheung et al. demonstrated the interplay between fat and muscle mass in INC in the murine $Ctns^{-/-}$ model, showing profound muscle wasting, together with inhibited myogenesis, stimulated proteolysis, overexpressed pro-inflammatory cytokines (among them interleukin 1α, interleukin 6, and TNFα) in brown adipose tissue, hypermetabolism, upregulated thermogenesis, and increased presence of beige adipocytes [17]. The authors also describe the potential value of both native and active vitamin D in improving adipose tissue browning and muscle wasting in their murine $Ctns^{-/-}$ model [51]. In this model, repletion of vitamin D improved (and sometimes normalized) weight gain, food intake, lean and fat mass; it also improved energy homeostasis as well as the size of skeletal muscle fibers and in vivo muscular function. From a molecular perspective, vitamin D repletion corrected abnormal expression of molecules, playing a key role in adipose tissue browning, and normalized the most important 20 differentially expressed genes in $Ctns^{-/-}$ mice, as evaluated by muscle RNA-seq [51]. Whether vitamin D may exert similar effects in patients with INC remains to be proven. These results are, nevertheless, particularly relevant in the field of INC for two main reasons: 1. most patients with INC receive native vitamin D supplementation and sometimes active vitamin D analogs; and, 2. vitamin D is an anti-inflammatory agent [52].

Indeed, Prencipe et al., reported an upregulation of the IL1 β receptor 1 and IL1 receptor 2 in the kidneys of LPS treated animal models and in INC patients, this stimulation being driven by caspase 1 in the inflammasome [53]. It should be born in mind, that patients with INC displayed elevated levels of Il1β, Il18, and caspase 1 compared to healthy controls, but they also displayed significantly elevated levels of Il18 compared to patients with Familial Mediterranean Fever, a prototypical autoinflammatory disease [54]. Recently, Cheung et al., demonstrated that by treating $Ctns^{-/-}$ mice with the Il1 receptor antagonist Anakinra they were able to attenuate the cachexia phenotype and correct the abnormal expression of the main biomarkers of beige adipose cells and adipocyte tissue browning, and to attenuate 12 of the 20 main, differentially expressed genes in $Ctns^{-/-}$ mice [55]. Anakinra treatment also normalized muscle weight and fiber size and decreased infiltration in muscle fat [55]. These results were close to those observed earlier by the same team using vitamin D [51], questioning again the role of vitamin D in inflammation regulation.

Several pro inflammatory cytokines have been described as substitutes for RANKL, the factor synthesized by osteoblasts to promote osteoclastic differentiation, and, notably, interleukin 1β (IL1β) or interleukin 6 (IL6) [56]. If the interleukin-1 deregulation observed in cystinotic muscle is also proven to be true in other target tissues, notably in bone, this may open up a new avenue for therapeutic perspectives in INC.

6. Conclusions: Perspectives in Research

CMBD has emerged over the last decade as a well-recognized, long-term complication, inducing significant morbidity and impaired quality of life in teenagers and adults with INC. Its underlying pathophysiology is complex, consisting of abnormal mineral regulation, intrinsic bone defects, cysteamine toxicity, muscle wasting, and likely interleukin-1 driven inflammation. In future, biotherapies targeting the IL1β and/or Il6 pathway may improve muscle wasting and, subsequently, CMBD, but this remains to be proven. In the meantime, the promising results of stem cells transplantation on muscular cystine content in the murine model [57], should be confirmed in the currently ongoing clinical trials.

Author Contributions: D.H., M.L.-N., C.A. and J.B. have written, reviewed, and edited the original draft preparation. All authors have read and agreed to the published version of the manuscript.

Funding: J.B. received research fees from the Cystinosis Research Foundation and the French Patients' Association AIRG for the CYSTEA-BONE project.

Acknowledgments: D.H. and J.B. are members of the European Reference Network for Rare Renal Diseases (ERKNet).

Conflicts of Interest: D.H. received speaker fees and research grants from Horizon and Chiesi. The other authors declare no conflict of interest.

References

1. Town, M.; Jean, G.; Cherqui, S.; Attard, M.; Forestier, L.; Whitmore, S.A.; Callen, D.F.; Gribouval, O.; Broyer, M.; Bates, G.P.; et al. A novel gene encoding an integral membrane protein is mutated in nephropathic cystinosis. *Nat. Genet.* **1998**, *18*, 319–324. [CrossRef]
2. Cherqui, S.; Courtoy, P.J. The renal Fanconi syndrome in cystinosis: Pathogenic insights and therapeutic perspectives. *Nat. Rev. Nephrol.* **2017**, *13*, 115–131. [CrossRef]
3. Markello, T.C.; Bernardini, I.M.; Gahl, W.A. Improved renal function in children with cystinosis treated with cysteamine. *N. Engl. J. Med.* **1993**, *328*, 1157–1162. [CrossRef] [PubMed]
4. Machuca-Gayet, I.; Quinaux, T.; Bertholet-Thomas, A.; Gaillard, S.; Claramunt-Taberner, D.; Acquaviva-Bourdain, C.; Bacchetta, J. Bone Disease in Nephropathic Cystinosis: Beyond Renal Osteodystrophy. *Int. J. Mol. Sci.* **2020**, *21*, 3109. [CrossRef]
5. Bacchetta, J.; Greco, M.; Bertholet-Thomas, A.; Nobili, F.; Zustin, J.; Cochat, P.; Emma, F.; Boivin, G. Skeletal implications and management of cystinosis: Three case reports and literature review. *BoneKEy Rep.* **2016**, *5*, 828. [CrossRef]
6. Bertholet-Thomas, A.; Claramunt-Taberner, D.; Gaillard, S.; Deschênes, G.; Sornay-Rendu, E.; Szulc, P.; Cohen-Solal, M.; Pelletier, S.; Carlier, M.C.; Cochat, P.; et al. Teenagers and young adults with nephropathic cystinosis display significant bone disease and cortical impairment. *Pediatr. Nephrol.* **2018**, *33*, 1165–1172. [CrossRef] [PubMed]
7. Florenzano, P.; Ferreira, C.; Nesterova, G.; Roberts, M.S.; Tella, S.H.; de Castro, L.F.; Brown, S.M.; Whitaker, A.; Pereira, R.C.; Bulas, D.; et al. Skeletal Consequences of Nephropathic Cystinosis. *J. Bone Miner. Res.* **2018**, *33*, 1870–1880. [CrossRef] [PubMed]
8. Langman, C.B. Bone Complications of Cystinosis. *J. Pediatr.* **2017**, *183S*, S2–S4. [CrossRef]
9. Langman, C.B. Oh cystinosin: Let me count the ways! *Kidney Int.* **2019**, *96*, 275–277. [CrossRef]
10. Santos, F.; Díaz-Anadón, L.; Ordóñez, F.A.; Haffner, D. Bone Disease in CKD in Children. *Calcif. Tissue Int.* **2021**, *108*, 423–438. [CrossRef]
11. Claramunt-Taberner, D.; Flammier, S.; Gaillard, S.; Cochat, P.; Peyruchaud, O.; Machuca-Gayet, I.; Bacchetta, J. Bone disease in nephropathic cystinosis is related to cystinosin-induced osteoclastic dysfunction. *Nephrol. Dial. Transpl.* **2018**, *33*, 1525–1532. [CrossRef]
12. Battafarano, G.; Rossi, M.; Rega, L.R.; Di Giovamberardino, G.; Pastore, A.; D'Agostini, M.; Porzio, O.; Nevo, N.; Emma, F.; Taranta, A.; et al. Intrinsic Bone Defects in Cystinotic Mice. *Am. J. Pathol.* **2019**, *189*, 1053–1064. [CrossRef] [PubMed]
13. Ewert, A.; Leifheit-Nestler, M.; Hohenfellner, K.; Büscher, A.; Kemper, M.J.; Oh, J.; Billing, H.; Thumfart, J.; Stangl, G.; Baur, A.C.; et al. Bone and mineral metabolism in children with nephropathic cystinosis compared to other CKD entities. *J. Clin. Endocrinol. Metab.* **2020**, *105*, e2738–e2752. [CrossRef] [PubMed]
14. Florenzano, P.; Jimenez, M.; Ferreira, C.R.; Nesterova, G.; Roberts, M.S.; Tella, S.H.; Fernandez de Castro, L.; Gafni, R.I.; Wolf, M.; Jüppner, H.; et al. Nephropathic Cystinosis: A Distinct Form of CKD-Mineral and Bone Disorder that Provides Novel Insights into the Regulation of FGF23. *J. Am. Soc. Nephrol. JASN* **2020**, *31*, 2184–2192. [CrossRef]
15. Quinaux, T.; Bertholet-Thomas, A.; Servais, A.; Boyer, O.; Vrillon, I.; Hogan, J.; Lemoine, S.; Gaillard, S.; Alioli, C.; Vasseur, S.; et al. Response to Cysteamine in Osteoclasts Obtained from Patients with Nephropathic Cystinosis: A Genotype/Phenotype Correlation. *Cells* **2021**, *10*, 2498. [CrossRef]

16. Gonzalez, A.; Cheung, W.W.; Perens, E.A.; Oliveira, E.A.; Gertler, A.; Mak, R.H. A Leptin Receptor Antagonist Attenuates Adipose Tissue Browning and Muscle Wasting in Infantile Nephropathic Cystinosis-Associated Cachexia. *Cells* **2021**, *10*, 1954. [CrossRef] [PubMed]
17. Cheung, W.W.; Cherqui, S.; Ding, W.; Esparza, M.; Zhou, P.; Shao, J.; Lieber, R.L.; Mak, R.H. Muscle wasting and adipose tissue browning in infantile nephropathic cystinosis. *J. Cachexia Sarcopenia Muscle* **2016**, *7*, 152–164. [CrossRef]
18. Hohenfellner, K.; Rauch, F.; Ariceta, G.; Awan, A.; Bacchetta, J.; Bergmann, C.; Bechtold, S.; Cassidy, N.; Deschenes, G.; Elenberg, E.; et al. Management of bone disease in cystinosis: Statement from an international conference. *J. Inherit. Metab. Dis.* **2019**, *42*, 1019–1029. [CrossRef]
19. Bertholet-Thomas, A.; Bacchetta, J.; Tasic, V.; Cochat, P. Nephropathic cystinosis–a gap between developing and developed nations. *N. Engl. J. Med.* **2014**, *370*, 1366–1367. [CrossRef]
20. Nesterova, G.; Gahl, W.A. Cystinosis: The evolution of a treatable disease. *Pediatr. Nephrol.* **2013**, *28*, 51–59. [CrossRef]
21. Besouw, M.T.P.; Bowker, R.; Dutertre, J.P.; Emma, F.; Gahl, W.A.; Greco, M.; Lilien, M.R.; McKiernan, J.; Nobili, F.; Schneider, J.A.; et al. Cysteamine toxicity in patients with cystinosis. *J. Pediatr.* **2011**, *159*, 1004–1011. [CrossRef] [PubMed]
22. Drube, J.; Wan, M.; Bonthuis, M.; Wühl, E.; Bacchetta, J.; Santos, F.; Grenda, R.; Edefonti, A.; Harambat, J.; Shroff, R.; et al. Clinical practice recommendations for growth hormone treatment in children with chronic kidney disease. *Nat. Rev. Nephrol.* **2019**, *15*, 577–589. [CrossRef]
23. Tiosano, D.; Hochberg, Z. Hypophosphatemia: The common denominator of all rickets. *J. Bone Miner. Metab.* **2009**, *27*, 392–401. [CrossRef]
24. Haffner, D.; Leifheit-Nestler, M.; Grund, A.; Schnabel, D. Rickets guidance: Part I-diagnostic workup. *Pediatr. Nephrol.* **2021**. Epub ahead of print. [CrossRef] [PubMed]
25. Bagga, A.; Sinha, A. Renal Tubular Acidosis. *Indian J. Pediatr.* **2020**, *87*, 733–744. [CrossRef] [PubMed]
26. Besouw, M.T.P.; Van Dyck, M.; Cassiman, D.; Claes, K.J.; Levtchenko, E.N. Management dilemmas in pediatric nephrology: Cystinosis. *Pediatr. Nephrol.* **2015**, *30*, 1349–1360. [CrossRef]
27. Besouw, M.T.P.; Schneider, J.; Janssen, M.C.; Greco, M.; Emma, F.; Cornelissen, E.A.; Desmet, K.; Skovby, F.; Nobili, F.; Lilien, M.R.; et al. Copper deficiency in patients with cystinosis with cysteamine toxicity. *J. Pediatr.* **2013**, *163*, 754–760. [CrossRef] [PubMed]
28. Nesterova, G.; Gahl, W. Nephropathic cystinosis: Late complications of a multisystemic disease. *Pediatr. Nephrol.* **2008**, *23*, 863–878. [CrossRef] [PubMed]
29. Winkler, L.; Offner, G.; Krull, F.; Brodehl, J. Growth and pubertal development in nephropathic cystinosis. *Eur. J. Pediatr.* **1993**, *152*, 244–249. [CrossRef]
30. Chik, C.L.; Friedman, A.; Merriam, G.R.; Gahl, W.A. Pituitary-testicular function in nephropathic cystinosis. *Ann. Intern. Med.* **1993**, *119*, 568–575. [CrossRef]
31. Rohayem, J.; Haffner, D.; Cremers, J.F.; Huss, S.; Wistuba, J.; Weitzel, D.; Kliesch, S.; Hohenfellner, K. Testicular function in males with infantile nephropathic cystinosis. *Hum. Reprod.* **2021**, *36*, 1191–1204. [CrossRef]
32. Wühl, E.; Haffner, D.; Offner, G.; Broyer, M.; van't Hoff, W.; Mehls, O.; European Study Group on Growth Hormone Treatment in Children with Nephropathic Cystinosis. Long-term treatment with growth hormone in short children with nephropathic cystinosis. *J. Pediatr.* **2001**, *138*, 880–887. [CrossRef] [PubMed]
33. Tönshoff, B.; Cronin, M.J.; Reichert, M.; Haffner, D.; Wingen, A.M.; Blum, W.F.; Mehls, O. Reduced concentration of serum growth hormone (GH)-binding protein in children with chronic renal failure: Correlation with GH insensitivity. The European Study Group for Nutritional Treatment of Chronic Renal Failure in Childhood. The German Study Group for Growth Hormone Treatment in Chronic Renal Failure. *J. Clin. Endocrinol. Metab.* **1997**, *82*, 1007–1013. [PubMed]
34. Vester, U.; Schubert, M.; Offner, G.; Brodehl, J. Distal myopathy in nephropathic cystinosis. *Pediatr. Nephrol.* **2000**, *14*, 36–38. [CrossRef]
35. Sadjadi, R.; Sullivan, S.; Grant, N.; Thomas, S.E.; Doyle, M.; Hammond, C.; Duong, R.; Corre, C.; David, W.; Eichler, F. Clinical myopathy in patients with nephropathic cystinosis. *Muscle Nerve* **2020**, *61*, 74–80. [CrossRef] [PubMed]
36. Sonies, B.C.; Almajid, P.; Kleta, R.; Bernardini, I.; Gahl, W.A. Swallowing dysfunction in 101 patients with nephropathic cystinosis: Benefit of long-term cysteamine therapy. *Medicine* **2005**, *84*, 137–146. [CrossRef] [PubMed]
37. Anikster, Y.; Lacbawan, F.; Brantly, M.; Gochuico, B.L.; Avila, N.A.; Travis, W.; Gahl, W.A. Pulmonary dysfunction in adults with nephropathic cystinosis. *Chest* **2001**, *119*, 394–401. [CrossRef]
38. Charnas, L.R.; Luciano, C.A.; Dalakas, M.; Gilliatt, R.W.; Bernardini, I.; Ishak, K.; Cwik, V.A.; Fraker, D.; Brushart, T.A.; Gahl, W.A. Distal vacuolar myopathy in nephropathic cystinosis. *Ann. Neurol.* **1994**, *35*, 181–188. [CrossRef]
39. Iyob-Tessema, H.; Wang, C.S.; Kennedy, S.; Reyes, L.; Shin, S.; Greenbaum, L.A.; Hogan, J. Grip Strength in Adults and Children with Cystinosis. *Kidney Int. Rep.* **2021**, *6*, 389–395. [CrossRef]
40. Frost, H.M.; Schönau, E. The "muscle-bone unit" in children and adolescents: A 2000 overview. *J. Pediatr. Endocrinol. Metab. JPEM* **2000**, *13*, 571–590. [CrossRef]
41. Graciolli, F.G.; Neves, K.R.; Barreto, F.; Barreto, D.V.; Dos Reis, L.M.; Canziani, M.E.; Sabbagh, Y.; Carvalho, A.B.; Jorgetti, V.; Elias, R.M.; et al. The complexity of chronic kidney disease-mineral and bone disorder across stages of chronic kidney disease. *Kidney Int.* **2017**, *91*, 1436–1446. [CrossRef] [PubMed]

42. Fang, Y.; Ginsberg, C.; Seifert, M.; Agapova, O.; Sugatani, T.; Register, T.C.; Freedman, B.I.; Monier-Faugere, M.-C.; Malluche, H.; Hruska, K.A. CKD-induced wingless/integration1 inhibitors and phosphorus cause the CKD-mineral and bone disorder. *J. Am. Soc. Nephrol. JASN* **2014**, *25*, 1760–1773. [CrossRef] [PubMed]
43. Carrillo-López, N.; Panizo, S.; Alonso-Montes, C.; Román-García, P.; Rodríguez, I.; Martínez-Salgado, C.; Dusso, A.S.; Naves, M.; Cannata-Andía, J.B. Direct inhibition of osteoblastic Wnt pathway by fibroblast growth factor 23 contributes to bone loss in chronic kidney disease. *Kidney Int.* **2016**, *90*, 77–89. [CrossRef] [PubMed]
44. Gattineni, J.; Alphonse, P.; Zhang, Q.; Mathews, N.; Bates, C.M.; Baum, M. Regulation of renal phosphate transport by FGF23 is mediated by FGFR1 and FGFR4. *Am. J. Physiol. Renal Physiol.* **2014**, *306*, F351–F358. [CrossRef] [PubMed]
45. Richter, B.; Faul, C. FGF23 Actions on Target Tissues—With and without Klotho. *Front. Endocrinol.* **2018**, *9*, 189. [CrossRef]
46. Robling, A.G.; Niziolek, P.J.; Baldridge, L.A.; Condon, K.W.; Allen, M.R.; Alam, I.; Mantila, S.M.; Gluhak-Heinrich, J.; Bellido, T.M.; Harris, S.E.; et al. Mechanical stimulation of bone in vivo reduces osteocyte expression of Sost/sclerostin. *J. Biol. Chem.* **2008**, *283*, 5866–5875. [CrossRef]
47. Haffner, D.; Leifheit-Nestler, M. CKD-MBD post kidney transplantation. *Pediatr. Nephrol. Berl. Ger.* **2021**, *36*, 41–50. [CrossRef]
48. Tönshoff, B. Immunosuppressive therapy post-transplantation in children: What the clinician needs to know. *Expert Rev. Clin. Immunol.* **2020**, *16*, 139–154. [CrossRef]
49. Conforti, A.; Taranta, A.; Biagini, S.; Starc, N.; Pitisci, A.; Bellomo, F.; Cirillo, V.; Locatelli, F.; Bernardo, M.E.; Emma, F. Cysteamine treatment restores the in vitro ability to differentiate along the osteoblastic lineage of mesenchymal stromal cells isolated from bone marrow of a cystinotic patient. *J. Transl. Med.* **2015**, *13*, 143. [CrossRef]
50. Festa, B.P.; Chen, Z.; Berquez, M.; Debaix, H.; Tokonami, N.; Prange, J.A.; van de Hoek, G.; Alessio, C.; Raimondi, A.; Nevo, N.; et al. Impaired autophagy bridges lysosomal storage disease and epithelial dysfunction in the kidney. *Nat. Commun.* **2018**, *9*, 161. [CrossRef]
51. Cheung, W.W.; Hao, S.; Wang, Z.; Ding, W.; Zheng, R.; Gonzalez, A.; Zhan, J.-Y.; Zhou, P.; Li, S.; Esparza, M.C.; et al. Vitamin D repletion ameliorates adipose tissue browning and muscle wasting in infantile nephropathic cystinosis-associated cachexia. *J. Cachexia Sarcopenia Muscle* **2020**, *11*, 120–134. [CrossRef] [PubMed]
52. Adams, J.S.; Hewison, M. Update in vitamin D. *J. Clin. Endocrinol. Metab.* **2010**, *95*, 471–478. [CrossRef] [PubMed]
53. Prencipe, G.; Caiello, I.; Cherqui, S.; Whisenant, T.; Petrini, S.; Emma, F.; De Benedetti, F. Inflammasome activation by cystine crystals: Implications for the pathogenesis of cystinosis. *J. Am. Soc. Nephrol. JASN* **2014**, *25*, 1163–1169. [CrossRef] [PubMed]
54. Ozen, S. Update in familial Mediterranean fever. *Curr. Opin. Rheumatol.* **2021**, *33*, 398–402. [CrossRef]
55. Cheung, W.W.; Hao, S.; Zheng, R.; Wang, Z.; Gonzalez, A.; Zhou, P.; Hoffman, H.M.; Mak, R.H. Targeting interleukin-1 for reversing fat browning and muscle wasting in infantile nephropathic cystinosis. *J. Cachexia Sarcopenia Muscle* **2021**, *12*, 1296–1311. [CrossRef]
56. Feng, W.; Guo, J.; Li, M. RANKL-independent modulation of osteoclastogenesis. *J. Oral Biosci.* **2019**, *61*, 16–21. [CrossRef]
57. Syres, K.; Harrison, F.; Tadlock, M.; Jester, J.V.; Simpson, J.; Roy, S.; Salomon, D.R.; Cherqui, S. Successful treatment of the murine model of cystinosis using bone marrow cell transplantation. *Blood* **2009**, *114*, 2542–2552. [CrossRef]

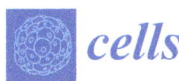

Review

Central Nervous System Complications in Cystinosis: The Role of Neuroimaging

Aude Servais [1,2,*], Jennifer Boisgontier [2,3], Ana Saitovitch [2,3], Aurélie Hummel [1] and Nathalie Boddaert [2,3]

[1] Department of Nephrology and Transplantation, Centre de référence des Maladies Rénales Héréditaires de l'Enfant et de l'Adulte, Necker Hospital, AP-HP, 75015 Paris, France; aurelie.hummel@aphp.fr
[2] INSERM U1163, Imagine Institute, Paris University, 75015 Paris, France; boisgontier.jennifer1414@gmail.com (J.B.); a.saitovitch@gmail.com (A.S.); nathalie.boddaert@aphp.fr (N.B.)
[3] Paediatric Radiology Department, INSERM U1299, Hôpital Necker Enfants Malades, AP-HP, 75015 Paris, France
* Correspondence: aude.servais@aphp.fr; Tel.: +33-1-4438-1515; Fax: +33-1-4449-5450

Abstract: Despite improvement in the specific treatment, clinical and anatomo-functional central nervous system (CNS) abnormalities of various severities are still observed in cystinosis patients. Patients who develop CNS complications today have a worse compliance to cysteamine treatment. Radiological studies have shown that cortical or central (ventriculomegaly) atrophy is observed in more than two thirds of cystinosis patients' magnetic resonance imaging (MRI) and correlates with the intelligence quotient score. Half of cystinosis patients have marked aspecific white matter hyperintensities. The development of advanced neuroimaging techniques provides new tools to further investigate CNS complications. A recent neuroimaging study using a voxel-based morphometry approach showed that cystinosis patients present a decreased grey matter volume in the left middle frontal gyrus. Diffusion tensor imaging studies have shown white matter microstructure abnormalities in children and adults with cystinosis, respectively in areas of the dorsal visual pathway and within the corpus callosum's body. Finally, leucocyte cystine levels are associated with decreased resting cerebral blood flow, measured by arterial spin labelling, in the frontal cortex, which could be associated with the neurocognitive deficits described in these patients. These results reinforce the relevance of neuroimaging studies to further understand the mechanisms that underline CNS impairments.

Keywords: cystinosis; central nervous system; cortical atrophy; arterial spin labelling; cysteamine; cystine blood level

1. Introduction

Cystinosis is a rare autosomal recessive disease caused by intracellular cystine accumulation [1,2]. Three clinical forms have been described based on the severity of symptoms and the age of onset: infantile cystinosis characterized by renal proximal tubulopathy and early progression to end-stage renal disease (ESRD), a juvenile form with a markedly slower rate of progression and an adult form with mainly, but not only, ocular abnormalities [3]. Over the last 20 years, specific treatment with cysteamine and progress in renal transplantation and dialysis have significantly improved the long-term outcome of cystinosis patients. However, extra-renal complications may still occur [4]. In particular, in historical cohorts, central nervous system complications (CNS) were observed in adolescents and young adults not fully treated with cysteamine, as this treatment became available only in the 1990s [5–7]. Today, in the era of early specific treatment with cysteamine, a high prevalence of mild to severe clinical and radiological CNS impairments is still observed in adult patients. Such complications may affect quality of life, academic function, and professional insertion. The development and availability of advanced neuroimaging techniques provides new tools to investigate the underlying neurophysiopathological mechanisms

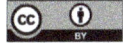

of metabolic diseases and further understand their impact on broader neurological and neurocognitive dysfunction [8]. However, studies in this domain are still scarce, and only two have specifically used such an approach.

2. Clinical Presentation

2.1. Clinical Data

Neurological symptoms have been reported in adolescents and young adults with cystinosis in historical cohorts [5–7]. Two main clinical forms have been observed. The first one is a cystinosis encephalopathy with cerebellar signs and/or motor difficulties, mainly of the lower limbs, a decrease of oral expression, and the progressive development of pyramidal symptoms, somnolence, epileptic seizures, and mental deterioration [7,9]. Motor coordination difficulties were initially described and have been further corroborated in more recent studies of motor performance [10–12]. The second form resembles a stroke-like episode, which could present itself with coma or hemiplegia or milder symptoms. In parallel, hydrocephalus has also been described in some patients [13], not necessarily associated with clinical symptoms [7]. Cerebrospinal fluid examination is normal except for elevated pressure, suggesting that the hydrocephalus might result from decreased cerebrospinal fluid absorption related to the deposition of cystine in choroidal plexuses and meninges [13,14].

CNS complications are a major concern since the long-term prognosis of adult cystinosis patients appears to be primarily related to neurological complications [15]. Indeed, in a French cohort, neurological disorders were globally reported in 37% of patients and included paresis in 75%, cognitive impairment in 56%, stroke in 37%, and seizures in 31% [15]. In addition, the cause of death was linked to neurological reason in one-third of cases in that series and in two patients out of thirty-three (6%) in the series of Gahl et al. [16]. These data further reinforce the relevance of investigating CNS complications in this disease. A more recent study, specifically focusing on CNS complications, included 18 adults with infantile cystinosis [17]. In that cohort, CNS complications were largely present, despite early diagnosis and treatment in most patients. Seven patients (39%) presented with at least one central nervous system clinical abnormality: 2 (11%) with seizures, 3 (17%) with memory impairment, and 5 (28%) with cognitive impairment. Of note, patients with renal diseases and in particular cystinosis patients may have electrolyte abnormalities that can also trigger seizures, without implying a central nervous system etiology. One patient (5%) presented with a stroke-like episode. Mini-mental state examination, which screens for cognitive function deficit, was assessed in twelve patients, and the median score was twenty-seven out of thirty, with four patients having a decreased score below twenty-five.

2.2. Risk Factors for the Development of Central Nervous System Complications

In historical publications, CNS complications' occurrence did not correlate with other extra-renal complications of cystinosis, but their frequency was directly correlated with age in the absence of early treatment [5–7]. Indeed, the impact of specific treatment on such complications has been described [7,15,16,18]. Interestingly, it has been demonstrated that cysteamine intake could decrease neurocognitive impairments in neurodegenerative diseases, such as Huntington's disease, supporting its action on neurological symptoms, even if the underlying mechanism may be different [19]. A more recent study has shown that patients who develop CNS complication today are those who have a lower compliance score and/or receive a lower cysteamine dose, without an effect of age [17]. In addition, even if other factors such as psychosocial struggle should be considered, all patients with at least one central nervous system symptom had poor compliance to treatment, further reinforcing the role of cysteamine treatment in preventing neurocognitive symptoms. Unfortunately, despite these results, compliance to treatment remains a major challenge in the context of cystinosis, in particular in adults [20]. The effect of treatment on already-existing neurological complications is less clear, but the early identification of such neurological symptoms could help in the adjustment of treatment and prompt referral to a specialized neurologist [7].

3. Pathophysiology

The underlying mechanisms of CNS complication remain poorly understood. Investigations using animal models have shown that cystinosin knockout mice, C57BL/6 *Ctns* $^{-/-}$ mice, have elevated cystine levels in the hippocampus, cerebellum, forebrain, and brainstem, which increase with age. In addition, cystine crystals have been detected within the choroid plexus and situated adjacent to capillaries. This has been associated with spatial reference and working memory deficits [21]. These results support the hypothesis that cystinosis-associated central nervous system anomalies are due, at least in part, to progressive cystine accumulation.

The exact pathogenic role of cystine crystals remains unknown. Several non-exclusive hypotheses have been formulated (Figure 1). Firstly, it could involve oligodendrocytes since cystine crystals have been observed in these cells [7,22,23]. A second hypothesis is the alteration of the blood–brain barrier based on the finding of abundant cystine deposits within the cerebral pericytes, which contribute to this barrier [22]. A third hypothesis is the progressive development of a microvascular disease of the brain. Indeed, cystine crystals have been observed in perivascular macrophages [7], and a cerebral cystine-crystal-associated vasculopathy with perivascular inflammatory infiltrates has been described [22,24], consistent with the inflammasome activation by cystine crystals already shown [25]. In addition to microvascular lesions, large vessel involvement has been reported, and this may be the cause of other types of cerebral complications [26–28]. Accumulation of intracellular cystine itself may be a risk factor for vascular calcifications, even if adult cystinotic patients usually have several other risk factors for vascular calcification and atherosclerosis since most patients have endured renal failure and have undergone at least one renal allograft procedure [18,29].

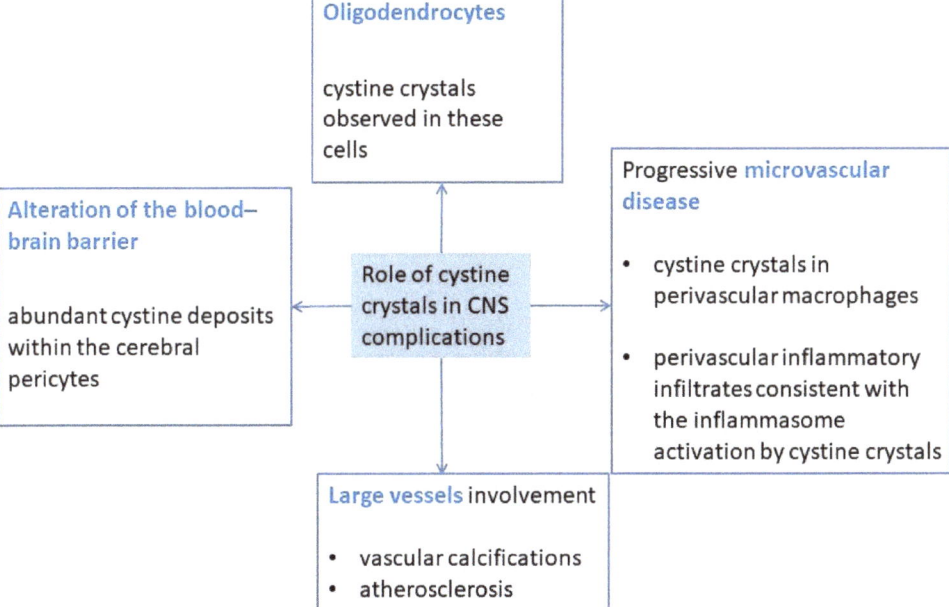

Figure 1. Role of cystine crystals in CNS complications: pathophysiological hypotheses.

4. Neurocognitive Impairments

The investigation of neurocognitive impairment in cystinosis patients has shown that even if they generally do not have intellectual disability, mild neurocognitive impairment can be present [10,12,30]. Indeed, specific impairments in the processing of visual information, as well as relative weakness in visual motor, visual spatial, and visual memory skills have been described, which may be associated with learning difficulties, primarily in arithmetic. Significant difficulties are observed in executive-function-related abilities [12,31–35]. A fine-motor coordination deficit in children and adolescents with cystinosis has also been documented [11]. In addition, abnormalities seem to increase with age, which may reflect a progressive cognitive impairment, possibly as a result of cystine accumulation in the brain over time [30]. Impaired working memory has also been described, with visual memory being more impaired than auditory memory in one study [35,36].

Interestingly, there is a significant correlation between the total intelligence quotient (IQ) and the age at cysteamine treatment start: the sooner cysteamine is started, the less the IQ is impacted [35]. Of note, all cystinosis patients from the mentioned study who started cysteamine before 2 y of age had an IQ within the normal range, which is in accordance with another study showing that cystinosis patients treated before 2 y of age had a better outcome [12].

5. Radiological Data

In adult cystinosis patients, there is a very high prevalence of abnormalities on clinical brain scans: 89% of patients have an abnormal exam using advanced imaging techniques [17].

5.1. Calcifications

In historical cohorts, mineralization of the basal ganglia seemed to be specific to severe encephalopathy. In some patients with profound neurological deficits, brain imaging or post-mortem examination revealed multifocal cystic necrosis, dystrophic calcifications of the basal ganglia and periventricular areas, extensive demyelination of the internal capsule, spongy changes in the brachium pontis, and vacuolization [22,37,38]. Cerebral calcifications were observed in 22–38% of cases, but in a more recent study, computed tomography scan found brain calcification in only one patient out of twenty-one who presented with a stroke-like episode [15–17].

5.2. Cortical Atrophy

Cortical atrophy is the most frequent radiological finding in cystinosis patients. By computed tomography (CT) scan or magnetic resonance imaging (MRI), cortical atrophy is observed in almost all patients with CNS symptoms [7]. Cerebral atrophy is also reported in patients without important CNS clinical abnormality and in patients with minor alterations in cognitive performance, in particular with impairment of visual memory [15,36,39]. In a recent study, among patients with infantile cystinosis, 72% showed evidence of cortical atrophy, 67% central atrophy (ventriculomegaly), and 50.0% demonstrated both (Figure 2) [17]. In that study, only two patients with infantile cystinosis had a normal brain MRI, both being the youngest patients included. Interestingly, no atrophy was observed in patients with late-onset cystinosis, even if the patients analyzed were older than the other cystinosis patients. Importantly, such atrophy was specifically observed in cystinosis patients, and not in controls with nephropathy. In another study, also including younger patients, cystinosis patients presented significantly more atrophy than age- and sex-matched healthy controls in the frontal, parietal, temporal, and occipital regions, the corpus callosum, and the cerebellum [35]. It is worth noticing that atrophy was localized in parieto-occipital regions, which is consistent with the visuo-spatial-specific impairment described in these patients.

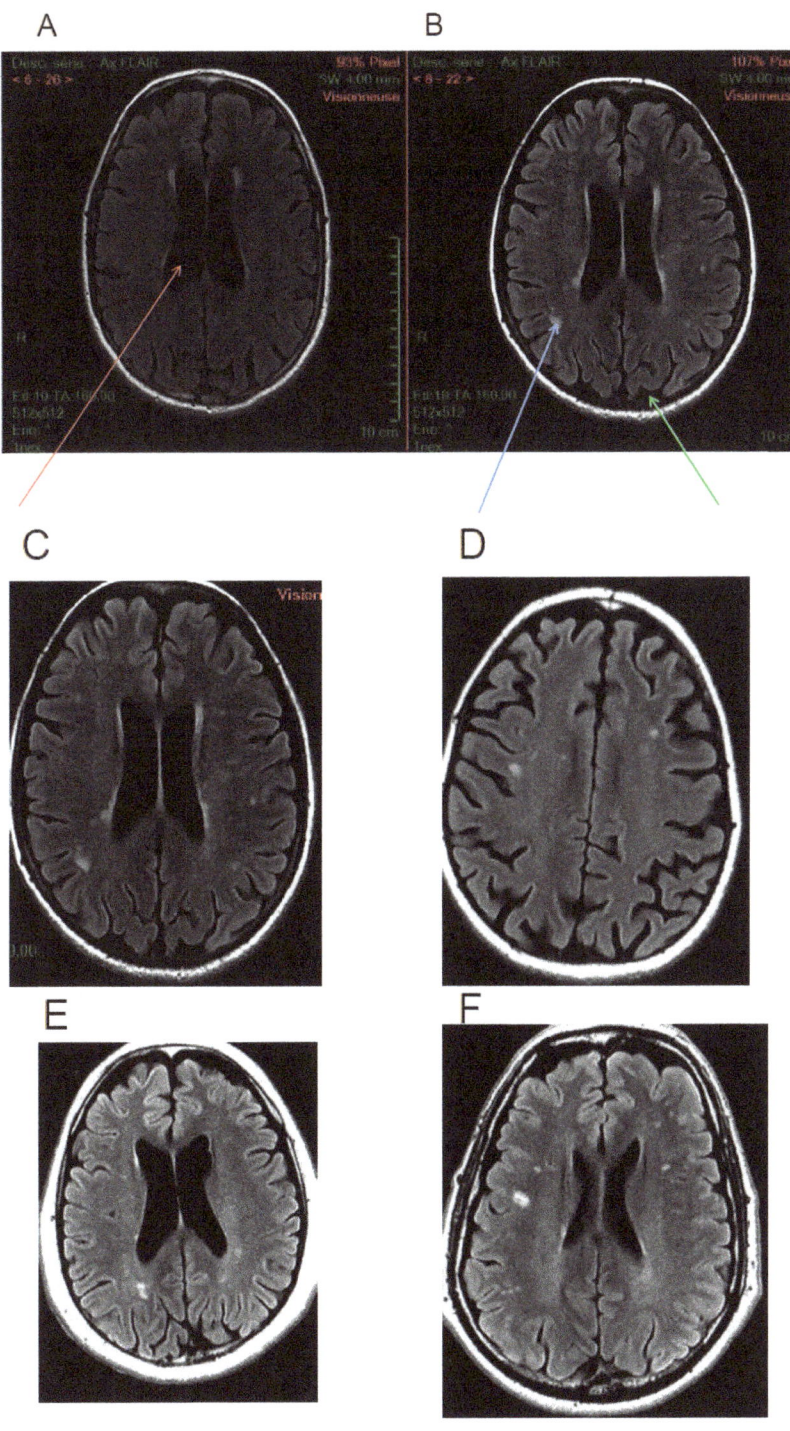

Figure 2. *Cont.*

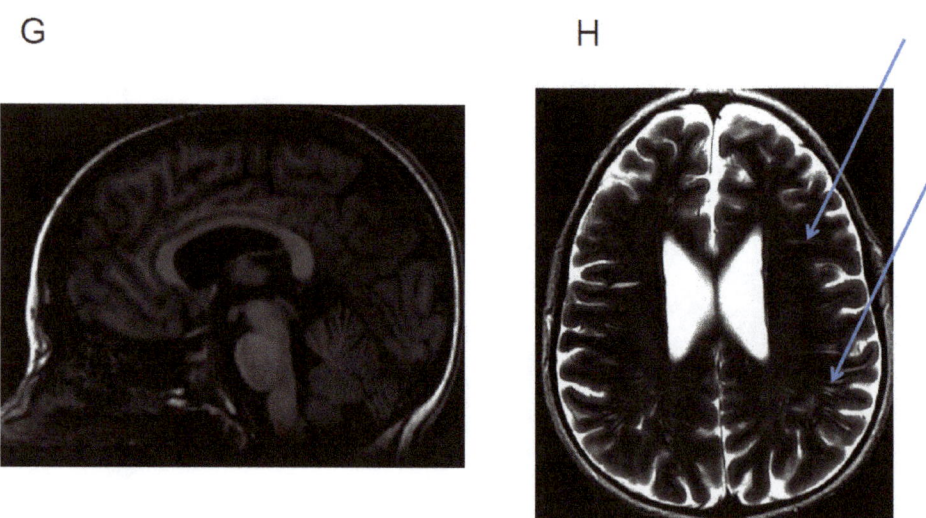

Figure 2. Axial FLAIR sequences. Examples of brain MRI anatomical images of cystinosis patients showing (**A**) an isolated ventricular dilatation (red arrow), (**B**) in another patient, cortical atrophy (green arrow) and diffuse white matter anomalies (blue arrow) associated with ventricular dilatation, (**C–F**) diffuse subcortical white matter hyperintensities, and (**G,H**) Wirshow or perivascular space enlargement (blue arrow)(images from N. Boddaert, Necker hospital).

In a study conducted with children and adolescents with cystinosis, Trauner et al. investigated brain volume loss and the correlation with motor coordination deficits. The results showed no significant differences in motor coordination scores between the group of patients who presented brain volume loss and the group who did not [11]. In a recent study, Curie et al. found a significant correlation between the degree of brain atrophy and the total IQ score [35]. Indeed, non-atrophic cystinosis patients had a significantly higher IQ than atrophic patients, which confirmed the previous findings [36].

5.3. White Matter Hyperintensities

White matter hyperintensities can be observed in 50% of cystinosis patients, including in patients with adolescent onset cystinosis (Figure 2) [17,35]. However, we have recently shown that these hyperintensities can also be observed in other patients with chronic renal failure [17]. White matter anomalies have been reported in some previous studies [7,40]. Interestingly, white matter abnormalities have been described in adults with chronic kidney disease compared to controls, suggesting that chronic kidney disease may result in a brain phenotype consistent with accelerated aging [35,41,42]. These results demonstrate the importance of adding a control group with renal failure when investigating brain abnormalities in cystinosis patients.

5.4. Others

It has been described that children with cystinosis have a 12-fold higher prevalence of Chiari I malformations than the general pediatric population. Indeed, Chiari malformation is observed in 9.5% to 18% of patients [17,43,44]. Even though there are usually no clinical manifestations, some patients may present with symptoms or signs thought to be related to the malformation. Surgical decompression is rarely needed [44].

Cazals et al. described a case of an adult patient with perivascular uptake of contrast associated with micronodular T2 hypointensity [45], which could represent microhemorragic lesions secondary to small vessel damage. In such situations, susceptibility weighted

(SWI) or gradient echo (GRE) imaging would be useful to add to MRI scans to further evaluate the presence of microhemorrhages. Finally, magnetic resonance spectroscopy sequences do not show any cystine peak or any other abnormal peak in patients with cystinosis [17].

6. Neuroimaging Investigations of Anatomo-Functional CNS Abnormalities

The development of advanced neuroimaging techniques has provided new tools to study the underlying neurophysiopathological mechanisms of metabolic diseases. Indeed, different MRI sequences allow noninvasively measuring anatomical and functional brain parameters. In addition, computational statistical software allows comparing these parameters between patients and controls, for instance, as well as to investigate putative correlations with clinical profiles or treatments, providing valuable knowledge in the field. However, so far, very few studies have used this approach to investigate CNS abnormalities in cystinosis patients.

6.1. Grey Matter

In the only study investigating grey matter abnormalities, we compared anatomical images from cystinosis patients to those from controls with nephropathy and from healthy controls [17]. We used a voxel-based morphometry (VBM) analysis to compare grey matter volume between groups in each and every voxel of the brain. This whole-brain approach allows investigating putative differences in grey matter without an a priori hypothesis. The results showed significantly decreased grey matter in the left middle frontal gyrus in cystinosis patients compared to healthy controls. Interestingly, brain abnormalities within this region could be associated with executive function deficits clinically described in these patients [10,12]. A significant decrease in grey matter in the same region was also observed in controls with nephropathy compared to healthy controls. No significant difference was observed between cystinosis patients and controls with nephropathy, which suggests that these abnormalities may not be specific to cystinosis patients and encourage brain imaging and neurocognitive investigations in a broader range of renal diseases.

6.2. White Matter

Beyond a radiological description of white matter abnormalities characterized by hyperintensities in MRI scans, which are largely described in cystinosis patients as presented earlier, the white matter microstructure can also be studied using diffusion tensor imaging MRI sequences. Diffusion tensor imaging measures the random motion, or diffusion, of water molecules in neural tissue and allows inferring the structural characteristics of the local tissue environment underlying the movement, i.e., the white matter itself. Two main indices have been investigated: the mean diffusivity (MD), a measurement of the overall magnitude of diffusional motion, and the fractional anisotropy (FA), as an index of the brain white matter microarchitecture [46].

In 2010, Bava et al. studied the cerebral white matter microstructure in 24 young children with cystinosis (age 3–7 years) and examined fractional anisotropy and mean diffusivity [43]. Children with cystinosis evidenced a decrease in fractional anisotropy and a corresponding elevation in mean diffusivity, indicating lower fiber integrity and therefore abnormal anatomical connectivity, in areas of the dorsal visual pathway. This suggests that abnormalities in cerebral white matter are present early on in development [43]. Older cystinosis children (>5 years) demonstrated stronger associations between cystine level and mean diffusivity in bilateral parietal regions, suggesting that, in addition to an early disruption in white matter maturation, there might be a secondary progressive effect of cystine accumulation on white matter organization and connectivity [43]. Recently, using tract-based spatial statistics analysis, we investigated white matter microstructure in adults with cystinosis [17]. Our results showed a significantly decreased fractional anisotropy in cystinosis patients compared to healthy controls in clusters within the corpus callosum's body, indicating a white matter microarchitecture abnormality, which suggests abnormal anatomical connectivity in this region (Figure 3). This bundle, which plays a central role in inter-hemispheric communication, has also recently been associated with cognitive processes [47,48]. However, controls with nephropathy also present with these abnormalities compared to healthy controls, suggesting that they may not be specific to cystinosis patients.

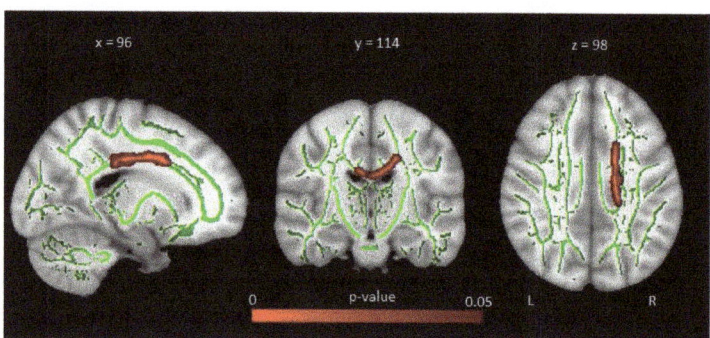

Figure 3. Results from tract-based spatial statistics analyses: voxelwise group differences in fractional anisotropy when comparing cystinosis patients and healthy controls. Sagittal, coronal, and axial slices of the tract-based spatial statistics contrasts between cystinosis patients and healthy controls. Red clusters indicate reduced fractional anisotropy in cystinosis patients compared to healthy individuals. Images of contrast are overlaid on a standard Montreal Neurological Institute (MNI) template 1 mm brain and a fractional anisotropy skeleton (in green) with a threshold set to range from 0.2 to 0.8. Tract-based spatial statistics results are thresholded at $p \leq 0.05$, corrected for multiple comparisons across space (FWE) using threshold-free cluster enhancement adjusted for age and sex.

6.3. Resting Brain Function

The study of resting brain function provides information on the level of activity of the different brain regions as a "baseline", outside task performance. Using arterial spin labelling MRI (ASL-MRI), cerebral blood flow (CBF) can be measured at the cerebral level using intrinsic physiological contrast by labelling water protons from cervical arteries and measuring them once they are at the cerebral level [49]. In a recent study, we compared arterial spin labelling images between patients with cystinosis and healthy controls, using a whole-brain approach [17]. We did not find any significant differences in resting cerebral blood flow values between groups. However, in cystinosis patients, the results showed a significant negative correlation between the cystine blood level and resting cerebral blood flow in the right superior frontal gyrus (Figure 4). Indeed, patients with higher levels of cystine were those presenting with lower resting cerebral blood flow values in the superior frontal cortex, which reinforces the link between cystinosis disease and abnormalities within frontal brain regions. Importantly, the superior frontal cortex is associated with executive functions, and the described abnormalities could underline the neurocognitive deficits described in cystinosis patients, such as memory impairments or further cognitive impairments.

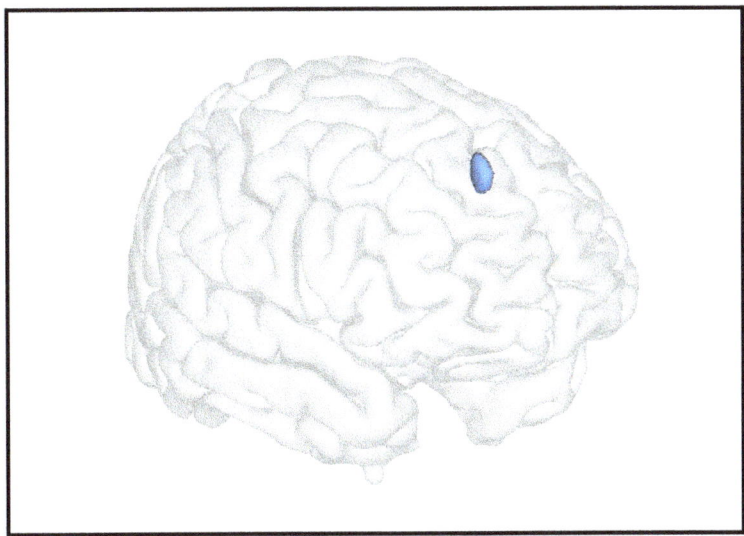

Figure 4. Advanced neuroimaging techniques can help in understanding the impact of cystinosis on the brain's anatomo-function and its link with neurocognitive impairments. For instance, here, we illustrate the results of Scheme 10 (y = 50 z = 40), a brain region strongly implicated in cognitive functions: the higher the cystine levels, the lower the resting CBF in this area, which is associated with cognitive functions. Maximum intensity projections of T statistics clusters that are significantly correlated with individual cystine blood level are superimposed on a 3D volume rendering on grey matter in the MNI space.

7. Electrophysiological Activity

Functional brain activity in cystinosis may be assessed by a high-density electroencephalogram (EEG) [50]. This non-invasive method provides information at the millisecond scale, measures functional brain activity, and thus, assesses the integrity of neural function. A case report tested visual processing in two children with cystinosis before and after kidney transplantation. Before transplantation (and during dialysis), both children showed delayed and decreased early visually evoked responses, compared to their age-matched peers, but with both amplitude and latency measures normalized two years after transplantation [51].

High-density EEG was used to analyze basic sensory processing in cystinosis, focusing on early auditory sensory processing (N1) and sensory memory (mismatch negativity) [50]. The auditory sensory processing is the first prominent negative auditorily evoked potential [52] and reflects neural activity generated in and around the primary auditory cortex [53]. The memory mismatch negativity, operating at the sensory memory level, occurs when a repeating stimulus (the standard) in an auditory stream is replaced by a deviant stimulus.

No anomalies have been found in the auditory sensory processing, suggesting that sensory transmission through the auditory system is largely intact in individuals with cystinosis. However, individuals with cystinosis present reduced responses for the longer stimulus onset asynchronies, which could indicate a reduced duration of auditory sensory memory traces, and thus sensory memory impairment, in children and adolescents diagnosed with cystinosis [50]. Adults with cystinosis produce highly similar sensory perceptual auditorily evoked potential responses to controls, suggesting intact early auditory cortical processing. However, significantly increased auditory sensory perceptual processing amplitudes, increased attentional orienting, and reduced sensory memory at slower stimulation rates are observed, suggesting mild-to-moderate changes in auditory sensory memory and attentional processing [54].

8. Conclusions

Despite an improvement in specific treatment and transplantation, CNS abnormalities of various severities are still present in adult cystinosis patients. In particular, neurocognitive impairment has been largely described. Unraveling the brain mechanisms that underline these abnormalities is essential to develop actions to improve long-term patient outcome. By MRI, cortical or central atrophy is observed in more than two-thirds of cystinosis patients and correlates with the total IQ score. The development of advanced neuroimaging techniques provides new tools to investigate CNS complications and the brain correlates of neurocognitive impairments. Therefore, future studies, in particular focusing on brain–behavior correlations, can bring new light to the subject. It is important to note that some findings may not be specific to cystinosis, supporting not only the importance of adding a control group with renal failure when investigating brain abnormalities in cystinosis patients, but also the relevance of neuroimaging investigations in patients with renal failure in general. It was recently shown that leucocyte cystine levels are associated with decreased resting cerebral blood flow in the frontal cortex, which could be related to the neurocognitive deficits described in cystinosis patients. These results further reinforce the importance of compliance to cysteamine treatment, which is a major concern in these adult patients, since it seems to play a major role in cognitive and neurological complications.

Author Contributions: Conceptualization, A.S. (Aude Servais), A.S. (Ana Saitovitch), and N.B.; methodology, A.S. (Aude Servais), A.S. (Ana Saitovitch), and N.B.; formal analysis, A.S. (Aude Servais), A.S. (Ana Saitovitch), and J.B.; investigation, A.S. (Aude Servais), A.S. (Ana Saitovitch), J.B., A.H., N.B.; writing—original draft preparation, A.S. (Aude Servais), A.S. (Ana Saitovitch), J.B.; writing—review and editing, A.S. (Aude Servais), A.S. (Ana Saitovitch), J.B., A.H., N.B.; supervision, A.S. (Aude Servais), A.S. (Ana Saitovitch), N.B. All authors have read and agreed to the published version of the manuscript.

Funding: The work on neuroimaging in cystinosis patients was supported by a grant from the Cystinosis Research Foundation.

Institutional Review Board Statement: Not applicable.

Informed Consent Statement: Not applicable.

Conflicts of Interest: The authors declare no conflict of interest.

References

1. Kalatzis, V.; Cherqui, S.; Antignac, C.; Gasnier, B. Cystinosin, the protein defective in cystinosis, is a H(+)-driven lyso-somal cystine transporter. *EMBO J.* **2001**, *20*, 5940–5949. [CrossRef] [PubMed]
2. Gahl, W.A.; Thoene, J.G.; Schneider, J.A. Cystinosis. *N. Engl. J. Med.* **2002**, *347*, 111–121. [CrossRef] [PubMed]
3. Servais, A.; Morinière, V.; Grünfeld, J.-P.; Noël, L.-H.; Goujon, J.-M.; Chadefaux-Vekemans, B.; Antignac, C. Late-Onset Nephropathic Cystinosis: Clinical Presentation, Outcome, and Genotyping. *Clin. J. Am. Soc. Nephrol.* **2008**, *3*, 27–35. [CrossRef]
4. Gahl, W.A.; Kaiser-Kupfer, M.I. Complications of nephropathic cystinosis after renal failure. *Pediatr. Nephrol.* **1987**, *1*, 260–268. [CrossRef] [PubMed]
5. Gahl, W.A.; Schneider, J.A.; Thoene, J.G.; Chesney, R. Course of nephropathic cystinosis after age 10 years. *J. Pediatr.* **1986**, *109*, 605–608. [CrossRef]
6. Theodoropoulos, D.S.; Krasnewich, D.; Kaiser-Kupfer, M.I.; Gahl, W.A. Classic nephropathic cystinosis as an adult disease. *JAMA J. Am. Med. Assoc.* **1993**, *270*, 2200–2204. [CrossRef]
7. Broyer, M.; Tete, M.J.; Guest, G.; Bertheleme, J.P.; Labrousse, F.; Poisson, M. Clinical polymorphism of cystinosis encephalopathy. Results of treatment with cysteamine. *J. Inherit. Metab. Dis.* **1996**, *19*, 65–75. [CrossRef]
8. Rossi, A.; Biancheri, R. Magnetic Resonance Spectroscopy in Metabolic Disorders. *Neuroimaging Clin. N. Am.* **2013**, *23*, 425–448. [CrossRef]
9. Fink, J.K.; Brouwers, P.; Barton, N.; Mohammed, H.M.; Sato, S.; Hill, S.; Cohen, W.E.; Fivush, B.; Gahl, W.A. Neurologic Complications in Long-standing Nephropathic Cystinosis. *Arch. Neurol.* **1989**, *46*, 543–548. [CrossRef]

10. Trauner, D.A.; Chase, C.; Scheller, J.; Katz, B.; Schneider, J.A. Neurologic and cognitive deficits in children with cystinosis. *J. Pediatr.* **1988**, *112*, 912–914. [CrossRef]
11. Trauner, D.A.; Williams, J.; Ballantyne, A.O.; Spilkin, A.M.; Crowhurst, J.; Hesselink, J. Neurological impairment in nephropathic cystinosis: Motor coordination deficits. *Pediatr. Nephrol.* **2010**, *25*, 2061–2066. [CrossRef] [PubMed]
12. Viltz, L.; Trauner, D.A. Effect of Age at Treatment on Cognitive Performance in Patients with Cystinosis. *J. Pediatr.* **2013**, *163*, 489–492. [CrossRef] [PubMed]
13. Dogulu, C.F.; Tsilou, E.; Rubin, B.; FitzGibbon, E.J.; Kaiser-Kupper, M.I.; Rennert, O.M.; Gahl, W.A. Idiopathic intracranial hypertension in cystinosis. *J. Pediatr.* **2004**, *145*, 673–678. [CrossRef]
14. Ross, D.L.; Strife, C.F.; Towbin, R.; Bove, K.E. Nonabsorptive hydrocephalus associated with nephropathic cystinosis. *Neurology* **1982**, *32*, 1330. [CrossRef] [PubMed]
15. Brodin-Sartorius, A.; Tête, M.; Niaudet, P.; Antignac, C.; Guest, G.; Ottolenghi, C.; Charbit, M.; Moyse, D.; Legendre, C.; Lesavre, P.; et al. Progression of Nephropathic Cystinosis in Late Adolescents and Adults: The Impact of Cysteamine Therapy. *Kidney Int.* **2012**, *81*, 179–189. [CrossRef] [PubMed]
16. Gahl, W.A.; Balog, J.Z.; Kleta, R. Nephropathic Cystinosis in Adults: Natural History and Effects of Oral Cysteamine Therapy. *Ann. Intern. Med.* **2007**, *147*, 242–250. [CrossRef]
17. Servais, A.; Saitovitch, A.; Hummel, A.; Boisgontier, J.; Scemla, A.; Sberro-Soussan, R.; Snanoudj, R.; Lemaitre, H.; Legendre, C.; Pontoizeau, C.; et al. Central nervous system complications in adult cystinosis patients. *J. Inherit. Metab. Dis.* **2020**, *43*, 348–356. [CrossRef]
18. Ueda, M.; O'brien, K.; Rosing, D.R.; Ling, A.; Kleta, R.; McAreavey, D.; Bernardini, I.; Gahl, W.A. Coronary Artery and Other Vascular Calcifications in Patients with Cystinosis after Kidney Transplantation. *Clin. J. Am. Soc. Nephrol.* **2006**, *1*, 555–562. [CrossRef]
19. Borrell-Pagès, M.; Canals, J.M.; Cordelières, F.P.; Parker, J.A.; Pineda, J.R.; Grange, G.; Bryson, E.A.; Guillermier, M.; Hirsch, E.; Hantraye, P.; et al. Cystamine and cysteamine increase brain levels of BDNF in Huntington disease via HSJ1b and transglutaminase. *J. Clin. Investig.* **2006**, *116*, 1410–1424. [CrossRef]
20. Ariceta, G.; Lara, E.; Camacho, J.A.; Oppenheimer, F.; Vara, J.; Santos, F.; Muñoz, M.A.; Cantarell, C.; Calvo, M.G.; Romero, R.; et al. Cysteamine (Cystagon(R)) adherence in patients with cystinosis in Spain: Successful in children and a challenge in adolescents and adults. *Nephrol. Dial. Transplant.* **2015**, *30*, 475–480. [CrossRef]
21. Maurice, T.; Hippert, C.; Serratrice, N.; Dubois, G.; Jacquet, C.; Antigna, C.; Kremer, E.J.; Kalatzis, V. Cystine accumulation in the CNS results in severe age-related memory deficits. *Neurobiol. Aging* **2009**, *30*, 987–1000. [CrossRef] [PubMed]
22. Vogel, D.G.; Malekzadeh, M.H.; Cornford, M.E.; Schneider, J.A.; Shields, W.D.; Vinters, H.V. Central nervous system involvement in nephropathic cystinosis. *J. Neuropathol. Exp. Neurol.* **1990**, *49*, 591–599. [CrossRef] [PubMed]
23. Nesterova, G.; Gahl, W. Nephropathic cystinosis: Late complications of a multisystemic disease. *Pediatr. Nephrol.* **2007**, *23*, 863–878. [CrossRef] [PubMed]
24. Berger, J.R.; Dillon, D.A.; Young, B.A.; Goldstein, S.J.; Nelson, P. Cystinosis of the brain and spinal cord with associated vasculopathy. *J. Neurol. Sci.* **2009**, *284*, 182–185. [CrossRef]
25. Prencipe, G.; Caiello, I.; Cherqui, S.; Whisenant, T.; Petrini, S.; Emma, F.; De Benedetti, F. Inflammasome Activation by Cystine Crystals: Implications for the Pathogenesis of Cystinosis. *J. Am. Soc. Nephrol.* **2014**, *25*, 1163–1169. [CrossRef]
26. Strayer, D.S. Cystinosis and a Dissecting Aortic Aneurysm in a 7-Year-Old Boy. *Arch. Pediatr. Adolesc. Med.* **1979**, *133*, 436–438. [CrossRef]
27. Jonas, A.J.; Conley, S.B.; Marshall, R.; Johnson, R.A.; Marks, M.; Rosenberg, H. Nephropathic cystinosis with central nervous system involvement. *Am. J. Med.* **1987**, *83*, 966–970. [CrossRef]
28. Neutel, D.; Geraldes, R.; Pereira, P.; Da Costa, A.G.; Pimentel, J.; Melo, T.P.E. Recurrent Ischemic Stroke in an Adult with Cystinosis: A Clinical–Pathological Case. *J. Stroke Cerebrovasc. Dis.* **2013**, *22*, e674–e675. [CrossRef]
29. Mitsnefes, M.M. Cardiovascular Disease in Children with Chronic Kidney Disease. *J. Am. Soc. Nephrol.* **2012**, *23*, 578–585. [CrossRef]
30. Scarvie, K.M.; Ballantyne, A.O.; Trauner, D.A. Visuomotor performance in children with infantile nephropathic cystinosis. *Percept. Mot. Skills* **1996**, *82*, 67–75. [CrossRef]
31. Ballantyne, A.O.; Spilkin, A.M.; Trauner, D.A. Executive Function in Nephropathic Cystinosis. *Cogn. Behav. Neurol.* **2013**, *26*, 14–22. [CrossRef] [PubMed]
32. Aly, R.; Makar, S.; El Bakri, A.; Soliman, N.A. Neurocognitive functions and behavioral profiles in children with nephropathic cystinosis. *Saudi. J. Kidney Dis. Transpl.* **2014**, *25*, 1224–1231. [PubMed]
33. Besouw, M.T.P.; Hulstijn-Dirkmaat, G.M.; van der Rijken, R.E.A.; Cornelissen, E.A.M.; van Dael, C.M.; Walle, J.V.; Lilien, M.R. Neurocognitive functioning in school-aged cystinosis patients. *J. Inherit. Metab. Dis.* **2010**, *33*, 787–793. [CrossRef]
34. Sathappan, A.; Trauner, D. Hierarchical processing of visual stimuli in nephropathic cystinosis. *J. Inherit. Metab. Dis.* **2019**, *42*, 545–552. [CrossRef] [PubMed]
35. Curie, A.; Touil, N.; Gaillard, S.; Galanaud, D.; Leboucq, N.; Deschênes, G.; Morin, D.; Abad, F.; Luauté, J.; Bodenan, E.; et al. Neuropsychological and neuroanatomical phenotype in 17 patients with cystinosis. *Orphanet J. Rare Dis.* **2020**, *15*, 1–22. [CrossRef] [PubMed]

36. Nichols, S.L.; Press, G.A.; Schneider, J.A.; Trauner, D.A. Cortical atrophy and cognitive performance in infantile nephropathic cystinosis. *Pediatr. Neurol.* **1990**, *6*, 379–381. [CrossRef]
37. Levine, S.; Paparo, G. Brain lesions in a case of cystinosis. *Acta Neuropathol.* **1982**, *57*, 217–220. [CrossRef]
38. Cochat, P.; Drachman, R.; Gagnadoux, M.F.; Pariente, D.; Broyer, M. Cerebral atrophy and nephropathic cystinosis. *Arch. Dis. Child.* **1986**, *61*, 401–403. [CrossRef]
39. Ehrich, J.; Stoeppler, L.; Offner, G.; Brodehl, J. Evidence for Cerebral Involvement in Nephropathic Cystinosis. *Neuropediatrics* **1979**, *10*, 128–137. [CrossRef]
40. Marquardt, L.; Kuramatsu, J.B.; Roesch, J.; Engelhorn, T.; Huttner, H.B. Posterior reversible encephalopathy syndrome in cystinosis. *Clin. Neurol. Neurosurg.* **2013**, *115*, 644–645. [CrossRef]
41. Chiu, Y.L.; Tsai, H.H.; Lai, Y.J.; Tseng, H.Y.; Wu, Y.; Peng, Y.; Chiu, C.; Chuang, Y. Cognitive impairment in patients with end-stage renal disease: Accelerated brain aging? *J. Formos. Med. Assoc.* **2019**, *118*, 867–875. [CrossRef] [PubMed]
42. Drew, D.A.; Koo, B.-B.; Bhadelia, R.; Weiner, D.E.; Duncan, S.; La Garza, M.M.-D.; Gupta, A.; Tighiouart, H.; Scott, T.; Sarnak, M.J. White matter damage in maintenance hemodialysis patients: A diffusion tensor imaging study. *BMC Nephrol.* **2017**, *18*, 1–7. [CrossRef]
43. Bava, S.; Theilmann, R.J.; Sach, M.; May, S.J.; Frank, L.R.; Hesselink, J.R.; Vu, D.; Trauner, D.A. Developmental changes in cerebral white matter microstructure in a disorder of lysosomal storage. *Cortex* **2010**, *46*, 206–216. [CrossRef] [PubMed]
44. Rao, K.I.; Hesselink, J.; Trauner, D.A.; Chiari, I. Malformation in Nephropathic Cystinosis. *J. Pediatr.* **2015**, *167*, 1126–1129. [CrossRef] [PubMed]
45. Cazals, X.; Lauvin, M.A.; Favelle, O.; Domengie, F.; Nivet, H.; Cottier, J.P. Cystinosis encephalopathy: MRI perivascular enhancement with micronodular T2* hypointensity. *Diagn. Interv. Imaging* **2013**, *94*, 653–655. [CrossRef]
46. Basser, P.J.; Pierpaoli, C. A simplified method to measure the diffusion tensor from seven MR images. *Magn. Reson. Med.* **1998**, *39*, 928–934. [CrossRef]
47. Doron, K.W.; Gazzaniga, M.S. Neuroimaging techniques offer new perspectives on callosal transfer and interhemispheric communication. *Cortex* **2008**, *44*, 1023–1029. [CrossRef]
48. Goldman, J.G.; Bledsoe, I.O.; Merkitch, D.; Dinh, V.; Bernard, B.; Stebbins, G.T. Corpus callosal atrophy and associations with cognitive impairment in Parkinson disease. *Neurology* **2017**, *88*, 1265–1272. [CrossRef]
49. Wu, W.-C.; Jiang, S.-F.; Yang, S.-C.; Lien, S.-H. Pseudocontinuous arterial spin labeling perfusion magnetic resonance imaging—A normative study of reproducibility in the human brain. *NeuroImage* **2011**, *56*, 1244–1250. [CrossRef]
50. Francisco, A.A.; Foxe, J.J.; Horsthuis, D.J.; Molholm, S. Impaired auditory sensory memory in Cystinosis despite typical sensory processing: A high-density electrical mapping study of the mismatch negativity (MMN). *Neuroimage Clin.* **2020**, *25*, 102170. [CrossRef]
51. Ethier, A.-A.; Lippé, S.; Merouani, A.; Lassonde, M.; Saint-Amour, D. Reversible Visual Evoked Potential Abnormalities in Uremic Children. *Pediatr. Neurol.* **2012**, *46*, 390–392. [CrossRef] [PubMed]
52. Näätänen, R.; Picton, T. The N1 Wave of the Human Electric and Magnetic Response to Sound: A Review and an Analysis of the Component Structure. *Psychophysiology* **1987**, *24*, 375–425. [CrossRef] [PubMed]
53. Giard, M.; Perrin, F.; Echallier, J.; Thévenet, M.; Froment, J.; Pernier, J. Dissociation of temporal and frontal components in the human auditory N1 wave: A scalp current density and dipole model analysis. *Electroencephalogr. Clin. Neurophysiol. Potentials Sect.* **1994**, *92*, 238–252. [CrossRef]
54. Francisco, A.A.; Berruti, A.S.; Kaskel, F.J.; Foxe, J.J.; Molholm, S. Assessing the integrity of auditory processing and sensory memory in adults with cystinosis (CTNS gene mutations). *Orphanet J. Rare Dis.* **2021**, *16*, 1–10. [CrossRef] [PubMed]

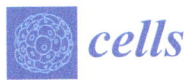 *cells*

Review

Fertility in Cystinosis

Ahmed Reda [1,*], Koenraad Veys [2,*] and Martine Besouw [3,*]

1. Lab of Developmental Biology and Reproductive Medicine, Department of Physiology and Pharmacology, Karolinska Institutet, 17165 Stockholm, Sweden
2. Division of Pediatric Nephrology, Department of Pediatrics, University Hospitals Leuven, 3000 Leuven, Belgium
3. Department of Pediatric Nephrology, University of Groningen, University Medical Center Groningen, 9700 RB Groningen, The Netherlands
* Correspondence: ahmed.reda@ki.se (A.R.); koenraad.veys@uzleuven.be (K.V.); m.t.p.besouw@umcg.nl (M.B.)

Abstract: Cystinosis is a rare inheritable lysosomal storage disorder characterized by cystine accumulation throughout the body, chronic kidney disease necessitating renal replacement therapy mostly during adolescence, and multiple extra-renal complications. The majority of male cystinosis patients are infertile due to azoospermia, in contrast to female patients who are fertile. Over recent decades, the fertility status of male patients has evolved from a primary hypogonadism in the era before the systematic treatment with cysteamine to azoospermia in the majority of cysteamine-treated infantile cystinosis patients. In this review, we provide a state-of-the-art overview on the available clinical, histopathological, animal, and in vitro data. We summarize current insights on both cystinosis males and females, and their clinical implications including the potential effect of cysteamine on fertility. In addition, we identify the remaining challenges and areas for future research.

Keywords: cystinosis; fertility; azoospermia; hypogonadism; cysteamine; histopathology; mouse model

Citation: Reda, A.; Veys, K.; Besouw, M. Fertility in Cystinosis. *Cells* **2021**, *10*, 3539. https://doi.org/10.3390/cells10123539

Academic Editor: Akito Maeshima

Received: 23 November 2021
Accepted: 13 December 2021
Published: 15 December 2021

Publisher's Note: MDPI stays neutral with regard to jurisdictional claims in published maps and institutional affiliations.

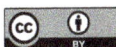

Copyright: © 2021 by the authors. Licensee MDPI, Basel, Switzerland. This article is an open access article distributed under the terms and conditions of the Creative Commons Attribution (CC BY) license (https://creativecommons.org/licenses/by/4.0/).

1. Introduction

Cystinosis is a rare autosomal metabolic disorder caused by bi-allelic mutations in the *CTNS* gene. This gene encodes the protein cystinosin, which is a lysosomal membrane protein responsible for transporting cystine, produced by the degradation of proteins in lysosomes, from the lysosome into the cytosol. Hence, mutations in *CTNS* cause the intralysosomal accumulation of cystine, leading to various effects in the body [1]. The age at presentation and the severity of the disease allows the classification of cystinosis into three clinical phenotypes: the most severe infantile form (95% of patients), the juvenile form (5%), and the adult ocular benign form (very rare) [2,3]. In the most severe form, the disease initially affects the kidneys, mostly causing end-stage kidney disease (ESKD) in adolescence or early adulthood. In addition, extra-renal complications develop, which most commonly affect the eyes and endocrine and neuromuscular systems [3]. Cysteamine is currently the only available disease-modifying treatment. It is an aminothiol that depletes the accumulated cystine in lysosomes [2,3]. One of the more recently reported unexpected extra-renal complications in male cystinosis patients is azoospermia. Female cystinosis patients, however, have normal fertility and can become pregnant, as reported earlier [4].

For clinical fertility management purposes, azoospermia is classified into obstructive (OA) and nonobstructive azoospermia (NOA), based on clinical sexual characteristics (testicular volume) and sex hormone levels [5]. In OA, the azoospermia is caused by an obstruction in the genital tract and testicular function is preserved, while in NOA, the azoospermia is caused by testicular dysfunction [5]. Hence, azoospermia combined with normal testicular function would most likely be diagnosed as OA, whilst azoospermia combined with impaired testicular function would most likely be diagnosed as NOA [6].

Due to the advances in the treatment of cystinosis patients over recent decades, their life expectancy has substantially increased, making fertility a new and important issue for both patients and their treating physicians [7]. In this review, we provide an overview of the fertility status in cystinosis patients (males and females) and of the possible effects of cysteamine on fertility.

2. Fertility in Female Cystinosis Patients

Women with cystinosis have been reported to suffer from delayed puberty, with a menarche around the age of 15–19 years, while a stable menstrual cycle is reached at least two years after menarche [8]. In accordance, the plasma levels of follicle-stimulating hormone (FSH), luteinizing hormone (LH), and estradiol were only rising long after the onset of puberty. However, most adult women with cystinosis showed normal levels of FSH, LH, and estradiol [8].

Unlike men suffering from cystinosis, fertility seems to be unaffected in female cystinosis patients. Several reports have described successful pregnancies in women with cystinosis [4,9–13]. The specific issues that can arise when women with cystinosis become pregnant were recently reviewed by Blakey et al. In summary, various maternal and fetal adverse events were reported, including cephalopelvic disproportion due to maternal short stature, gestational diabetes, hypothyroidism, and respiratory muscle weakness, on top of the complications of a pregnancy following a kidney transplantation [4,14]. The latter include a higher incidence of pre-eclampsia, gestational diabetes, Cesarean section, and pre-term delivery [14].

Another important issue in female cystinosis patients who want children is the teratogenicity of cysteamine. Since this is a lifesaving treatment, the timing of its discontinuation should be well thought out. The current advice is to stop cysteamine as soon as a pregnancy test is found to be positive [13]. However, in one case study, a woman with cystinosis on cysteamine was informed about her pregnancy, being 12 weeks pregnant, but cysteamine treatment had to be discontinued. Later, the patient had a Cesarean section, giving birth to a healthy baby [15]. Since it remains uncertain whether or not cysteamine is excreted into breast milk, breastfeeding is currently not recommended [4].

In general, it is advised for women with cystinosis who want to become pregnant to seek medical advice in advance, preferably in a clinic with expertise in pregnancies in patients with chronic kidney disease or kidney transplantation. By doing so, teratogenic medications can be switched before conception and a plan can be made when cysteamine has to be stopped. Since cystinosis is an autosomal recessive disorder, the chances for the child to develop cystinosis are very low if the father is unaffected. However, since he could be an asymptomatic carrier, pre-conceptional genetic counselling should be offered [16,17]. If the patient's partner does not carry a mutation in the *CTNS* gene, the chances that the child will develop cystinosis are minimal. Importantly, some mutations can be difficult to detect (such as deep intronic mutations), so couples should be counseled that there is still a very small likelihood that the child will have cystinosis if such a mutation remains undetected in the patient's partner.

In our expert opinion, we do not advise performing prenatal genetic testing to exclude cystinosis in an unborn child given the risk of miscarriage caused by the procedure. If early genetic testing is warranted, DNA can be extracted from cord blood or from the baby after birth to perform urgent analysis of the *CTNS* gene. The delay of a few weeks in the diagnosis of cystinosis is unlikely to influence long-term prognosis, since the diagnosis will still be made very early, and treatment can be started accordingly.

3. Fertility in Male Cystinosis Patients

3.1. Sexual Hormone Levels

Primary hypogonadism in male cystinosis patients was first described in 1993 [18]. In those days, treatment with cysteamine was not prescribed and monitored as strictly as it is nowadays, and it was often stopped after kidney transplantation. Hypogonadism with delayed puberty and delayed bone age was found to be very common, but it was not reported whether the men studied (all of whom had been transplanted) were treated with cysteamine or not. Over the years, primary hypogonadism with increased levels of the gonadotropins LH and FSH was reported very frequently in male cystinosis patients [18–21], and also in those investigated in the current era when treatment with cysteamine is started early in life and continued after kidney transplantation [19–21]. In addition, inhibin B is a hormone secreted by Sertoli cells that has an important role in spermatogenesis [22,23]. Since inhibin B was suggested to be a good marker for Sertoli cell function [24], it was added to the panel of hormones to be investigated in more recent studies. Inhibin B levels were found to be reduced in several men [19], a finding that was confirmed in subsequent studies [20,21]. This was a valuable addition to the panel of hormones since for the first time it showed clear evidence for Sertoli cell dysfunction in male cystinosis patients, in addition to Leydig cell dysfunction, which is characterized by low testosterone levels [25].

Reduced kidney function or immunosuppressive treatment for kidney transplantation did not seem to be the cause for these hormone disturbances [18–20]. In fact, in the original study by Chik et al. hormone levels in cystinosis patients were compared to a group of men of similar age who underwent a kidney transplant for a disease other than cystinosis, with a comparable renal function and immunosuppressive treatment regimen [18]. Interestingly, secondary hypogonadism, characterized by reduced FSH and LH levels with normal testicular function [18,19], and even normal sex hormone levels have been reported sporadically as well, the latter being more frequently observed in younger men [18–21].

3.2. Testicular Volume and Histology

In the early cohort described by Chik et al., who were likely to be treated with cysteamine less vigorously compared to current practice, testicular volume was reduced in all 10 studied men [18]. In more recent cohorts, it was strikingly found that testicular volume was generally normal in younger men but tended to decrease with increasing age, indicating progressive testicular atrophy [20,21].

There are sporadic reports of testicular biopsy samples, the first being a postmortem investigation showing fibrosis, germinal dysplasia and Leydig cell hyperplasia with numerous cystine crystals, but seminiferous tubules were still visible [18]. Later, histology reports in patients treated with cysteamine confirmed fibrosis, but showed no germinal dysplasia and the Johnson score (a measure for spermatogenesis in the seminiferous tubules [26]) ranged between 7 and 9, indicating intact spermatogenesis [19,20]. Interestingly, while biopsy samples from the central part of the testes showed intact spermatogenesis, more damage was observed, including spermatogonial arrest on light microscopy and enlarged lysosomes in both Leydig and Sertoli cells on transmission electron microscopy in samples taken from the periphery, indicating that the progressive testicular damage seen in male cystinosis patients starts in the periphery at the end of the arterial blood supply [21].

In addition, the infiltration of activated macrophages was found in the interstitial testicular tissues, as well as the presence of perturbed blood–testis barrier in infantile cystinosis patients using histological analysis and Zonula occludens-1 as a marker for the quality of the blood–testis barrier. This could indicate that inflammation might be a common cause for both the primary hypogonadism and for epididymal dysfunction, ultimately causing obstruction [20].

3.3. Semen Analysis

In the first paper that mentions semen analysis in cystinosis patients, azoospermia was found in all three investigated men, including one patient with normal sex hormone levels [18].

Years later, semen analysis in five male cystinosis patients confirmed azoospermia in all subjects, even in those with normal sex hormone levels, and normal ejaculate volumes and pH in four of them. In this report, for the first time, concerns were raised regarding male fertility in cystinosis patients treated with cysteamine [19].

Later studies confirmed azoospermia in most men suffering from infantile cystinosis; however, oligozoospermia was found in 1 out of 10 male infantile cystinosis patients in a subsequent investigation [20] and another study in 15 men showed oligozoospermia in two of them, while one man was even reported to have normozoospermia [21]. The ages of these four men with either oligo- or normozoospermia, ranged between 18 and 28 years [20,21]. It remains intriguing as to why this small proportion of men retained viable sperm in their ejaculate, while azoospermia was found in all other men with the infantile phenotype who were of the same age or even younger. The type of *CTNS* mutation did not seem to play a role, since all four men harbored severe mutations in *CTNS* [20,21]. Even more fascinating is the fact that sperm cells could also be demonstrated in the semen of three cystinosis patients with a noninfantile phenotype: oligozoospermia was found in two subjects with juvenile cystinosis (29 and 35 years old), and one man with ocular cystinosis (48 years old) was reported to have normozoospermia and has children [20].

Since male cystinosis patients with a normal Johnson score in their testicular biopsies were often reported to also suffer from primary hypogonadism, this primary hypogonadism could not have been the cause of the observed azoospermia. On the other hand, no sperm could be retrieved by percutaneous epididymal sperm aspiration (PESA) on several occasions in a man with a normal Johnson score, which could indicate a nonobstructive due to his azoospermia. Since testicular ultrasound also showed no signs of obstruction in two additional men, a nonobstructive cause of the azoospermia was initially suspected [19]. However, a few years later, a successful PESA was performed in another male cystinosis patient who had suffered from azoospermia in the previous study [19,27]. The PESA was followed by intracytoplasmic sperm injection (ICSI) and led to the first successful pregnancy induced by a male infantile cystinosis patient, resulting in the birth of healthy twins [27]. Later, viable sperm cells could be extracted by PESA in another patient [20] and by microsurgical testicular sperm extraction (mTESE) in another two men with infantile cystinosis [21], all of whom had azoospermia in their semen analysis, again confirming adequate spermatogenesis in these men. Thus, the evidence for an obstructive cause of cystinosis-related azoospermia with sufficient spermatogenesis started to accumulate.

3.4. Scrotal Ultrasound Imaging

Since the finding that there seemed to be no signs of obstruction on testicular ultrasound in two men with cystinosis [19], it has been published how more detailed scrotal ultrasounds could be used to predict obstruction in the genital tract [28]. In order to further investigate the hypothesis of OA in cystinosis, detailed scrotal ultrasound studies were subsequently performed. In one study, it was found that all six male infantile cystinosis patients showed signs of vasal obstruction with an enlarged caput epididymis relative to the ipsilateral testicular volume, of whom one patient with the youngest age had an oligozoospermia (see Figure 1). Interestingly, two male juvenile cystinosis patients with oligozoospermia and one male ocular cystinosis patient with normozoospermia all had a normal scrotal ultrasound [20]. Additionally, in another study, signs of obstruction with dilatation of the rete testis were found in 12 out of 18 investigated male infantile cystinosis patients, two of whom showed oligozoospermia [21].

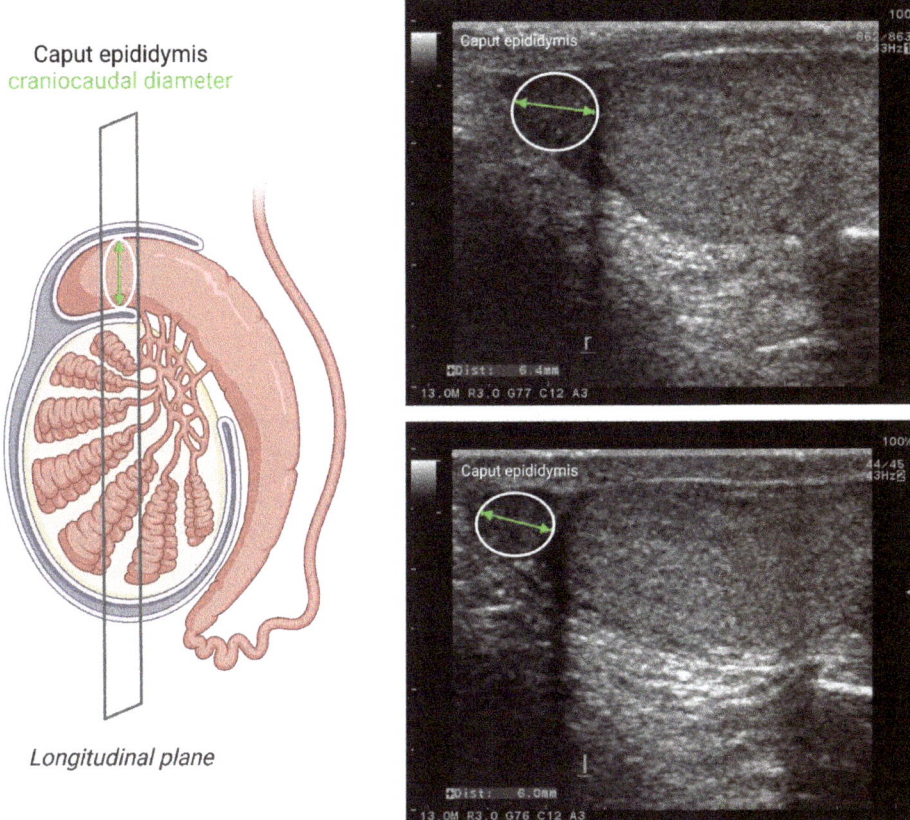

Figure 1. Use of scrotal ultrasound to diagnose obstructive azoospermia. On the left side, a schematic diagram illustrating the hypothesized dilatation in caput epididymis due to obstruction in the male genital tract. The craniocaudal diameter of caput epididymis is determined and normalized to the ipsilateral testicular volume (calculated by the formula radius 1 × radius 2 × radius 3 × 4/3 × π, where radii 1, 2, and 3 are the different axial radii of testis determined by ultrasonic imaging). On the right side, the upper figure shows an example for a scrotal ultrasound image for an adult infantile cystinosis patient, illustrating a dilated caput epididymis. The lower figure shows an example for a scrotal ultrasound image for an adult healthy male, with no signs of dilated caput epididymis [20]. Green arrows in the two ultrasound images represent the craniocaudal diameter of caput epididymis (6.4 mm in upper panel figure; 6.0 mm in lower panel figure).

3.5. Seminal Plasma Markers

Several markers in seminal plasma have been studied in order to confirm an obstructive due to the azoospermia observed in infantile cystinosis. One study aimed to perform semen analysis in 15 male infantile cystinosis patients, although semen volume was too small (<0.3 mL) in two of them for seminal markers to be determined. In the remaining patients, normal levels of neutral α-glucosidase (NAG), secreted mainly by epididymis, were found in all except one patient, and the authors concluded that the epididymal secretory capacity and flux of secretions was not affected. They found reduced levels of both fructose (which is the most important source of energy for the spermatozoa and helps to maintain the alkaline pH of the semen), and zinc in 33% of the studied patients. The authors hypothesized that reduced fructose levels could be a sign of obstruction at the level of the excretory ducts of the vesicular glands and that reduced zinc levels could represent an obstruction at the level of the prostate. These abnormalities, however, did not explain all cases of azoospermia or oligozoospermia, since the remaining 67% of patients had normal levels of these seminal plasma markers [21].

In another study, the seminal plasma levels of the epididymal secreted markers Extracellular Matrix protein-1 (ECM-1), which is highly expressed in the epididymis, and NAG, which is a specific and established marker for epididymal secretion used in the previous study as a seminal marker [21], were analyzed. ECM-1 and NAG have been identified as good markers of obstruction of the male genital tract [29–31]. These markers were subsequently tested in nine male cystinosis patients (6 with the infantile subtype, 2 with the juvenile subtype and 1 with the ocular subtype) and compared to nine healthy men following vasectomy, and to another seven healthy men without vasectomy. It was found that all infantile cystinosis patients had reduced levels of ECM-1 when compared to healthy controls without vasectomy. Moreover, the levels of NAG were comparable to those in men following vasectomy, which was lower when compared to the levels measured in the men without vasectomy. This seems to contrast to the fact that normal levels of α-glucosidase have been found in the other study of seminal plasma markers of male infantile cystinosis patients. However, the fact that the reported levels were not compared to a normal standard but to two control groups containing healthy men both with and without vasectomy strengthen these results. The combination of reduced ECM-1 and NAG in all studied patients further confirmed the hypothesis of OA as the cause of fertility problems in male infantile cystinosis patients [20] (see Figure 2).

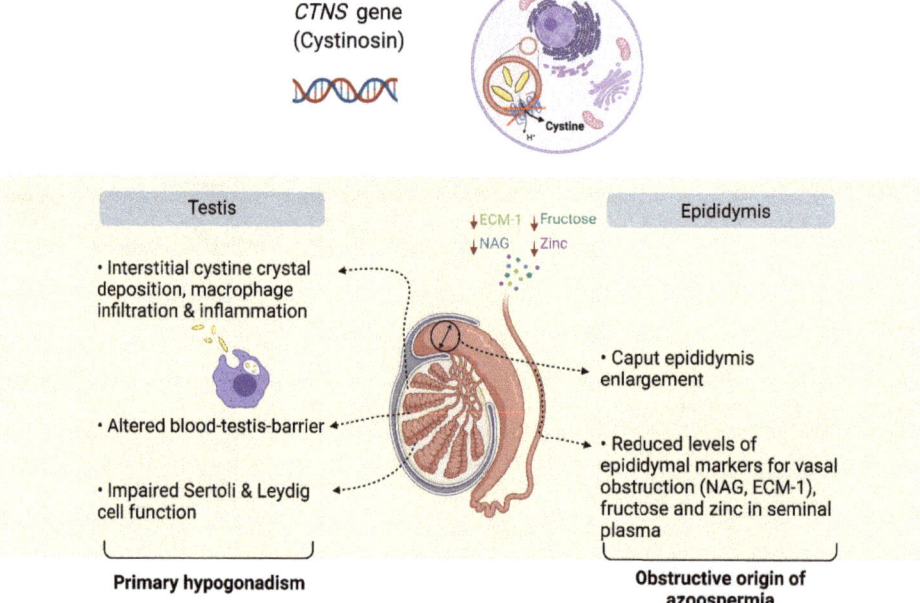

Figure 2. Plausible mechanism of infertility in male infantile cystinosis patients. Bi-allelic mutations in the *CTNS* gene lead to accumulation of cystine in the lysosomes, cell apoptosis, phagocytosis of cell debris and cystine crystals, and inflammation. In kidneys, it is known to be associated with an increased shedding of epithelial cells. In infantile type male cystinosis cystinosis patients, an enlarged caput epididymis, and reduction in seminal plasma markers, including zinc, fructose, extracellular matrix protein-1 (ECM-1) and neutral α glucosidase (NAG), point towards obstruction of the male genital tract as the primary cause for azoospermia. In parallel, cystine accumulation and macrophage infiltration results in interstitial inflammation in the testis, which is associated with alterations at the blood–testis barrier, and Sertoli and Leydig cell impairment, leading to a progressive primary hypogonadism.

4. Fertility in Cystinosis Animal Models

Unequivocally, animal studies can be of great importance to understand mechanisms and pathophysiology of diseases. In this context, male fertility in cystinosis was studied using a $Ctns^{-/-}$ knockout mouse model [32] that was generated on a C57BL/6 background, replacing the last four exons of $Ctns$ gene with an IRES-β$galneo$ cassette [33]. The results showed that male $Ctns^{-/-}$ knockout mice showed normal fertility compared to their wild-type litter mates, represented by a similar litter size, testicular morphology, and semen analysis. This meant that the knockout model, albeit showing a renal but mild phenotype, cannot be used to investigate male fertility in cystinosis in absence of the reproductive phenotype [32]. It was not an exception for a mouse model not to exhibit the full clinical phenotype of a disease, since earlier mouse models for similar metabolic disorders, such as Pompe's disease and Gitelman's syndrome, could not replicate the full phenotype as well [34–36]. Later, it was shown that the male $Ctns^{-/-}$ knockout mice had a perturbed blood–testis barrier [20]. A possible explanation behind the absence of the full human phenotype is that the presence of the genetic modifiers can compensate for the absence of a specific gene in mice, and that the renal phenotype in the $Ctns^{-/-}$ knockout mice, as well as the reproductive phenotype, is less pronounced compared to humans.

In an attempt to find a more suitable animal model for cystinosis, zebrafish were proposed as an alternative [37,38]. In a study by Berlingerio et al., the authors found that both male and female $Ctns^{-/-}$ zebrafish were fertile. However, female $Ctns^{-/-}$ zebrafish showed reduced egg production and percentage of fertilized eggs compared to wild-type zebrafish [38]. In addition, a histological analysis of the testicular tissue showed the accumulation of spermatozoa in the spermatogenic cysts when compared to wild-type zebrafish [38]. Interestingly, the accumulation of spermatozoa in the spermatogenic cysts could be a sign of obstruction, which potentiate the hypothesis that azoospermia in male infantile cystinosis patients is obstructive in origin.

In Vitro Studies in Cystinosis

In addition to these studies on men and mice, a human epididymal epithelial cell line [39] was studied in which the *CTNS* gene was downregulated by siRNA silencing [20]. A transcriptomic analysis revealed altered processes such as fluid shear stress, interleukin-6 production, actin cytoskeleton reorganization, and modified amino acids and sulfur compounds transport [20]. Since these biological processes are important to maintain a healthy epithelial layer, it would be expected that alterations in these processes would lead to a loss of the epithelial layer and shedding of cells, which could play a role in the development of obstruction [20].

5. Effect of Cysteamine on Fertility

Cysteamine is a cystine-depleting agent and the only available lifesaving treatment for nephropathic cystinosis. In early studies, it was proven to be a protective agent for spermatogonial stem cells (SSCs) in rats, following X-ray irradiation [40,41]. In addition, studies using cysteamine in sperm cryopreservation in bulls, ram, and goat showed increased sperm motility after thawing [42–44]. Nonetheless, there are several reports that suggest a potential negative impact of cysteamine on fertility. When added to the fresh sperm of bulls and buffalos, cysteamine was shown to reduce sperm quality, analyzed by computer assisted sperm analysis system [45,46]. In addition, cysteamine was shown to act as a contraceptive when added to rabbit fresh sperm, inhibiting in vivo fertilization [47]. In one recent study, oral cysteamine treatment in sheep for 6 months at a dose of 20 mg/kg/day reduced sperm count and motility and disturbed blood–testis barrier [48].

In contrast, there are no clear studies on the effects of cysteamine on sperm quality in men. It had been hypothesized that cysteamine could, in theory, cause increased ghrelin levels, which in turn could have a negative effect on Leydig and Sertoli cell function [19]. However, this has never been confirmed. In addition, as explained earlier, over time, the hypothesis of the pathogenesis of azoospermia moved from likely to be nonobstructive towards likely to be obstructive. In addition, when analyzing the age at onset of, and adherence to cysteamine treatment, it was concluded that cysteamine could slow down the testicular degeneration, although it still cannot be fully stopped [21].

Recently, the effect of cysteamine in the previously described cystinosis mouse model was studied, using wild-type C57BL/6 mice and $Ctns^{-/-}$ knockout mice that were fed with food mixed with cysteamine at a high dose of 500 mg/kg/day for 6 months [20]. Following the different fertility parameters, no negative effect of cysteamine on epididymal sperm count, litter size, plasma LH, FSH, and testosterone, and seminal vesicle weight was detected in both wild-type and knockout mice. Moreover, a histological analysis of murine testicular tissues showed no effect of cysteamine in both wild-type and knockout mice. The disturbance in the blood–testis barrier that was found in the knockout mice could not be restored by cysteamine. A separate bioavailability study was performed to investigate the availability of cysteamine in testicular tissue, along with cystine accumulation, using wild-type and knockout mice. The results showed that cysteamine did cross the blood–testis barrier but could not reduce cystine accumulation in testicular tissue to the extent that is seen in other organs, such as the kidneys. This could explain to a large extent the absence of an effect of cysteamine on the testis of male cystinosis patients and their fertility in general, even if they were strictly compliant on cysteamine treatment.

In accordance, in a previous study investigating the effect of oral cysteamine on female reproduction in wild-type rats, the authors showed that cysteamine had no adverse effects on conception and early embryonic development [49]. Hence, it is believed that cysteamine would not have a negative impact on reproduction in both male and female cystinosis patients. However, clinical studies investigating the effect of cysteamine in cystinosis patients treated with the drug would have great value.

6. Future Perspectives

Even though female infantile cystinosis patients seem to have normal fertility, there is room for future research to focus on neonatal outcomes in these children. To our knowledge, there are no reports of intrauterine growth retardation caused by placental dysfunction in cystinotic women, although in theory placental cystine accumulation could adversely influence its function. However, this has never been studied in a systematic manner. Additionally, it would be interesting to study whether or not compliance to cysteamine treatment prior to pregnancy improves pregnancy outcomes.

Given the obstructive origin of azoospermia, preserving gonadal function in male cystinosis patients, if possible, is of the utmost importance to safeguard the possibility to father their own offspring via assisted reproductive technology. Therefore, future research should be aimed at further elucidating the exact pathogenesis of hypogonadism, which is now presumed to be related to inflammation and fibrosis caused by cystine deposition. More specifically, studying Leydig and Sertoli cell function in cystinosis and how to preserve it, could be of interest. In addition, it remains unclear why regular cysteamine dosages have subtherapeutic effects in testicular tissue and future studies could focus on different treatment strategies that have more of an effect on testicular cystine accumulation. In this regard, a cystinosis animal model more resembling human disease and in vitro models are indispensable.

Additionally, it would be interesting to investigate the inflammatory aspect of cystinosis and its role in the reproductive phenotype, since this could open the door to study the use of anti-inflammatory agents to alleviate the reproductive symptoms. In addition, the use of medications that can lower the seminal plasma viscosity has not been studied thus far.

Furthermore, semen analysis and sperm cryopreservation should be offered to all post-pubertal cystinosis males and hence be included as a recommendation in the standard clinical management guidelines for cystinosis. Once implemented, a large-scale registry-based observational study could provide the most reliable data on the proportion of infantile male cystinosis patients that show oligo- instead of azoospermia and give a better insight into their clinical determinants.

7. Conclusions

In conclusion, female cystinosis patients seem to have a normal fertility, although complications during pregnancy that are secondary to the disease and kidney transplantation frequently occur. In contrast, most male infantile cystinosis patients suffer from azoospermia due to obstructive causes, with intact spermatogenesis in early adulthood. This renders them able to father their own biological children using epididymal or testicular sperm, followed by ICSI. Given the fact that cystinosis is an autosomal recessive disorder, the chances for the child to develop cystinosis are extremely small when the partner is confirmed not to be carrier of a *CTNS* mutation.

Surprisingly, oligozoospermia or even normozoospermia can be found sporadically in male infantile cystinosis patients (mainly in those <30 years of age), which may be due to the presence of another yet unidentified factor that mitigates the effect of cystinosis on fertility. Moreover, oligozoospermia and normozoospermia have been reported in juvenile and ocular cystinosis, respectively. Based on this specific finding, we recommend performing a semen analysis at the earliest age possible for (post-pubertal) male cystinosis patients to confirm the presence or absence of azoospermia, since some patients could still have a few sperm cells in their semen which could be cryopreserved. This will increase their opportunities to father their own biological children. Importantly, compliance to cysteamine treatment does not negatively affect the clinical fertility phenotype in male cystinosis patients, albeit it is not able to restore fertility.

Author Contributions: All authors have contributed to the first draft and the final revised manuscript. All authors have read and agreed to the published version of the manuscript.

Funding: This research received no external funding.

Conflicts of Interest: The authors have no conflict of interest to report.

References

1. Town, M.; Jean, G.; Cherqui, S.; Attard, M.; Forestier, L.; Whitmore, S.A.; Callen, D.F.; Gribouval, O.; Broyer, M.; Bates, G.P.; et al. A novel gene encoding an integral membrane protein is mutated in nephropathic cystinosis. *Nat. Genet.* **1998**, *18*, 319–324. [CrossRef]
2. Gahl, W.A.; Thoene, J.G.; Schneider, J.A. Cystinosis. *N. Engl. J. Med.* **2002**, *347*, 111–121. [CrossRef]
3. Emma, F.; Nesterova, G.; Langman, C.; Labbe, A.; Cherqui, S.; Goodyer, P.; Janssen, M.C.; Greco, M.; Topaloglu, R.; Elenberg, E.; et al. Nephropathic cystinosis: An international consensus document. *Nephrol. Dial. Transplant.* **2014**, *29* (Suppl. 4), iv87–iv94. [CrossRef] [PubMed]
4. Blakey, H.; Proudfoot-Jones, J.; Knox, E.; Lipkin, G. Pregnancy in women with cystinosis. *Clin. Kidney J.* **2019**, *12*, 855–858. [CrossRef]
5. Wosnitzer, M.; Goldstein, M.; Hardy, M.P. Review of Azoospermia. *Spermatogenesis* **2014**, *4*, e28218. [CrossRef]
6. Wosnitzer, M.S.; Goldstein, M. Obstructive azoospermia. *Urol. Clin. N. Am.* **2014**, *41*, 83–95. [CrossRef]
7. Elmonem, M.A.; Veys, K.R.; Soliman, N.A.; van Dyck, M.; van den Heuvel, L.P.; Levtchenko, E. Cystinosis: A review. *Orphanet J. Rare Dis.* **2016**, *11*, 47. [CrossRef] [PubMed]
8. Winkler, L.; Offner, G.; Krull, F.; Brodehl, J. Growth and pubertal development in nephropathic cystinosis. *Eur. J. Pediatr.* **1993**, *152*, 244–249. [CrossRef]
9. Reiss, R.E.; Kuwabara, T.; Smith, M.L.; Gahl, W.A. Successful pregnancy despite placental cystine crystals in a woman with nephropathic cystinosis. *N. Engl. J. Med.* **1988**, *319*, 223–226. [CrossRef] [PubMed]
10. Andrews, P.A.; Sacks, S.H.; van't Hoff, W. Successful pregnancy in cystinosis. *JAMA* **1994**, *272*, 1327–1328. [CrossRef]
11. Haase, M.; Morgera, S.; Bamberg, C.; Halle, H.; Martini, S.; Dragun, D.; Neumayer, H.H.; Budde, K. Successful pregnancies in dialysis patients including those suffering from cystinosis and familial Mediterranean fever. *J. Nephrol.* **2006**, *19*, 677–681. [PubMed]
12. Ramappa, A.J.; Pyatt, J.R. Pregnancy-associated cardiomyopathy occurring in a young patient with nephropathic cystinosis. *Cardiol. Young* **2010**, *20*, 220–222. [CrossRef] [PubMed]
13. Chuang, Y.W.; Wen, M.C.; Wu, M.J.; Shu, K.H.; Cheng, C.H.; Yu, T.M.; Huang, S.T.; Chen, C.H. Follow-up and treatment of renal transplantation with nephropathic cystinosis in central Taiwan. *Transplant. Proc.* **2012**, *44*, 80–82. [CrossRef]

14. Deshpande, N.A.; James, N.T.; Kucirka, L.M.; Boyarsky, B.J.; Garonzik-Wang, J.M.; Montgomery, R.A.; Segev, D.L. Pregnancy outcomes in kidney transplant recipients: A systematic review and meta-analysis. *Am. J. Transplant.* **2011**, *11*, 2388–2404. [CrossRef]
15. Kuczborska, K.; Gozdowska, J.; Lewandowska, D.; Grenda, R.; Galazka, Z.; Nazarewski, S.; Durlik, M. Therapeutic Problems and Pregnancy in a Patient With Infantile Nephropathic Cystinosis: A Case Report. *Transplant. Proc.* **2019**, *51*, 545–547. [CrossRef]
16. Ariceta, G.; Camacho, J.A.; Fernandez-Obispo, M.; Fernandez-Polo, A.; Gamez, J.; Garcia-Villoria, J.; Lara Monteczuma, E.; Leyes, P.; Martin-Begue, N.; Oppenheimer, F.; et al. Cystinosis in adult and adolescent patients: Recommendations for the comprehensive care of cystinosis. *Nefrologia* **2015**, *35*, 304–321. [CrossRef] [PubMed]
17. Boman, H.; Schneider, J.A. Prenatal diagnosis of nephropathic cystinosis. Pregnancy at risk ascertained through heterozygote diagnosis of parents. *Acta Paediatr. Scand.* **1981**, *70*, 389–393. [CrossRef] [PubMed]
18. Chik, C.L.; Friedman, A.; Merriam, G.R.; Gahl, W.A. Pituitary-testicular function in nephropathic cystinosis. *Ann. Intern. Med.* **1993**, *119*, 568–575. [CrossRef] [PubMed]
19. Besouw, M.T.; Kremer, J.A.; Janssen, M.C.; Levtchenko, E.N. Fertility status in male cystinosis patients treated with cysteamine. *Fertil. Steril.* **2010**, *93*, 1880–1883. [CrossRef]
20. Reda, A.; Veys, K.; Kadam, P.; Taranta, A.; Rega, L.R.; Goffredo, B.M.; Camps, C.; Besouw, M.; Cyr, D.; Albersen, M.; et al. Human and animal fertility studies in cystinosis reveal signs of obstructive azoospermia, an altered blood-testis barrier and a subtherapeutic effect of cysteamine in testis. *J. Inherit. Metab. Dis.* **2021**, *44*, 1393–1408. [CrossRef]
21. Rohayem, J.; Haffner, D.; Cremers, J.F.; Huss, S.; Wistuba, J.; Weitzel, D.; Kliesch, S.; Hohenfellner, K. Testicular function in males with infantile nephropathic cystinosis. *Hum. Reprod.* **2021**, *36*, 1191–1204. [CrossRef]
22. O'Connor, A.E.; De Kretser, D.M. Inhibins in normal male physiology. *Semin. Reprod. Med.* **2004**, *22*, 177–185. [CrossRef]
23. Pierik, F.H.; Vreeburg, J.T.; Stijnen, T.; De Jong, F.H.; Weber, R.F. Serum inhibin B as a marker of spermatogenesis. *J. Clin. Endocrinol. Metab.* **1998**, *83*, 3110–3114. [CrossRef] [PubMed]
24. Bordallo, M.A.; Guimaraes, M.M.; Pessoa, C.H.; Carrico, M.K.; Dimetz, T.; Gazolla, H.M.; Dobbin, J.; Castilho, I.A. Decreased serum inhibin B/FSH ratio as a marker of Sertoli cell function in male survivors after chemotherapy in childhood and adolescence. *J. Pediatr. Endocrinol. Metab.* **2004**, *17*, 879–887. [CrossRef]
25. Gurung, P.; Yetiskul, E.; Jialal, I. Physiology, Male Reproductive System. In *StatPearls*; StatPearls Publishing: Treasure Island, FL, USA, 2021.
26. Johnsen, S.G. Testicular biopsy score count—A method for registration of spermatogenesis in human testes: Normal values and results in 335 hypogonadal males. *Hormones* **1970**, *1*, 2–25. [CrossRef] [PubMed]
27. Veys, K.R.; D'Hauwers, K.W.; van Dongen, A.; Janssen, M.C.; Besouw, M.T.P.; Goossens, E.; van den Heuvel, L.P.; Wetzels, A.; Levtchenko, E.N. First Successful Conception Induced by a Male Cystinosis Patient. *JIMD Rep.* **2018**, *38*, 1–6. [CrossRef] [PubMed]
28. Pezzella, A.; Barbonetti, A.; Micillo, A.; D'Andrea, S.; Necozione, S.; Gandini, L.; Lenzi, A.; Francavilla, F.; Francavilla, S. Ultrasonographic determination of caput epididymis diameter is strongly predictive of obstruction in the genital tract in azoospermic men with normal serum FSH. *Andrology* **2013**, *1*, 133–138. [CrossRef] [PubMed]
29. Drabovich, A.P.; Dimitromanolakis, A.; Saraon, P.; Soosaipillai, A.; Batruch, I.; Mullen, B.; Jarvi, K.; Diamandis, E.P. Differential diagnosis of azoospermia with proteomic biomarkers ECM1 and TEX101 quantified in seminal plasma. *Sci. Transl. Med.* **2013**, *5*, 212ra160. [CrossRef]
30. Lei, B.; Xing, R.; Zhou, X.; Lv, D.; Wan, B.; Shu, F.; Zhong, L.; Wu, H.; Mao, X. Neutral alpha-1,4-glucosidase and fructose levels contribute to discriminating obstructive and nonobstructive azoospermia in Chinese men with azoospermia. *Andrologia* **2016**, *48*, 670–675. [CrossRef]
31. Eertmans, F.; Bogaert, V.; Van Poecke, T.; Puype, B. An Improved Neutral a-Glucosidase Assay for Assessment of Epididymal Function-Validation and Comparison to the WHO Method. *Diagnostics* **2014**, *4*, 1–11. [CrossRef]
32. Besouw, M.T.; van Pelt, A.M.; Gaide Chevronnay, H.P.; Courtoy, P.J.; Pastore, A.; Goossens, E.; Devuyst, O.; Antignac, C.; Levtchenko, E.N. Studying nonobstructive azoospermia in cystinosis: Histologic examination of testes and epididymis and sperm analysis in a Ctns(-)/(-) mouse model. *Fertil. Steril.* **2012**, *98*, 162–165. [CrossRef] [PubMed]
33. Nevo, N.; Chol, M.; Bailleux, A.; Kalatzis, V.; Morisset, L.; Devuyst, O.; Gubler, M.C.; Antignac, C. Renal phenotype of the cystinosis mouse model is dependent upon genetic background. *Nephrol. Dial. Transplant.* **2010**, *25*, 1059–1066. [CrossRef] [PubMed]
34. Janne, P.A.; Suchy, S.F.; Bernard, D.; MacDonald, M.; Crawley, J.; Grinberg, A.; Wynshaw-Boris, A.; Westphal, H.; Nussbaum, R.L. Functional overlap between murine Inpp5b and Ocrl1 may explain why deficiency of the murine ortholog for OCRL1 does not cause Lowe syndrome in mice. *J. Clin. Investig.* **1998**, *101*, 2042–2053. [CrossRef] [PubMed]
35. Bijvoet, A.G.; van de Kamp, E.H.; Kroos, M.A.; Ding, J.H.; Yang, B.Z.; Visser, P.; Bakker, C.E.; Verbeet, M.P.; Oostra, B.A.; Reuser, A.J.; et al. Generalized glycogen storage and cardiomegaly in a knockout mouse model of Pompe disease. *Hum. Mol. Genet.* **1998**, *7*, 53–62. [CrossRef] [PubMed]
36. Schultheis, P.J.; Lorenz, J.N.; Meneton, P.; Nieman, M.L.; Riddle, T.M.; Flagella, M.; Duffy, J.J.; Doetschman, T.; Miller, M.L.; Shull, G.E. Phenotype resembling Gitelman's syndrome in mice lacking the apical Na+-Cl- cotransporter of the distal convoluted tubule. *J. Biol. Chem.* **1998**, *273*, 29150–29155. [CrossRef]

37. Elmonem, M.A.; Khalil, R.; Khodaparast, L.; Khodaparast, L.; Arcolino, F.O.; Morgan, J.; Pastore, A.; Tylzanowski, P.; Ny, A.; Lowe, M.; et al. Cystinosis (ctns) zebrafish mutant shows pronephric glomerular and tubular dysfunction. *Sci. Rep.* **2017**, *7*, 42583. [CrossRef]
38. Berlingerio, S.P.; He, J.; De Groef, L.; Taeter, H.; Norton, T.; Baatsen, P.; Cairoli, S.; Goffredo, B.; de Witte, P.; van den Heuvel, L.; et al. Renal and Extra Renal Manifestations in Adult Zebrafish Model of Cystinosis. *Int. J. Mol. Sci.* **2021**, *22*, 9398. [CrossRef]
39. Dube, E.; Dufresne, J.; Chan, P.T.; Hermo, L.; Cyr, D.G. Assessing the role of claudins in maintaining the integrity of epididymal tight junctions using novel human epididymal cell lines. *Biol. Reprod.* **2010**, *82*, 1119–1128. [CrossRef]
40. Mandl, A.M. The Effect of Cysteamine on the Survival of Spermatogonia after X-irradiation. *Int. J. Radiat. Biol. Relat. Stud. Phys. Chem. Med.* **1959**, *1*, 131–142. [CrossRef]
41. Starkie, C.M. The effect of cysteamine on the survival of foetal germ cells after irradiation. *Int. J. Radiat. Biol. Relat. Stud. Phys. Chem. Med.* **1961**, *3*, 609–617. [CrossRef]
42. Sariozkan, S.; Tuncer, P.B.; Buyukleblebici, S.; Bucak, M.N.; Canturk, F.; Eken, A. Antioxidative effects of cysteamine, hyaluronan and fetuin on post-thaw semen quality, DNA integrity and oxidative stress parameters in the Brown Swiss bull. *Andrologia* **2015**, *47*, 138–147. [CrossRef]
43. Bucak, M.N.; Atessahin, A.; Varisli, O.; Yuce, A.; Tekin, N.; Akcay, A. The influence of trehalose, taurine, cysteamine and hyaluronan on ram semen Microscopic and oxidative stress parameters after freeze-thawing process. *Theriogenology* **2007**, *67*, 1060–1067. [CrossRef] [PubMed]
44. Bucak, M.N.; Tuncer, P.B.; Sariozkan, S.; Ulutas, P.A.; Coyan, K.; Baspinar, N.; Ozkalp, B. Effects of hypotaurine, cysteamine and aminoacids solution on post-thaw microscopic and oxidative stress parameters of Angora goat semen. *Res. Vet. Sci.* **2009**, *87*, 468–472. [CrossRef] [PubMed]
45. Tuncer, P.B.; Buyukleblebici, S.; Eken, A.; Tasdemir, U.; Durmaz, E.; Buyukleblebici, O.; Coskun, E. Comparison of cryoprotective effects of lycopene and cysteamine in different cryoprotectants on bull semen and fertility results. *Reprod. Domest. Anim.* **2014**, *49*, 746–752. [CrossRef] [PubMed]
46. Swami, D.S.; Kumar, P.; Malik, R.K.; Saini, M.; Kumar, D.; Jan, M.H. Cysteamine supplementation revealed detrimental effect on cryosurvival of buffalo sperm based on computer-assisted semen analysis and oxidative parameters. *Anim. Reprod. Sci.* **2017**, *177*, 56–64. [CrossRef] [PubMed]
47. Anderson, R.A.; Feathergill, K.; Kirkpatrick, R.; Zaneveld, L.J.D.; Coleman, K.T.; Spear, P.G.; Cooper, M.D.; Waller, D.P.; Thoene, J.G. Characterization of cysteamine as a potential contraceptive anti-HIV agent. *J. Androl.* **1998**, *19*, 37–49. [PubMed]
48. Wang, Y.; Zhao, Y.; Yu, S.; Feng, Y.; Zhang, H.; Kou, X.; Chu, M.; Cui, L.; Li, L.; Zhang, P.; et al. Regulation of steroid hormones and energy status with cysteamine and its effect on spermatogenesis. *Toxicol. Appl. Pharmacol.* **2016**, *313*, 149–158. [CrossRef] [PubMed]
49. Assadi, F.K.; Mullin, J.J.; Beckman, D.A. Evaluation of the reproductive and developmental safety of cysteamine in the rat: Effects on female reproduction and early embryonic development. *Teratology* **1998**, *58*, 88–95. [CrossRef]

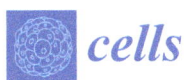

Review

In Vitro and In Vivo Models to Study Nephropathic Cystinosis

Pang Yuk Cheung [1], Patrick T. Harrison [2], Alan J. Davidson [1] and Jennifer A. Hollywood [1,*]

1. Department of Molecular Medicine and Pathology, The University of Auckland, Auckland 1142, New Zealand; pang.cheung@auckland.ac.nz (P.Y.C.); a.davidson@auckland.ac.nz (A.J.D.)
2. Department of Physiology, BioSciences Institute, University College Cork, T12 XF62 Cork, Ireland; p.harrison@ucc.ie
* Correspondence: j.hollywood@auckland.ac.nz

Abstract: The development over the past 50 years of a variety of cell lines and animal models has provided valuable tools to understand the pathophysiology of nephropathic cystinosis. Primary cultures from patient biopsies have been instrumental in determining the primary cause of cystine accumulation in the lysosomes. Immortalised cell lines have been established using different gene constructs and have revealed a wealth of knowledge concerning the molecular mechanisms that underlie cystinosis. More recently, the generation of induced pluripotent stem cells, kidney organoids and tubuloids have helped bridge the gap between in vitro and in vivo model systems. The development of genetically modified mice and rats have made it possible to explore the cystinotic phenotype in an in vivo setting. All of these models have helped shape our understanding of cystinosis and have led to the conclusion that cystine accumulation is not the only pathology that needs targeting in this multisystemic disease. This review provides an overview of the in vitro and in vivo models available to study cystinosis, how well they recapitulate the disease phenotype, and their limitations.

Keywords: cystinosis; lysosomal storage disease; cell and animal models

Citation: Cheung, P.Y.; Harrison, P.T.; Davidson, A.J.; Hollywood, J.A. In Vitro and In Vivo Models to Study Nephropathic Cystinosis. *Cells* **2022**, *11*, 6. https://doi.org/10.3390/cells11010006

Academic Editor: Elena N. Levtchenko

Received: 6 November 2021
Accepted: 19 December 2021
Published: 21 December 2021

Publisher's Note: MDPI stays neutral with regard to jurisdictional claims in published maps and institutional affiliations.

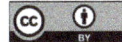

Copyright: © 2021 by the authors. Licensee MDPI, Basel, Switzerland. This article is an open access article distributed under the terms and conditions of the Creative Commons Attribution (CC BY) license (https://creativecommons.org/licenses/by/4.0/).

1. Introduction

Infantile nephropathic cystinosis is a rare, hereditary, autosomal recessive, lysosomal storage disease affecting 1 in 100,000–200,000 live births [1]. It is caused by mutations in the gene *CTNS* which encodes for cystinosin, a cystine-proton cotransporter found on the lysosomal membrane [2,3]. Worldwide, the most common mutation is a homozygous 57 kb deletion that eliminates the first nine exons and part of exon 10 of the gene and part/all of neighbouring genes *TRPV1* and *CARKL*, respectively [4]. Cystinotic patients are usually asymptomatic at birth and develop normally until the first 6 months of life, when they present with failure to thrive, excessive thirst and urination, dehydration, and sometimes rickets. These symptoms result from Fanconi syndrome, which is the excessive urinary loss of electrolytes such as glucose, phosphate, amino acids, bicarbonate, and low molecular weight proteins, as a consequence of renal proximal tubule dysfunction [5,6]. Schneider et al. (1967), were the first to show that cystinosis is characterised by the accumulation of cystine within lysosomes [7], and today the disease is recognised as the most common cause of inherited renal Fanconi syndrome [8]. The Fanconi syndrome in cystinosis is accompanied by the presence of "swan-neck" lesions in the kidney cortex, which are caused by atrophy of the epithelial cells of the proximal tubule. Cystinotic children later develop glomerular dysfunction with progressive glomerular podocyte injury, as well as multinucleated podocytes. If untreated, cystinosis progresses to end-stage kidney disease (ESKD) by the end of the first decade of life [9,10]. Other non-renal symptoms include photophobia due to cystine crystal deposition in the cornea, hypothyroidism, bone deformities, stunted growth, cognitive impairment, muscle wasting and, in males, infertility due to hypogonadism [5,11,12]. In addition to infantile nephropathic cystinosis, which is the most frequent form of the disease, there are two milder forms: late-onset juvenile nephropathic cystinosis and ocular cystinosis. The former patients are usually diagnosed at an older age and develop photophobia, mild proximal tubule dysfunction, and ESKD at a slower rate compared to infantile nephropathic cystinosis [6]. In the latter, patients display ocular symptoms with no renal phenotype and are generally diagnosed in adulthood [13]. In this review, we will focus on infantile nephropathic cystinosis.

Currently, the only treatment available for cystinosis is cysteamine, an aminothiol that depletes lysosomal cystine by entering the lysosome and generating cysteine and a cysteine-cysteamine mixed disulfide [14]. The cysteine-cysteamine mixed disulfide exits the lysosome by the cationic amino acid transporter, PQLC2, while free cysteine has been found to be freely removed, most likely via a cysteine-specific lysosomal transport system, thus by-passing the need for cystinosin [5,15,16]. Long-term use and compliance of cysteamine has been shown to improve the prognosis of cystinosis with early and continuous treatment delaying progression to ESKD by six to ten years [1,17,18] and improving glomerular function, quality of life and decreasing the incidence of nonrenal complications [18–22]. However, while cysteamine therapy has substantially improved patient outcomes, it does not reverse the Fanconi syndrome, and most patients eventually require a kidney transplant. The suboptimal benefit of cysteamine has been attributed to its low compliance due to severe side-effects such as unpleasant body odour, gastrointestinal problems such as nausea and vomiting, and requirement for large (1.95 g/m^2/day) and frequent dosing (every 6 h) [23]. A slow-release form of cysteamine was approved by the FDA in 2013 that requires dosing every 12 h, thus improving the quality of life of patients. However, the impact of the delayed released form of the drug on the disease is similar to cysteamine and does not prevent Fanconi syndrome [24,25]. It is clear that cysteamine cannot reverse the renal manifestations, suggesting that cystinosin may have alternative cellular functions beyond its role as a cystine transporter. Indeed, it has been shown that some of the cellular defects observed in cytsinotic cells, such as autophagy and endocytosis, are not rescued with cysteamine treatment [26–29]. The development of better therapies that also target these alternative pathways necessitates in vitro and in vivo models that closely mimic the human disease. Over the years, several models have been developed, including in vitro systems that use cells from individuals with cystinosis, as well as genetically modified animal models (Figure 1). In this review, we examine the current models available for the study of cystinosis and evaluate how well they recapitulate the human disease. Furthermore, we explore how these models are helping researchers gain a better understanding of the disease and develop improved therapies.

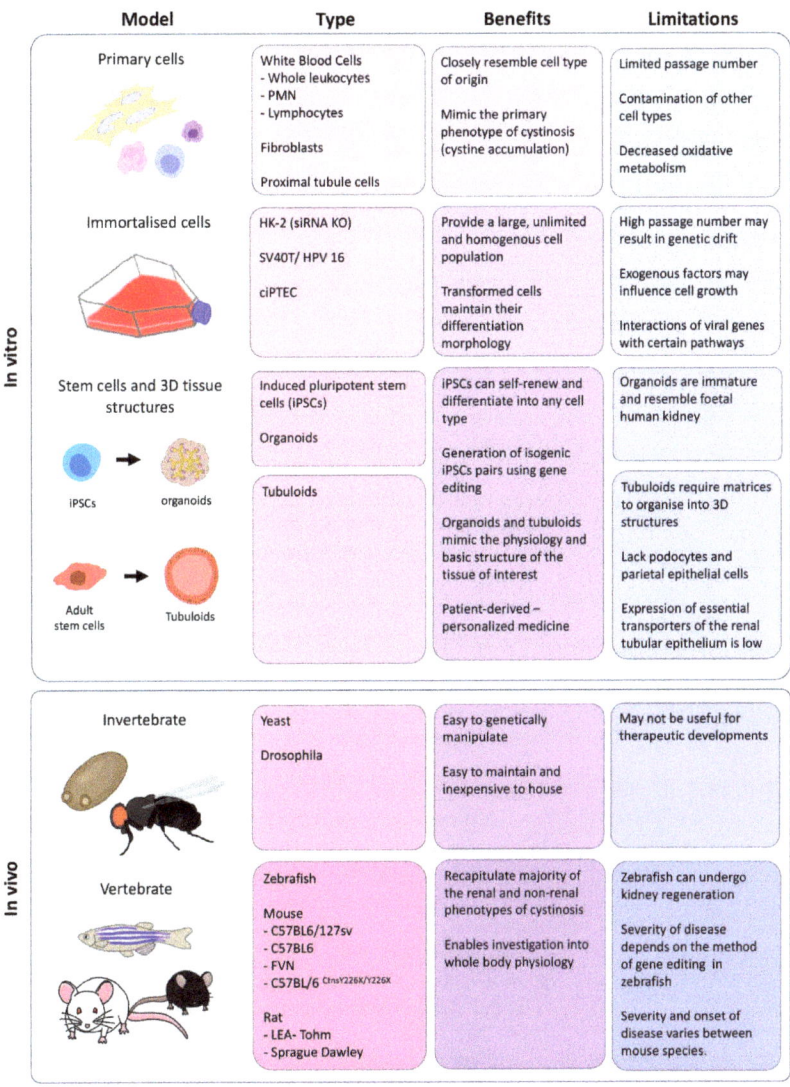

Figure 1. Schematic overview summarising the different in vitro and in vivo cystinotic models. PMN = polymorphonuclear; HK-2 = human kidney-2; SV40T = simian virus 40 large T antigen; HPV 16= human papillomavirus type 16; ciPTEC = conditionally immortalised proximal tubule epithelial.

2. In Vitro Models

2.1. Primary Human Cells

The pioneering studies of the 1960s and 1970s were performed on human cystinotic white blood cells, fibroblasts, or lymph nodes, as these were easily attainable. This early work was pivotal in discovering the basic underlying cause of cystinosis. Whole leukocytes, polymorphonuclear (PMN) leukocytes or lymphocytes obtained from cystinotic patients as well as fibroblasts from skin biopsies showed that cystine levels in these cells were 80–100 times greater than in control subjects [7,30]. In 1968, examination of lymph nodes from cystinotic patients using electron microscopy revealed that cystine accumulation occurred in lysosomes, as seen by the presence of cystine crystals [31]. An early model of cystinosis was the use of cystine dimethylester (CDME) to artificially load lysosomes with cystine, thereby mimicking the primary phenotype of this disease [32]. Using this method, studies on lysosomes from isolated leukocytes demonstrated that cystinosis arises, at least in part, from an absence of cystine exodus from the lysosome as a result of defective transport [33–36]. However, CDME loading is now largely discredited as a method to model cystinosis as it does not take into account the lack of a functional cystinosin transporter, it exerts direct toxicity on cells, inhibits mitochondrial ATP production and does not accurately mimic the pathophysiology of cystinosis in vivo [37,38].

Further studies conducted in primary fibroblasts showed that the source of the cystine is from the degradation of cystine-rich proteins and not from oxidised cysteine [39]. However, a recent study by Adelmann et al. (2020) showed that, in fact, a substantial amount of cystine derives from oxidised cytosolic cysteine imported into the lysosomes via the MFSD12 transporter [40]. Interestingly, they found that knockdown of MFSD12 resulted in reduced cystine accumulation in cystinotic fibroblasts. Further investigations are needed to determine if this is a potential therapeutic target for future treatments. The use of polymorphonuclear leukocytes and fibroblasts were critical in the testing of possible treatments for cystinosis. Early studies with reducing agents such as ascorbic acid and dithiothreitol showed that these were ineffective at removing excess lysosomal cystine from fibroblasts and were toxic to the cells [41]. In 1976, Thoene et al. showed that cystine accumulation in fibroblasts and PMN leukocytes could be dramatically decreased when cells were treated with the aminothiol, cysteamine [14,42]. The efficacy of cysteamine is still assessed and monitored in patients today by measuring cystine levels in PMN leukocytes. Primary fibroblasts have also been used to study other mechanisms that may contribute to the pathogenesis of cystinosis, such as mitochondrial dysfunction, glutathione (GSH) production and apoptosis [43–45]. Despite cystine accumulation, cystine crystals are not present in primary fibroblasts or leukocytes derived from patients. This could be explained by the fact that these cells are relatively fast growing and short-lived; therefore, there is insufficient time for crystal formation.

Cystinosis is a multisystemic disease with accumulation of cystine in lysosomes throughout the body. However, the kidney is the first organ affected and, therefore, renal cell models have been widely utilised. Renal biopsies and cadavers are good sources of renal cells; however, methods to obtain these cells are invasive or not widely available, respectively [46,47]. Alternatively, methods have been developed to harvest exfoliated proximal tubule cells (PTCs) from urine. Cystinotic PTCs, cultured from urine samples, show a ~100-fold increase in cystine levels compared to control PTCs collected from healthy donors [48,49]. These primary cystinotic PTCs were also found to display a decrease in total GSH levels when compared to control PTCs, whereas this difference was not seen in primary fibroblasts [43,45,50]. The reason for this discrepancy is unknown but may be caused by metabolic differences between each cell type [51].

Investigations by Sansanwal et al. using cystinotic proximal tubule cells and kidney biopsies found high levels of the autophagosome marker LC3-II, and the autophagic substrate p62, compared to healthy controls or cells from patients with non-cystinotic renal defects [52,53]. The colocalisation of LC3-II and p62 in cystinotic cells suggested that there is a block in the autophagy pathway, involved in the recycling of intracellular constituents, a finding that has since been confirmed by other groups [26,29].

Overall, the use of primary cells derived from individuals with cystinosis have been a valuable tool. However, primary cells when grown in vitro can be influenced by external factors. They are slow growing and can only be passaged a limited number of times before losing their epithelial phenotype and undergoing senescence [54]. Regarding primary PTCs, there is the potential for contamination by other cell types such as distal tubule cells and fibroblasts, which might complicate the interpretation of findings. Renal cells in culture have also been shown to decrease oxidative metabolism and rely on glycolytic activity, and this may make any extrapolations to the in vivo setting difficult [55]. Finally, there may be variability between samples due to differences in the patient background, such as age, genetics, and environmental factors.

2.2. Immortalised Cell Lines

Immortalised cell lines offer many advantages over primary cells as they are homogeneous and easy to maintain indefinitely, thus overcoming the limitations of cellular senescence seen with primary cells. A number of immortalised PTCs have been established, most notably by transfecting cells with human papillomavirus type 16 (HPV 16) E6/E7 and simian virus 40 large T antigen (SV40T) genes. Both HPV 16 E6/E7 and SV40T achieve immortalisation by deregulating cell cycle checkpoints and preventing growth arrest [56,57].

The human kidney-2 (HK-2) cell line, generated by immortalising healthy human PTCs with HPV 16 E6/E7, has been used in numerous studies including cystinosis [58–61]. HK-2 cells were employed to explore the notion that Cystinosin may have additional functions outside of the lysosome. HK-2 cells were transfected with a construct encoding green fluorescence protein (GFP) fused to the CTNS-LKG isoform, revealing that this variant of Cystinosin was localised to the plasma membrane [62]. Zhang et al. (2019), used gene editing to disrupt *CTNS* in HK-2 cells and found that these cells accumulate cystine and have impaired chaperone-mediated autophagy (CMA) [63], in agreement with similar observations made in cystinotic mouse fibroblasts [26]. In addition, Zhang et al. (2019), showed that *CTNS* knockout HK-2 cells display decreased expression of *LRP2* and *LC3-II* along with defective LAMP2A and Rab11 trafficking and expression, consistent with disruptions in the endolysosomal compartment [63]. These defects could not be rescued by cysteamine treatment but instead by upregulating CMA using small-molecule activators [63]. These observations provided further evidence that defects in autophagy and endolysosomal trafficking play an important role in the cystinotic phenotype.

Urine-derived cystinotic PTCs that were immortalised with HPV 16 E6/E7, were found to have elevated oxidised glutathione, while total GSH, free cysteine and ATP were all normal, leading to the suggestion that increased oxidative stress may contribute to tubular dysfunction in cystinosis [64]. In later studies, Ivanova et al. (2015) showed that cystinotic PTCs exhibit disorganisation of the endolysosomal compartment, with defective LRP2-dependant endocytosis of proteins and delayed processing of ligands. These latter two cellular phenotypes can be partially restored following treatment with cysteamine [59].

With regards to cystine levels, immortalised cystinotic PTCs load cystine (~0.9 nmol/mg protein) within the range seen in SV40T-immortalised cystinotic fibroblasts (~1.75 nmol/mg protein) and transformed cystinotic lymphoblasts (~0.23 nmol/mg protein) [35,64,65]. However, these levels are lower than those reported in primary cystinotic fibroblasts (2.0 to 6.1 nmol/mg protein), primary cystinotic PTCs (3.48 to 13.8 nmol/mg protein) and in situ kidney (16.7 to 101.7 nmol/mg protein; [1,4,45,48,49,66]. One reason for this variability could be due to the high proliferation rate of immortalised cells, which may limit the amount of cystine that can accumulate within the lysosome [5]. Another cause may be the method used to measure cystine. Earlier studies used protein binding assays and radiolabeling which requires radioactivity, limiting its use, while in later years there has been a shift to more accessible high-performance liquid-based chromatography.

To limit the proliferation rate, a temperature sensitive SV40T variant (SV40tsA58U19) was used to generate conditionally immortalised cystinotic proximal tubule epithelial cells (ciPTECs). This SV40T variant permits cells to proliferate only at lower temperatures of 33 °C. At 37 °C, the large T antigen becomes inactive, and proliferation is halted, allowing cells to mature and differentiate [67]. The use of a temperature sensitive SV40T variant was later combined with transfection of human telomerase (hTERT), which prevents the cells from undergoing replicative senescence [68]. The cystine levels of these cystinotic ciPTECs are 37-fold higher than healthy ciPTECs (~5 vs. 0.14 nmol/mg protein, respectively) and 6-fold higher than PTCs immortalised with HPV16 E6/E7 [64]. Rega et al. (2016), used ciPTECs to investigate the role of transcription factor EB (TFEB), a master regulator of lysosomal biogenesis and autophagy genes [27]. By knocking down *CTNS* with short interfering RNAs they found that cystinotic ciPTECs displayed reduced *TFEB* expression and delayed endocytic cargo processing, and these defects could not be restored with cysteamine. However, inducing TFEB activity reduced cystine accumulation and stimulated cargo processing, further supporting the notion that Cystinosin plays roles beyond cystine transport [27].

Despite their ease of use and availability, caution must be taken when interpreting results with immortalised cell lines. The 2-D environment is not equivalent to the in vivo setting, and this can greatly affect cell behaviour and gene expression [69]. Furthermore, immortalisation can have a profound effect on cell biology. For example, HPV oncoproteins interfere with autophagy, potentially as a way to promote viral replication [70]. In the case of HPV16 oncoproteins, these have been found to activate mTOR complex 1 (mTORC1), a negative regulator of autophagy, and impair autophagosome-lysosome fusion [71]. As cystinosis has been found to impair autophagy, care must be taken with cells immortalized with HPV to avoid confounding effects on the autophagy pathway.

2.3. Modelling Cystinosis by siRNA Knockdown

Several groups have used siRNA to transiently knock down *CTNS* in human and animal cells. The first reported study achieved a 50% decrease in Cystinosin protein in HK-2 cells, resulting in increased levels of cysteine and cystine, as well as decreases in both GSH and the oxidised form (GSSG), and a mild increase in the redox state of the Cys/CySS-couple [72]. In a subsequent study looking at aspects of mitochondrial dysfunction, Bellomo et al. (2018) found similar results when comparing *CTNS*-null ciPTECs (homozygous for the 57-kb deletion) and HK-2 cells transiently transfected with siRNA [60]. Their findings included the observation that both cells showed altered mitochondrial function. Specifically, they found that *CTNS*-deficient cells display significantly lower levels of mitochondrial cAMP and a reduction in complex I and V activities and mitochondrial membrane potential [60]. These observations are in keeping with the finding that cystinotic human kidneys show abnormal mitochondrial morphology and increased mitophagy [52]. These defects may be related to the interorganelle communication that occurs between mitochondria and the endolysosomal compartment and the quality control role of lysosomes in degrading defective mitochondria [73]. In support of this, Bellomo et al. found that cysteamine could restore most of the mitochondrial functions [60].

Using rabbit renal proximal tubules, Taub and colleagues (2011) used siRNA-mediated knockdown to investigate the effect of Cystinosin deficiency on epithelial transport, with the goal of understanding the cause of the Fanconi syndrome [74]. They found that knocking down *CTNS* resulted in a 50% decrease in ATP levels, consistent with cystinotic cells having compromised mitochondrial function. They investigated the activity of the basolateral Na^+/K^+-ATPase, a major consumer of ATP in PTCs and a prerequisite for driving Na^+-dependent cotransport at the apical membrane but detected no decrease in activity. Instead, they found a major reduction in the surface localization of the phosphate transport (Slc34A1 aka NaPi2a), accounting for the reduced renal phosphate uptake in cystinosis. However, this defect was not generalizable to all PTC apical proteins, as dipeptidyl peptidase IV was unaffected [74].

In a follow-up study [75], Taub et al. (2012) used the same siRNA knockdown approach to investigate a link between ATP levels and apoptosis in cystinotic cells. They found that AMP-activated protein kinase (AMPK), a sensor of cellular energy change that acts to increase ATP, was activated in *CTNS*-knockdown cells, in keeping with the ATP deficit. Their cystinosin-deficient cells showed an increased sensitivity to apoptosis in response to the nephrotoxin cisplatin, and this could be abrogated by inhibiting AMPK. As AMPK activation has been implicated as an inducer of apoptosis, for instance via phosphorylation of the tumor suppressor p53 [76] they concluded that the ATP deficit seen in *CTNS*-knockdown cells may sensitize these cells to toxicant-induced cell death.

Using siRNA-mediated knockdown of Cystinosin in HK-2, Sumayao et al. (2013) found a similar decrease in ATP levels [38]. They also identified an increase in intracellular O_2^- and NO production, although there was no increase in the overall oxidative stress of the cells in response to H_2O_2 challenge. Unlike in other studies, they did not detect a perturbation in autophagy, which led to the suggestion that cystine accumulation may not be obligatory for perturbing autophagy. Alternatively, the discrepancy in their findings may be due to their partial knockdown of Cystinosin (40% reduction in protein) and a corresponding low level of cystine accumulation (only 3-fold higher than control cells), which may be insufficient to illicit a complete cystinotic phenotype.

McEvoy et al. (2015) used siRNA to knock down Cystinosin in a rat pancreatic β-cell line and reported a reduction in ATP production, an increase in oxidative stress and an attenuation of nutrient-stimulated insulin secretion [77]. Although the effect of cysteamine treatment on these cells was not examined, it has been reported that early cysteamine therapy can reduce the incidence of diabetes in individuals with cystinosis and delay the age of onset [18,19].

2.4. Induced Pluripotent Stem Cells and Kidney Organoids

Induced pluripotent stem cells (iPSCs) are a valuable tool in disease modelling and have been essential in advancing our understanding of the pathophysiology of other lysosomal storage diseases [78]. Reprogramming of somatic cells such as fibroblasts, with ectopic expression of pluripotent genes, *Sox2*, *Oct4*, *Klf4* and *c-Myke*, was first described in 2006 [79]. iPSCs have the ability to self-renew and, under proper conditions, can differentiate into any cell type of the body and produce self-organised three-dimensional tissue structures called organoids. [79–81]. Kidney organoids resemble mini organs, mimicking the physiology and the basic structures of the tissue of interest such as the nephron, thus bridging the gap between traditional monolayer cell cultures and in vivo animal models for disease modelling [82]. Using gene-editing technologies such as CRISPR-Cas 9, it is possible to generate isogenic pairs of disease-specific and control iPSC lines and organoids, thus allowing a comparison between identical genetic and epigenetic backgrounds with the only difference being the introduced mutation [83]. This is important, as there can be large variations between iPSC lines, even when they are derived from the same donor cell population.

Hollywood et al., (2020), knocked out *CTNS* (*CTNS*-KO) in human iPSCs using CRISPR-Cas9 with these cells showing ~50-fold higher levels of cystine compared to the isogenic control (~2.5 vs. 0.05 nmol/mg protein) [29]. In addition, this group also generated patient-derived cystinotic iPSCs (*CTNS*$^{-/-}$) by reprogramming stromal cells originating from a cystinotic kidney. Kidney organoids made from these cystinotic iPSC lines showed differential loading of cystine (~9 vs 2.5 nmol/mg protein for cystinotic vs. control, respectively), enlarged lysosomes, increased apoptosis and increased numbers of autophagosomes indicative of a basal autophagy defect, compared to the controls [29]. Unlike prior cell culture studies, no differences were detected in GSH, ATP or mitochondria morphology. This discrepancy may be due to iPSC metabolism, which relies on glycolysis rather than oxidative phosphorylation for their energy needs [84]. Cysteamine treatment was able to mitigate the cystine and enlarged lysosome phenotypes but failed to correct the apoptosis and basal autophagy defects. While the latter observation may indicate a non-cystine related function of Cystinosin for autophagy, we have found that cysteamine suppresses basal autophagy in iPSCs (unpublished observations). Therefore, more experiments are needed to resolve this issue. Regardless, these data raise important considerations for treating cystinosis with cysteamine, as autophagy is critically important in proximal tubule cells, where it protects them from injury and apoptosis [85]. Hollywood et al., went on to show that treating cystinotic iPSCs and kidney organoids with cysteamine in combination with an mTOR inhibitor, everolimus, which activates autophagy, successfully rescued all of the cystinotic phenotypes. This work paves the way to developing a combination therapy for cystinosis that may be therapeutically superior to cysteamine alone.

While kidney organoids are a promising tool for modelling cystinosis and preclinical drug development, there are some limitations of the system. Most protocols generate kidney organoids that are similar in maturation to second trimester human fetal kidneys. In addition, off-target cell types such as neural, glial and muscle progenitor cells can arise in various proportions and are subject to significant batch-to-batch variation [86]. Extended time in culture does not significantly improve maturation but instead, in some cases, causes undesirable changes such as reduced expression of nephron markers and fibrosis [86–88]. Transplantation of kidney organoids into mice leads to improved maturation and vascularisation by the host, but this is technically challenging and limited by the overgrowth of off-target cell types [89,90]. As a result of these drawbacks, cystinotic kidney organoids do not model the tubular degeneration seen in cystinosis including the formation of swan-neck lesions, and further optimisation of organoid protocols are needed [29].

2.5. Tubuloids

Tubuloids were first described by Schutgens and colleagues (2019) and represent 3-D clusters of cells derived from primary renal epithelial cells originating from kidney tissue or urine samples. They are of lower complexity than organoids derived from iPSCs and appear as cystic, highly polarised epithelial structures [91]. Nevertheless, tubuloids contain differentiated, functional epithelial cells that express markers of the proximal tubule, loop of Henle, distal tubule and collecting duct, but not podocytes [91,92]. Jamalpoor et al. (2021) generated cystinotic tubuloids and identified high levels of alpha-ketoglutarate (αKG) as a contributing cause of the autophagy and proximal tubule defects [93]. They went on to show that bicalutamide, an antiandrogen medication that is primarily used to treat prostate cancer, significantly reduces αKG levels in cystinotic tubuloids. When bicalutamide was combined with cysteamine, it caused a two-fold more potent reduction in the level of cystine than cysteamine alone. This study demonstrated the power of the tubuloid system to model cystinosis, and as a new platform to undertake preclinical drug testing and develop new therapies for cystinosis [93].

Similar to iPSC-derived kidney organoids, there are some limitations to working with tubuloids. Glomerular cells are lacking and cannot be examined, some transporters are expressed at low levels, suggestive of dedifferentiation or loss of function, and there is a need to culture the cells within an extracellular matrix for their assembly, which adds an additional level of technical complexity compared to kidney organoids [91,92].

3. In Vivo Models

Unlike in vitro systems, animal models of cystinosis are able to recapitulate many aspects of the human disease with far greater complexity and in the physiological setting of a whole organism. As cystinosis affects multiple organs and progresses in severity over time, in vivo models are critical for gaining greater insights into the pathophysiology of the disease and for testing the efficacy and side-effects of new therapies. The most widely used in vivo models of cystinosis to date have been mice, rats and zebrafish (see Table 1 for a comparison).

Table 1. Comparison of cystinotic in vivo models PTC = proximal tubule cells, dpf = days post fertilisation, N.I = not investigated.

Species	Strain	Mutation in Ctns	Phenotypes									Reference
			Cystine Accumulation	Cystine Crystal	Renal Failure	Glomerulus Changes	PTC Lesions	PTC Dysfunction	Ocular Abnormalities	Bone Deformities	
Mouse	C57Bl6	IRES-βgal-neo cassette to remove the last 4 exon of Ctns	Yes	Yes	Yes (mild, onset at 10 months of age)	No	Yes (onset at 6 months of age)	Yes (partial, onset at 2 months of age)	Yes	Yes	[94–96]
	FVN	IRES-βgal-neo cassette to remove the last 4 exon of Ctns	Yes	Yes (but mild)	No	No	No	No	N.I	N.I	[95]
Zebrafish	larvae	homozygous nonsense mutation in exon 8	Yes	No	Yes (decreased inulin clearance)	Yes (podocyte foot effacement)	No	Yes (loss of megalin expression in PTCs)	N.I	N.I	[97]
	Adult	homozygous nonsense mutation in exon 8	Yes	Yes	N.I	Partial	Partial	Suggested	Yes	N.I	[97,98]
	larvae	TALEN-drive 8 bp deletion in exon 3	Yes	N.I	N.I	N.I	No	No	N.I	N.I	[99]
Rat	F344	13-bp deletion in exon 7	Yes	Yes (only in kidney cortex)	N.I	N.I	Yes	N.I (glucosuria was detected)	N.I	N.I	[100]
	Sprague Dawley	Indel mutations exon 3	Yes	Yes	Yes	Yes	Yes	Yes	Yes	Yes	[101]

3.1. Yeast

The first in vivo model of loss of Cystinosin function was the *Saccharomyces cerevisiae* strain *ers1D*. However, the relevance of this to cystinosis was not appreciated until the human *CTNS* gene was identified as a potential homologue. Full length *CTNS*, but not two cystinosis-causing variants (G308R and L338P), was found to complement the yeast mutant's sensitivity to the antibiotic hygromycin B [102–104]. A variant of *CTNS* that lacks the first 121 amino acids, which are located in the lysosomal lumen, was also able to complement *ERS1* deficiency, demonstrating the importance of the 7-transmembrane region for function. However, the yeast mutant does not abnormally load intracellular cystine and shows no differences in growth and survival compared to wild-type cells, although it is sensitive to oxidative stress [105]. Not unexpectedly then, cysteamine does not chemically complement the defect [104]. Thus, there are some limitations in using the yeast mutant in terms of studying cystinosis. Nevertheless, yeast is genetically tractable, and the complementation assay is well-suited to interrogate Cystinosin variants such as I133F and S298N, which cause severe disease but yet retain 80–100% cystine transport activity, or G197R, which has 20% cystine transport activity but only gives rise to the ocular form of cystinosis [106]. The yeast model has also been used to identify MEH1, a potential regulator of ERS1; therefore, it could be a useful tool to identify new interactors that may play a yet uncharacterised role in cystinosis [104].

3.2. Mouse

3.2.1. C57BL6/129sv-

The first *Ctns* knockout ($Ctns^{-/-}$) mouse model was generated on a mixed C57BL6/129sv background using a "promoter trap" approach that resulted in a truncated nonfunctional protein which failed to localise to the lysosome [94]. $Ctns^{-/-}$ mice display a ~40-fold increase in cystine levels in several organs, including the kidney, with loading increasing with age, compared to wild-type littermates [94]. Mild cystine crystal deposition is observed in interstitial cells of various tissues at 6-months of age including focal crystal deposits within proximal tubule cells. At this stage, behavioural anomalies also become apparent, with reduced motility compared to wild-type littermates. Slit lamp examination of 8-month-old $Ctns^{-/-}$ mice revealed cystine crystals in the cornea and bone abnormalities including decreased bone density and cortical width were observed. Additional bone deformities involving the tibia and femur are seen in the knockouts at 9-months of age [94]. However, despite accumulating high levels of cystine and the formation of cystine crystals in the kidney, no signs of proximal tubulopathy are detected either histologically or biochemically, and renal failure does not manifest in the knockouts up to 18-months of age [94]. The lack of correspondence between the mouse knockout and the progression and severity seen in the human disease was disappointing and suggested that the mixed C57BL6/129sv background may not be optimal for modelling cystinosis due to modifier genes.

3.2.2. C57BL/6 and FVB/N-

By backcrossing the C57BL6/129sv $Ctns^{-/-}$ strain onto the C57BL/6 and FVB/N backgrounds, two new cystinotic mouse models were subsequently developed [95]. Characterisation of these mice confirmed that the genetic background has a profound effect on the cystinotic phenotype [107]. While both C57BL/6 and FVB/N $Ctns^{-/-}$ mouse models display cystine loading in various organs, significant differences in phenotype severity exist between the two lines. For instance, on the C57BL/6 background the *Ctns* mutation results in higher kidney cystine levels compared to the FVB/N background, and manifests with "failure to thrive" and renal dysfunction phenotypes that are not seen with the FVB/N line [95]. Thus, the most severe cystinotic phenotype is observed on a pure C57BL/6 background, with much milder pathologies arising on the mixed (C57BL6/129sv) and FVB/N backgrounds.

The kidney abnormalities in C57BL/6 $Ctns^{-/-}$ mice are first apparent at 2-months of age with polyuria and the onset of Fanconi syndrome (increased excretion of glucose, phosphate, potassium, and low molecular weight proteins). Starting at 6-months of age, the renal cortex shows a loss of expression of proximal tubule apical transporters such as *LRP2*, reduced tight junction integrity, and "swan neck" lesions. By 9-months of age, the histological defects also include tubular atrophy, denuding of the proximal tubule epithelium and thickening of the tubular basement membranes. Renal function, as measured by urine levels of urea and creatinine, declines steadily from 10–18 months of age, consistent with chronic renal disease progressing to kidney failure [95,96,108].

Despite these morphological changes, the C57BL/6 *Ctns*$^{-/-}$ model does not completely recapitulate the human disease. Notably, the Fanconi syndrome does not include a loss of bicarbonate, amino acids and sodium. In addition, C57BL/6 *Ctns*$^{-/-}$ mice do not show podocytes abnormalities, unlike cystinotic patients where glomerular defects include foot process effacement and multinucleated podocytes [10,95,109]. In addition, C57BL/6 *Ctns*$^{-/-}$ mice develop Fanconi syndrome prior to the histological signs of proximal tubule atrophy whereas in human patients, Fanconi syndrome is concomitant with proximal tubule atrophy and the formation of "swan-neck" lesions [9,96]. This difference in timing may reflect a greater resolution of disease progression in mice and could be exploited to better understand the molecular changes governing the transition from dysfunctional transport activity to tubular atrophy. It should also be noted that subsequent publications by different groups using the C57BL/6 *Ctns*$^{-/-}$ mice have reported varying degrees of Fanconi syndrome, from mild/incomplete to nonexistent [110]. This variation may be due to inbreeding at different facilities.

Despite these differences, this mouse model has been instrumental in expanding our understanding of the pathogenesis of cystinosis [26,96,108,111]. Gaide Chevronnay et al. (2014) showed that cystine loading resulted in early loss of the SLC5A2 (SGLT-2) and SLC34A3 (NaPi-11a) transporters, the brush border receptors LRP2 and Cubilin, and the LT-lectin, suggestive of proximal tubule apical dedifferentiation [96]. As this dedifferentiation occurred before overt histological lesions in the proximal tubule, it suggests that apical dedifferentiation, rather than cellular atrophy, causes the Fanconi syndrome.

Galaretta et al. (2015) used C57BL/6 *Ctns*$^{-/-}$ mice to study the formation of the "swan neck" lesion and suggested it was an adaptive response to oxidative stress [112]. Subsequent in vitro studies using mouse primary proximal tubule cells from C57BL/6 *Ctns*$^{-/-}$ animals provided further evidence to indicate that the source of the oxidative stress are defective mitochondria that have not been removed due to lysosome dysfunction and the block in autophagy [99]. It was also discovered that increased oxidative stress promotes the phosphorylation of the tight junction protein ZO-1, providing an explanation for the disruption in tight junction integrity. Furthermore, phosphorylation of ZO-1 results in this protein no longer being able to sequester the Y-box transcription factor ZONAB, which moves into the nucleus and promotes proximal tubule cell proliferation and dedifferentiation [99]. These observations help establish a model of cystinotic kidney damage in which (1) cystine accumulation causes lysosomal and autophagic dysfunction, (2) the failure to clear defective mitochondria results in increased oxidative stress (sensitizing the cell to apoptosis), and (3) compensatory proliferation and dedifferentiation induces Fanconi syndrome, compromised epithelial integrity and tubular atrophy. A key protein facilitating this process in proximal tubule cells is LRP2, the multiligand receptor that is responsible for the endocytosis of filtered proteins including albumin, which is cystine rich due to several disulphide bonds [110]. Deleting *LRP2* in C57BL/6 *Ctns*$^{-/-}$ mice via a conditional Cre/Lox approach prevents cystine accumulation, crystal deposition, apical dedifferentiation in the kidney, and the subsequent formation of "swan neck" lesions [110].

Co-immunoprecipitation studies by Andrzejewska et al. (2016), using *Ctns*$^{-/-}$ mouse proximal tubule cells immortalised using the SV40 T antigen, revealed that Cystinosin interacts with components of the vascuolar H$^+$-ATPase-regulator complex that controls mTORC1 signalling [28]. This raised the possibility that the mTORC pathway, which is critical for cell proliferation and survival may be altered in cystinosis. They also report that the mTORC pathway is downregulated in these cells and was not rescued with cysteamine treatment. Interestingly, an earlier study by Napolitano et al. (2015), using *Ctns*$^{-/-}$ mouse primary fibroblasts showed no mTORC1 downregulation [26]. This discrepancy may be due to the viral antigens used for immortalisation as these can influence mTORC1 levels [113].

The C57BL/6 $Ctns^{-/-}$ mouse model has also been used to gather new insights into non-renal pathologies caused by cystinosis such as bone deformities, thyroid dysfunction, ocular abnormalities and muscle atrophy.

A study by Battafarano et al. (2019) showed that C57BL/6 $Ctns^{-/-}$ mice display intrinsic bone deformities as early as 1-month without any renal tubulopathy [111]. They found that cystinotic animals at this age show a reduction in trabecular bone volume, bone mineral density, and number and thickness, as well as an impairment in osteoblasts and osteoclasts, compared with wild-type animals. Gaide Chevronnay et al. (2016) used C57BL/6 $Ctns^{-/-}$ mice to investigate the early thyroid changes that lead to the hypothyroidism seen in cystinotic children [114]. They found that 9-month-old cystinotic mice recapitulate key features of human cystinosis-associated hypothyroidism, such as chronically increased levels of thyroid stimulating hormone, follicular activation and proliferation, and eventual thyrocyte lysosomal crystals. They also gathered important insights into the underlying mechanisms by linking impaired thyroglobulin production/processing to ER stress and activation of the unfolded protein response [114].

A characterisation of the ocular abnormalities in $Ctns^{-/-}$ mice found that cystine accumulates in a spatiotemporal pattern that closely resembles that of cystinotic patients [115]. The highest levels of cystine were observed in the cornea and iris with corneal crystals observed abundantly from 7-months of age (although mild photophobia was noted from 3-months of age). Only rare retinal crystals were detected (at 19-months of age), coinciding with degeneration of the retinal pigmented epithelium. By contrast, in humans this phenotype can be observed as early as infancy and can precede corneal changes [115,116].

Investigations by Cheung et al. (2016) found that the lower total body mass observed in $Ctns^{-/-}$ mice when compared to wild-type littermates was due to increased muscle wasting and energy expenditure. They observed a decrease in muscle mass as well as muscle fibre size along with muscle weakness as indicated by the reduced grip strength and rotarod activity in 12-month-old $Ctns^{-/-}$ mice. The authors also observed profound adipose tissue browning as well as the upregulation of genes associated with thermogenesis in both muscle and adipose tissues, both of which contribute to an increase in energy expenditure [117]. Furthermore, these mice were $25(OH)D_3$ and $1,25(OH)_2D_3$ insufficient, and treatment with vitamin D attenuated the adipose tissue browning and muscle wasting [118].

Finally, the C57BL/6 $Ctns^{-/-}$ mouse model has been a critical tool to develop and test new gene and cell-based therapies for cystinosis. Hippert et al. (2008) transduced $Ctns^{-/-}$ mice with an adenovirus vector that expresses the wild-type human *CTNS* cDNA and showed that long-term gene transfer (4 weeks) led to a reduction in hepatic cystine levels in young mice (2–3-months old) but not in older mice (>5-months) despite equal transduction efficiencies [119]. As older animals have higher cystine levels and more crystal deposits, they may be either refractory to this kind of therapeutic approach or they may need much longer treatment windows to reduce cystine loads. This study highlighted the importance of early intervention in patients.

Another study showed that transplantation of bone marrow cells from wild-type mice (with normal Cystinosin function) into C57BL/6 $Ctns^{-/-}$ mice leads to a >50% reduction in cystine levels in the kidney, eye, heart, liver, spleen and brain, 2 months post-transplantation [120]. Furthermore, the transplanted mice displayed improved renal function as seen by a decrease in serum creatinine and urea compared to nontreated $Ctns^{-/-}$ mice. Importantly, these benefits were observed for 13 months, indicating that this approach can confer long-term benefits [120,121]. The effectiveness of this cell-based therapy was found to be dependent on the level of wild-type bone marrow engraftment, with improved kidney function only observed in $Ctns^{-/-}$ mice that had >50% donor engraftment [121]. In a follow-up study, hematopoietic stem and progenitor cells from C57BL/6 $Ctns^{-/-}$ mice were genetically modified ex vivo to express functional *Ctns* via a lentiviral vector and then transplanted back into knockout animals. This led to abundant integration of transduced blood cells in a range of tissues and, in the highly engrafted animals, this was associated with a reduction in cystine content and improved kidney function compared to nontreated $Ctns^{-/-}$ mice [122]. It was subsequently shown that macrophages derived from the transduced blood stem and progenitor cells can generate intercellular bridges called tunnelling nanotubes. These structures are able to transfer lysosomes with functional Cystinosin from the donor cells into the Ctns-deficient proximal tubule and thyroid cells, thus explaining the mechanism of rescue [114,123]. As a result of these ground-breaking, proof-of-principle studies, this gene and cell-based therapy approach has begun phase 1/2 clinical testing (NCT03897361) in individuals with cystinosis.

3.2.3. C57BL/6 $Ctns^{Y226X/Y226X}$ Nonsense Mutant Mouse

A nonsense mutation that creates a premature stop codon in exon 7 of *CTNS* (W138X) is commonly found in cystinosis patients in Canada, making this variant a key therapeutic target for this population. To facilitate this, Brasell et al. (2019) used zinc finger nucleases to generate the equivalent mouse model ($Ctns^{Y226X/Y226X}$) on the C57BL/6 background [124]. These animals show a significant reduction in Ctns transcript levels and an eight-fold increase in cystine levels in the kidney compared to controls. Prior to 6-months the mutant mice appeared normal, with proteinuria detected at 9-months of age. The renal phenotype was very mild with only male mice showing occasional atrophy of the cells in the Bowman's capsule. Despite the partial phenotype of these animals, they proved useful to test a novel therapy involving an aminoglycoside (ELX-02) that promotes translational readthrough of the stop codon. $Ctns^{Y226X/Y226X}$ mice treated with ELX-02 were found to have a 30% reduction in kidney cystine levels compared to untreated controls, indicating the therapeutic potential of this approach [124].

3.3. Zebrafish

The zebrafish is a valuable model for modelling human diseases as it is inexpensive to house, undergoes rapid organogenesis and the pronephric kidney of the larval zebrafish has some structural and functional similarities to the mammalian nephron [125]. Two zebrafish *ctns* mutants have been generated, both displaying high levels of cystine at the larval stage compared to wild-type controls and responding to cysteamine added to the swimming water [97,99]. Other characteristics of $ctns^{-/-}$ larvae (seen in either one or both mutant lines) that agree with mammalian models of cystinosis include increased rate of apoptosis in proximal tubule cells, reduced LRP2 (and a corresponding impairment in proximal tubule cell endocytosis), enlarged lysosomes, increased autophagosomes in the proximal tubule cells and partial podocyte foot process effacement. This latter phenotype was associated with a leaky glomerular filtration barrier. Given that podocytopathy is not observed in C57BL/6 $Ctns^{-/-}$ mice, even in advanced age, the zebrafish model may be particularly suited to studying the effect of cystinosis on podocytes [97].

Follow-on analysis of adult $ctns^{-/-}$ zebrafish found that the highest level of cystine accumulation was in the kidney [98]. This result differs from C57BL/6 $Ctns^{-/-}$ mice where greatest cystine loading is seen in the liver and spleen. However, the zebrafish mesonephric kidney is also the site of hematopoiesis, which may explain the species difference [95]. Surprisingly, adult $ctns^{-/-}$ zebrafish do not show podocyte foot process effacement and only a mild enlargement of Bowman's capsule and the glomerular tuft [98]. This difference compared to the larval mutants may be related to differences in glomerular filtration rates, as larval zebrafish have a single glomerulus that may operate under greater stress compared to adult glomeruli. Adult $ctns^{-/-}$ zebrafish displayed some additional phenotypes that were not seen at the larval stage, which included ocular anomalies (increased thickness of the corneal stromal layer), decreased fertility and decreased locomotor activity. Unexpectedly, unlike human individuals with cystinosis and the C57BL/6 $Ctns^{-/-}$ mouse, the zebrafish mutant showed increased body weight and length compared to healthy controls.

One limitation of the zebrafish *ctns* mutant is a lack of "swan neck" lesions and widespread cystine crystal deposition, although cytoplasmic vacuoles with rectangular polymorphous shapes suggestive of cystine crystals are observed in the proximal tubule cells of adult mutants [98]. It is worth noting that zebrafish, unlike mammals, are able to undergo considerable renal regeneration following injury, and grow new nephrons throughout adult life [126]. Thus, it may not be possible for the full extent of the cystinotic renal pathology to be manifested in this model. Another limitation of the zebrafish in terms of preclinical drug development is their aquatic habit, which make it challenging to deliver compounds and perform pharmacokinetic analyses.

3.4. Rat

3.4.1. LEA/Tohm-

The Long-Evans Agouti (LEA/Tohm) rat spontaneous develops renal glucosuria and is used as a model of type 2 diabetes [127]. Using genetic linkage analysis, the causative locus was mapped to a region containing the *Ctns* gene with subsequent sequencing revealing a 13-bp deletion in exon 7 that truncates the protein [100]. The mutation was then bred onto the F344 (F344-$Ctns^{ug1}$) and characterised. At 10 months of age, abnormally high levels of cystine were present in several organs including the kidney (4.5-fold over controls). Histopathological signs of proximal tubular atrophy and cystine crystal deposition were found at one year of age, although the precise location of the crystals is unclear. A major drawback of this model is that the phenotype has not been comprehensively characterised. Renal function, LRP2 levels, apoptosis, oxidative stress, and autophagy have not been evaluated, therefore the degree of renal dysfunction and Fanconi syndrome is unknown. In addition, the onset of the disease and its progression were not reported, making it difficult to compare this model to the human disease.

3.4.2. Sprague Dawley

Hollywood et al., generated a new *Ctns* knockout rat model that closely recapitulates the human disease phenotype. Using CRISPR-Cas9 gene editing, frameshift indel mutations were introduced into exon 3 of the *Ctns* gene in the Sprague Dawley (SD) background, resulting in a truncated and non-functional Cystinosin protein [101]. These $Ctns^{-/-}$ rats show cystine loading and lysosomal crystal formation in various organs from 3-months of age. Fanconi syndrome manifests from 3–6-months of age as indicated by polyuria and polydipsia and increased urinary excretion of total protein, glucose, albumin and calcium. Histologically, $Ctns^{-/-}$ rats display kidney lesions, such as proximal tubule atrophy, basement membrane thickening, and the presence of "swan neck" lesions from 3-months of age, likely coinciding with the onset of Fanconi syndrome. Loss of LRP2 is observed starting in the superficial kidney cortex from 6-months of age, with a progressive decline towards the medulla until LRP2 is only found in the juxtamedullary tubules by 17-months of age [101]. This loss appears to be proceeded by injury, as determined by the upregulation of the proximal tubule injury marker, Harvcr1, in tubules lacking LRP2 [101]. Increased urinary levels of phosphate, as well as the decreased urea and creatinine excretion, are detected from 9-months of age onwards, together with increased levels of plasma creatinine, signifying impaired renal function. At this stage, $Ctns^{-/-}$ rats also show glomerular lesions, such as multinucleated podocytes and podocyte effacement, which are not seen in C57BL/6 $Ctns^{-/-}$ mice but are a feature of the human disease [109]. By 12-months of age, most of the glomerular tufts appear shrunken [10,101]. $Ctns^{-/-}$ rats display other non-renal pathophenotypes, such as failure to thrive, crystal deposition in the cornea and changes in the bone microstructure including cortical bone cross-sectional thickness, trabecular thickness, and cortical tissue mineral density [101]. Unlike the mouse knockout, behavioural defects are not observed in $Ctns^{-/-}$ rats. Overall, the phenotype of this new $Ctns^{-/-}$ rat model closely recapitulates the time course and severity of cystinosis in humans, making it a valuable new tool for the field.

3.5. Drosophila

CRISPR-Cas9 gene editing was used to create a fruit fly mutant in *CG17119*, the *Drosophila melanogaster* ortholog of *CTNS*, as part of a larger effort to understand the mTOR pathway and the growth requirements for different amino acids [128,129]. *Drosophila* Cystinosin localizes to lysosomes, and mutant larvae accumulate intracellular cystine. Under starvation conditions, cells lacking *Ctns* in the fat body (similar to white adipose tissue and the liver in humans) show increased mTORC1 signaling and decreased autophagy [129]. In addition, fasted mutants display a developmental delay and a shortened life span. This phenotype can be rescued by treatment with cysteamine, linking it to cystine accumulation. However, the mutants can also be rescued with rapamycin, which inhibits mTORC1 and activates autophagy. These observations agree well with the study of Hollywood et al. (2020), where the mTORC1 inhibitor Everolimus was used in combination with cysteamine to completely rescue cystinotic iPSCs [29], thus providing further evidence to indicate the importance of abnormal autophagy in the cystinotic phenotype.

4. Conclusions

The development of iPSC, primary and immortalised cell cultures, as well as a wide spectrum of animal models (yeast, *Drosophila*, zebrafish, mouse and rat), have all contributed to our current understanding of the molecular basis of cystinosis. The emerging consensus is that cystine accumulation in lysosomes leads to disruptions in the endocytic, autophagic and mitochondrial compartments, with varying levels of oxidative stress, energy deficit and sensitivity to apoptosis, depending on the tissue. Additional data suggests that cystine accumulation may not be responsible for all of the phenotypes observed in cystinosis. There is still much to be understood about the nontransport functions of Cystinosin, such as its involvement in the mTORC1 pathway, and it is hoped that these non-cystine-related functions will lead to better treatments. It is clear that no one model of cystinosis is perfect and each has its own associated benefits and limitations. The choice of model will depend on the aspect of the disease being studied and how well it is recapitulated relative to the cystinotic phenotype seen in humans. Care needs to be taken with interpreting the findings, as the levels of cystine loading and degree of cellular dysfunction varies between cell types (fibroblasts vs. renal; primary vs. immortalised) and is subject to genetic modifiers (mouse and potentially rat). Ultimately, the use of these models should inform the development of new treatments for cystinosis. Underscoring this need is the fact that despite long-term cystine depleting therapy, the Fanconi syndrome is not prevented or reversed, and kidney function continues to progressively decline in patients with nephropathic cystinosis. The C57BL/6 *Ctns*$^{-/-}$ mouse has been critical in this regard, as it was instrumental for the preclinical testing of the new gene therapy treatment that is in clinical trials. The SD *Ctns*$^{-/-}$ rat, with its phenotype closely mirroring the human disease, and the physiological advantages of rats for pre-clinical testing, should greatly facilitate the development of additional novel treatments for cystinosis.

Author Contributions: Conceptualization, P.Y.C. and J.A.H.; writing—original draft preparation, P.Y.C.; P.T.H.; A.J.D.; J.A.H.; writing—review and editing, P.Y.C.; P.T.H.; A.J.D.; J.A.H. All authors have read and agreed to the published version of the manuscript.

Funding: This work was supported by Cystinosis Ireland, Cystinosis Research Foundation (USA) and The University of Auckland.

Conflicts of Interest: The authors declare no conflict of interest.

References

1. Gahl, W.; Thoene, J.; Schneider, J. Cystinosis. *N. Engl. J. Med.* **2002**, *347*, 111–121. [CrossRef] [PubMed]
2. Town, M.; Jean, G.; Cherqui, S.; Attard, M.; Forestier, L.; Whitmore, S.A.; Callen, D.F.; Gribouval, O.; Broyer, M.; Bates, G.P.; et al. A novel gene encoding an integral membrane protein is mutated in nephropathic cystinosis. *Nat. Genet.* **1998**, *18*, 319–324. [CrossRef]
3. Kalatzis, V.; Cherqui, S.; Antignac, C.; Gasnier, B. Cystinosin, the protein defective in cystinosis, is a H$^+$-driven lysosomal cystine transporter. *EMBO J.* **2001**, *20*, 5940–5949. [CrossRef]

4. Forster, S.; Scarlett, L.; Lloyd, J.B. Mechanism of cystine reaccumulation by cystinotic fibroblasts in vitro. *Biosci. Rep.* **1990**, *10*, 225–229. [CrossRef]
5. Cherqui, S.; Courtoy, P.J. The renal Fanconi syndrome in cystinosis: Pathogenic insights and therapeutic perspectives. *Nat. Rev. Nephrol.* **2017**, *13*, 115–131. [CrossRef]
6. Bäumner, S.; Weber, L.T. Nephropathic cystinosis: Symptoms, treatment, and perspectives of a systemic disease. *Front. Pediatrics* **2018**, *6*, 1–8. [CrossRef]
7. Schneider, J.A.; Bradley, K.; Seegmiller, J.E. Increased cystine in leukocytes from individuals homozygous and heterozygous for cystinosis. *Science* **1967**, *157*, 1321–1322. [CrossRef]
8. Monnens, L.; Levtchenko, E. Evaluation of the proximal tubular function in hereditary renal Fanconi syndrome. *Nephrol. Dial. Transpl.* **2008**, *23*, 2719–2722. [CrossRef]
9. Mahoney, C.P.; Striker, G.E. Early development of the renal lesions in infantile cystinosis. *Pediatric Nephrol.* **2000**, *15*, 50–56. [CrossRef] [PubMed]
10. Stokes, M.B.; Jernigan, S.; D'Agati, V.D. Infantile nephropathic cystinosis. *Kidney Int.* **2008**, *73*, 782–786. [CrossRef] [PubMed]
11. Elmonem, M.A.; Veys, K.R.; Soliman, N.A.; Van Dyck, M.; Van Den Heuvel, L.P.; Levtchenko, E. Cystinosis: A review. *Orphanet J. Rare Dis.* **2016**, *11*, 1–17. [CrossRef] [PubMed]
12. Trauner, D. Neurocognitive Complications of Cystinosis. *J. Pediatrics* **2017**, *183*, S15–S18. [CrossRef] [PubMed]
13. Servais, A.; Morinière, V.; Grünfeld, J.P.; Noël, L.H.; Goujon, J.M.; Chadefaux-Vekemans, B.; Antignac, C. Late-onset nephropathic cystinosis: Clinical presentation, outcome, and genotyping. *Clin. J. Am. Soc. Nephrol.* **2008**, *3*, 27–35. [CrossRef] [PubMed]
14. Gahl, W.A.; Tietze, F.; De Butler, B.J.; Schulman, J.D. Cysteamine depletes cystinotic leucocyte granular fractions of cystine by the mechanism of disulphide interchange. *Biochem. J.* **1985**, *228*, 545–550. [CrossRef]
15. Jézégou, A.; Llinares, E.; Anne, C.; Kieffer-jaquinod, S.; O'Regan, S.; Aupetit, J.; Chabli, A.; Sagńe, C.; Debacker, C.; Chadefaux-Vekemans, B.; et al. Heptahelical protein PQLC2 is a lysosomal cationic amino acid exporter underlying the action of cysteamine in cystinosis therapy. *Proc. Natl. Acad. Sci. USA* **2012**, *109*, E3434–E3443. [CrossRef]
16. Pisoni, R.L.; Acker, T.L.; Lisowski, K.M.; Lemons, R.M.; Thoene, J.G. A cysteine-specific lysosomal transport system provides a major route for the delivery of thiol to human fibroblast lysosomes: Possible role in supporting lysosomal proteolysis. *J. Cell Biol.* **1990**, *110*, 327–335. [CrossRef]
17. Van Stralen, K.J.; Emma, F.; Jager, K.J.; Verrina, E.; Schaefer, F.; Laube, G.F.; Lewis, M.A.; Levtchenko, E.N. Improvement in the renal prognosis in nephropathic cystinosis. *Clin. J. Am. Soc. Nephrol.* **2011**, *6*, 2485–2491. [CrossRef]
18. Brodin-Sartorius, A.; Tête, M.J.; Niaudet, P.; Antignac, C.; Guest, G.; Ottolenghi, C.; Charbit, M.; Moyse, D.; Legendre, C.; Lesavre, P.; et al. Cysteamine therapy delays the progression of nephropathic cystinosis in late adolescents and adults. *Kidney Int.* **2012**, *81*, 179–189. [CrossRef]
19. Gahl, W.A.; Balog, J.Z.; Kleta, R. Nephropathic cystinosis in adults: Natural history and effects of oral cysteamine therapy. *Ann. Intern. Med.* **2007**, *147*, 242–250. [CrossRef]
20. Kleta, R.; Bernardini, I.; Ueda, M.; Varade, W.S.; Phornphutkul, C.; Krasnewich, D.; Gahl, W.A. Long-term follow-up of well-treated nephropathic cystinosis patients. *J. Pediatr.* **2004**, *145*, 555–560. [CrossRef]
21. Markello, T.C.; Bernardini, I.M.; Gahl, W.A. Improved renal function in children with cystinosis treated with cysteamine. *N. Engl. J. Med.* **1993**, *329*, 977–986. [CrossRef] [PubMed]
22. Nesterova, G.; Williams, C.; Bernardini, I.; Gahl, W.A. Cystinosis: Renal glomerular and renal tubular function in relation to compliance with cystine-depleting therapy. *Pediatric Nephrol.* **2015**, *30*, 945–951. [CrossRef] [PubMed]
23. Gahl, W.A.; Reed, G.F.; Thoene, J.G.; Schulman, J.D.; Rizzo, W.B.; Jonas, A.J.; Denman, D.W.; Schlesselman, J.J.; Corden, B.J.; Schneider, J.A. Cysteamine therapy for children with nephropathic cystinosis. *N. Engl. J. Med.* **1987**, *316*, 971–977. [CrossRef] [PubMed]
24. Dohil, R.; Fidler, M.; Gangoiti, J.A.; Kaskel, F.; Schneider, J.A.; Barshop, B.A. Twice-daily cysteamine bitartrate therapy for children with cystinosis. *J. Pediatr.* **2010**, *156*, 71–75. [CrossRef]
25. Dohil, R.; Cabrera, B.L. Treatment of cystinosis with delayed-release cysteamine: 6-year follow-up. *Pediatr. Nephrol.* **2013**, *28*, 507–510. [CrossRef] [PubMed]
26. Napolitano, G.; Johnson, J.L.; He, J.; Rocca, C.J.; Monfregola, J.; Pestonjamasp, K.; Cherqui, S.; Catz, S.D. Impairment of chaperone-mediated autophagy leads to selective lysosomal degradation defects in the lysosomal storage disease cystinosis. *EMBO Mol. Med.* **2015**, *7*, 158–174. [CrossRef]
27. Rega, L.R.; Polishchuk, E.; Montefusco, S.; Napolitano, G.; Tozzi, G.; Zhang, J.; Bellomo, F.; Taranta, A.; Pastore, A.; Polishchuk, R.; et al. Activation of the transcription factor EB rescues lysosomal abnormalities in cystinotic kidney cells. *Kidney Int.* **2016**, *89*, 862–873. [CrossRef]
28. Andrzejewska, Z.; Nevo, N.; Thomas, L.; Bailleux, A.; Chauvet, V.; Courtoy, P.J.; Chol, M.; Guerrera, I.C.; Antignac, C. Cystinosin is a Component of the Vacuolar H+-ATPase-Ragulator-Rag Complex Controlling Mammalian Target of Rapamycin Complex 1 Signaling. *J. Am. Soc. Nephrol.* **2016**, *27*, 1678–1688. [CrossRef]
29. Hollywood, J.A.; Przepiorski, A.; D'Souza, R.F.; Sreebhavan, S.; Wolvetang, E.J.; Harrison, P.T.; Davidson, A.J.; Holm, T.M. Use of Human Induced Pluripotent Stem Cells and Kidney Organoids To Develop a Cysteamine/mTOR Inhibition Combination Therapy for Cystinosis. *J. Am. Soc. Nephrol.* **2020**, *31*, 962–982. [CrossRef]
30. Schneider, J.A.; Rosenbloom, F.M.; Bradley, K.H.; Seegmiller, J.E. Increased free-cystine content of fibroblasts cultured from patients with cystinosis. *Biochem. Biophys. Res. Commun.* **1967**, *29*, 527–531. [CrossRef]

31. Patrick, A.D.; Lake, B.D. Cystinosis: Electron microscopic evidence of lysosomal storage of cystine in lymph node. *J. Clin. Pathol.* **1968**, *21*, 571–575. [CrossRef]
32. Reeves, J.P. Accumulation of amino acids by lysosomes incubated with amino acid methyl esters. *J. Biol. Chem.* **1979**, *254*, 8914–8921. [CrossRef]
33. Gahl, W.A.; Bashan, N.; Tietze, F.; Bernardini, I.; Schulman, J.D. Cystine transport is defective in isolated leukocyte lysosomes from patients with cystinosis. *Science* **1982**, *217*, 1263–1265. [CrossRef] [PubMed]
34. Gahl, W.A.; Tietze, F.; Bashan, N.; Steinherz, R.; Schulman, J.D. Defective cystine exodus from isolated lysosome-rich fractions of cystinotic leucocytes. *J. Biol. Chem.* **1982**, *257*, 9570–9575. [CrossRef]
35. Jonas, A.J.; Greene, A.A.; Smith, M.L.; Schneider, J.A. Cystine accumulation and loss in normal, heterozygous, and cystinotic fibroblasts. *Proc. Natl. Acad. Sci. USA* **1982**, *79*, 4442–4445. [CrossRef]
36. Jonas, A.; Smith, M.; Allison, W.; Laikind, P.; Greene, A.; Schneider, J. Proton translocating ATPase and lysosomal cystine transport. *J. Biol. Chem.* **1983**, *258*, 11727–11730. [CrossRef]
37. Wilmer, M.J.; Willems, P.H.; Verkaart, S.; Visch, H.J.; Graaf-Hess, D.E.; Blom, H.J.; Monnens, L.A.; van den Heuvel, L.P.; Levtchenko, E.N. Cystine dimethylester model of cystinosis: Still reliable? *Pediatr. Res.* **2007**, *62*, 151–155. [CrossRef]
38. Sumayao, R.; Mcevoy, B.; Martin-Martin, N.; Mcmorrow, T.; Newsholme, P. Cystine dimethylester loading promotes oxidative stress and a reduction in ATP independent of lysosomal cystine accumulation in a human proximal tubular epithelial cell line. *Exp. Physiol.* **2013**, *98*, 1505–1517. [CrossRef]
39. Thoene, J.G.; Lemons, R.M. Cystine accumulation in cystinotic fibroblasts from free and protein-linked cystine but not cysteine. *Biochem. J.* **1982**, *208*, 823–830. [CrossRef] [PubMed]
40. Adelmann, C.H.; Traunbauer, A.K.; Chen, B.; Condon, K.J.; Chan, S.H.; Kunchok, T.; Lewis, C.A.; Sabatini, D.M. MFSD12 mediates the import of cysteine into melanosomes and lysosomes. *Nature* **2020**, *588*, 699–704. [CrossRef]
41. Kroll, W.A.; Schneider, J.A. Decrease in Free Cystine Content of Cultured Cystinotic Fibroblasts by Ascorbic Acid. *Science* **1974**, *186*, 1040–1042. [CrossRef] [PubMed]
42. Thoene, J.G.; Oshima, R.G.; Crawhall, J.C. Intracellular cystine depletion by aminothiols in vitro and in vivo. *J. Clin. Investig.* **1976**, *58*, 180–189. [CrossRef]
43. Levtchenko, E.; de Graaf-Hess, A.; Wilmer, M.; van den Heuvel, L.; Monnens, L.; Blom, H. Altered status of glutathione and its metabolites in cystinotic cells. *Nephrol. Dial. Transplant.* **2005**, *20*, 1828–1832. [CrossRef]
44. Mannucci, L.; Pastore, A.; Rizzo, C.; Piemonte, F.; Rizzoni, G.; Emma, F. Impaired activity of the γ-glutamyl cycle in nephropathic cystinosis fibroblasts. *Pediatric Res.* **2006**, *59*, 332–335. [CrossRef] [PubMed]
45. Vitvitsky, V.; Witcher, M.; Banerjee, R.; Thoene, J. The redox status of cystinotic fibroblasts. *Mol. Genet. Metab.* **2010**, *99*, 384–388. [CrossRef] [PubMed]
46. Trifillis, A.L.; Regec, A.L.; Trump, B.F. Isolation, culture and characterization of human renal tubular cells. *J. Urol.* **1985**, *133*, 324–329. [CrossRef]
47. Pellett, O.L.; Smith, M.L.; Thoene, S.J.G.; Schneider, J.A.; Jonas, A.J. Renal cell culture using autopsy material from children with cystinosis. *In Vitro* **1984**, *20*, 53–58. [CrossRef]
48. Racusen, L.C.; Fivush, B.A.; Andersson, H.; Gahl, W.A. Culture of Renal with Nephropathic from the Urine of Patients. *J. Am. Soc. Nephrol.* **1991**, *1*, 1028–1033. [CrossRef]
49. Laube, G.F.; Haq, M.R.; van't Hoff, W.G. Exfoliated human proximal tubular cells: A model of cystinosis and Fanconi syndrome. *Pediatric Nephrol.* **2005**, *20*, 136–140. [CrossRef]
50. Laube, G.F.; Shah, V.; Stewart, V.C.; Hargreaves, I.P.; Haq, M.R.; Heales, S.J.R.; von't Hoff, W.G. Glutathione depletion and increased apoptosis rate in human cystinotic proximal tubular cells. *Pediatric Nephrol.* **2006**, *21*, 503–509. [CrossRef]
51. Bhargava, P.; Schnellmann, R.G. Mitochondrial energetics in the kidney. *Nat. Rev. Nephrol.* **2017**, *13*, 629–646. [CrossRef]
52. Sansanwal, P.; Yen, B.; Gahl, W.A.; Ma, Y.; Ying, L.; Wong, L.C.; Sarwal, M.M. Mitochondrial autophagy promotes cellular injury in nephropathic cystinosis. *J. Am. Soc. Nephrol.* **2010**, *21*, 272–283. [CrossRef] [PubMed]
53. Sansanwal, P.; Sarwal, M.M. P62/SQSTM1 prominently accumulates in renal proximal tubules in nephropathic cystinosis. *Pediatric Nephrol.* **2012**, *27*, 2137–2144. [CrossRef] [PubMed]
54. Qi, W.; Johnson, D.W.; Vesey, D.A.; Pollock, C.A.; Chen, X. Isolation, propagation and characterization of primary tubule cell culture from human kidney. *Nephrology* **2007**, *12*, 155–159. [CrossRef]
55. Dickman, K.G.; Mandel, L.J. Glycolytic and oxidative metabolism in primary renal proximal tubule cultures. *Am. J. Physiol.* **1989**, *257*, C333–C340. [CrossRef] [PubMed]
56. Münger, K.; Howley, P.M. Human papillomavirus immortalization and transformation functions. *Virus Res.* **2002**, *89*, 213–228. [CrossRef]
57. Ahuja, D.; Sáenz-Robles, M.T.; Pipas, J.M. SV40 large T antigen targets multiple cellular pathways to elicit cellular transformation. *Oncogene* **2005**, *24*, 7729–7745. [CrossRef]
58. Ryan, M.J.; Johnson, G.; Kirk, J.; Fuerstenberg, S.M.; Zager, R.A.; Torok-Storb, B. HK-2: An immortalized proximal tubule epithelial cell line from normal adult human kidney. *Kidney Int.* **1994**, *45*, 48–57. [CrossRef]
59. Ivanova, E.A.; De Leo, M.G.; Van Den Heuvel, L.; Pastore, A.; Dijkman, H.; De Matteis, M.A.; Levtchenko, E.N. Endo-lysosomal dysfunction in human proximal tubular epithelial cells deficient for lysosomal cystine transporter cystinosin. *PLoS ONE* **2015**, *10*, 1–18. [CrossRef]

60. Bellomo, F.; Signorile, A.; Tamma, G.; Ranieri, M.; Emma, F.; De Rasmo, D. Impact of atypical mitochondrial cyclic-AMP level in nephropathic cystinosis. *Cell Mol. Life Sci.* **2018**, *75*, 3411–3422. [CrossRef] [PubMed]
61. Sumayao, R.; McEvoy, B.; Newsholme, P.; McMorrow, T. Lysosomal cystine accumulation promotes mitochondrial depolarization and induction of redox-sensitive genes in human kidney proximal tubular cells. *J. Physiol.* **2016**, *594*, 3353–3370. [CrossRef] [PubMed]
62. Taranta, A.; Petrini, S.; Palma, A.; Mannucci, L.; Wilmer, M.J.; De Luca, V.; Diomedi-Camassei, F.; Corallini, S.; Bellomo, F.; van den Heuvel, L.P.; et al. Identification and subcellular localization of a new cystinosin isoform. *Am. J. Physiol. Renal. Physiol.* **2008**, *294*, F1101–F1108. [CrossRef] [PubMed]
63. Zhang, J.; He, J.; Johnson, J.L.; Rahman, F.; Gavathiotis, E.; Cuervo, A.M.; Catz, S.D. Chaperone-Mediated Autophagy Upregulation Rescues Megalin Expression and Localization in Cystinotic Proximal Tubule Cells. *Front. Endocrinol.* **2019**, *10*, 21. [CrossRef]
64. Wilmer, M.J.G.; De Graaf-Hess, A.; Blom, H.J.; Dijkman, H.B.P.M.; Monnens, L.A.; Van Den Heuvel, L.P.; Levtchenko, E.N. Elevated oxidized glutathione in cystinotic proximal tubular epithelial cells. *Biochem. Biophys. Res. Commun.* **2005**, *337*, 610–614. [CrossRef]
65. Chol, M.; Nevo, N.; Cherqui, S.; Antignac, C.; Rustin, P. Glutathione precursors replenish decreased glutathione pool in cystinotic cell lines. *Biochem. Biophys. Res. Commun.* **2004**, *324*, 231–235. [CrossRef] [PubMed]
66. Levtchenko, E.N.; Wilmer, M.J.G.; Janssen, A.J.M.; Koenderink, J.B.; Visch, H.J.; Willems, P.H.G.M.; de Graaf-Hess, A.; Blom, H.J.; van den Heuvel, L.P.; Monnens, L.A. Decreased intracellular ATP content and intact mitochondrial energy generating capacity in human cystinotic fibroblasts. *Pediatric Res.* **2006**, *59*, 287–292. [CrossRef]
67. Racusen, L.C.; Wilson, P.D.; Hartz, P.A.; Fivush, B.A.; Burrow, C.R. Renal proximal tubular epithelium from patients with nephropathic cystinosis: Immortalized cell lines as in vitro model systems. *Kidney Int.* **1995**, *48*, 536–543. [CrossRef]
68. Wilmer, M.J.; Saleem, M.A.; Masereeuw, R.; Ni, L.; van der Velden, T.J.; Russel, F.G.; Mathieson, P.W.; Monnens, L.A.; van den Heuvel, L.P.; Levtchenko, E.N. Novel conditionally immortalized human proximal tubule cell line expressing functional influx and efflux transporters. *Cell Tissue Res.* **2010**, *339*, 449–457. [CrossRef]
69. Bens, M.; Vandewalle, A. Cell models for studying renal physiology. *Pflug. Arch* **2008**, *457*, 1–15. [CrossRef]
70. Mattoscio, D.; Medda, A.; Chiocca, S. Human papilloma virus and autophagy. *Int. J. Mol. Sci.* **2018**, *19*, 1775. [CrossRef]
71. Mattoscio, D.; Casadio, C.; Miccolo, C.; Maffini, F.; Raimondi, A.; Tacchetti, C.; Gheit, T.; Tagliabue, M.; Galimberti, V.E.; De Lorenzi, F.; et al. Autophagy regulates UBC9 levels during viral-mediated tumorigenesis. *PLoS Pathog.* **2017**, *13*, e1006262. [CrossRef]
72. Bellomo, F.; Corallini, S.; Pastore, A.; Palma, A.; Laurenzi, C.; Emma, F.; Taranta, A. Modulation of CTNS gene expression by intracellular thiols. *Free Radic. Biol. Med.* **2010**, *48*, 865–872. [CrossRef] [PubMed]
73. Soto-Heredero, G.; Baixauli, F.; Mittelbrunn, M. Interorganelle Communication between Mitochondria and the Endolysosomal System. *Front. Cell Dev. Biol.* **2017**, *7*, 95. [CrossRef]
74. Taub, M.L.; Springate, J.E.; Cutuli, F. Reduced phosphate transport in the renal proximal tubule cells in cystinosis is due to decreased expression of transporters rather than an energy defect. *Biochem. Biophys. Res. Commun.* **2011**, *407*, 355–359. [CrossRef] [PubMed]
75. Taub, M.; Cutuli, F. Activation of AMP kinase plays a role in the increased apoptosis in the renal proximal tubule in cystinosis. *Biochem. Biophys. Res. Commun.* **2012**, *426*, 516–521. [CrossRef]
76. Okoshi, R.; Ozaki, T.; Yamamoto, H.; Ando, K.; Koida, N.; Ono, S.; Koda, T.; Kamijo, T.; Nakagawara, A.; Kizaki, H. Activation of AMP-activated protein kinase induces p53-dependent apoptotic cell death in response to energetic stress. *J. Biol. Chem.* **2008**, *283*, 3979–3987. [CrossRef]
77. McEvoy, B.; Sumayao, R.; Slattery, C.; McMorrow, T.; Newsholme, P. Cystine accumulation attenuates insulin release from the pancreatic β-cell due to elevated oxidative stress and decreased ATP levels. *J. Physiol.* **2015**, *593*, 5167–5182. [CrossRef] [PubMed]
78. Borger, D.K.; McMahon, B.; Lal, T.R.; Serra-Vinardell, J.; Aflaki, E.; Sidransky, E. Induced pluripotent stem cell models of lysosomal storage disorders. *DMM Dis. Models Mech.* **2017**, *10*, 691–704. [CrossRef]
79. Takahashi, K.; Yamanaka, S. Induction of Pluripotent Stem Cells from Mouse Embryonic and Adult Fibroblast Cultures by Defined Factors. *Cell* **2006**, *126*, 663–676. [CrossRef]
80. Song, B.; Smink, A.M.; Jones, C.V.; Callaghan, J.M.; Firth, S.D.; Bernard, C.A.; Laslett, A.L.; Kerr, P.G.; Ricardo, S.D. The Directed Differentiation of Human iPS Cells into Kidney Podocytes. *PLoS ONE* **2012**, *7*, 1–9. [CrossRef]
81. Lam, A.Q.; Freedman, B.S.; Morizane, R.; Lerou, P.H.; Valerius, M.T.; Bonventre, J.V. Rapid and efficient differentiation of human pluripotent stem cells into intermediate mesoderm that forms tubules expressing kidney proximal tubular markers. *J. Am. Soc. Nephrol.* **2014**, *25*, 1211–1225. [CrossRef]
82. Tian, P.; Lennon, R. The myriad possibility of kidney organoids. *Curr. Opin. Nephrol. Hypertens.* **2019**, *28*, 211–218. [CrossRef]
83. Lau, Y.K.; Du, X.; Rayannavar, V.; Hopkins, B.; Shaw, J.; Bessler, E.; Thomas, T.; Pires, M.M.; Keniry, M.; Parsons, R.E.; et al. Metformin and erlotinib synergize to inhibit basal breast cancer. *Oncotarget* **2014**, *5*, 10503–10517. [CrossRef]
84. Varum, S.; Rodrigues, A.S.; Moura, M.B.; Momcilovic, O.; Easley, C.A., 4th; Ramalho-Santos, J.; van Houten, B.; Schatten, G. Energy metabolism in human pluripotent stem cells and their differentiated counterparts. *PLoS ONE* **2011**, *6*, e20914. [CrossRef]
85. Kimura, T.; Takabatake, Y.; Takahashi, A.; Kaimori, J.Y.; Matsui, I.; Namba, T.; Kitamura, H.; Niimura, F.; Matsusaka, T.; Soga, T.; et al. Autophagy protects the proximal tubule from degeneration and acute ischemic injury. *J. Am. Soc. Nephrol.* **2011**, *22*, 902–913. [CrossRef]
86. Combes, A.N.; Zappia, L.; Er, P.X.; Oshlack, A.; Little, M.H. Single-cell analysis reveals congruence between kidney organoids and human fetal kidney. *Genome Med.* **2019**, *11*, 1–15. [CrossRef]
87. Wu, H.; Uchimura, K.; Donnelly, E.L.; Kirita, Y.; Morris, S.A.; Humphreys, B.D. Comparative Analysis and Refinement of Human PSC-Derived Kidney Organoid Differentiation with Single-Cell Transcriptomics. *Cell Stem. Cell* **2018**, *23*, 869–881. [CrossRef]

88. Przepiorski, A.; Sander, V.; Tran, T.; Hollywood, J.A.; Sorrenson, B.; Shih, J.H.; Wolvetang, E.J.; McMahon, A.P.; Holm, T.M.; Davidson, A.J. A Simple Bioreactor-Based Method to Generate Kidney Organoids from Pluripotent Stem Cells. *Stem. Cell Rep.* **2018**, *11*, 470–484. [CrossRef] [PubMed]
89. van den Berg, C.W.; Ritsma, L.; Avramut, M.C.; Wiersma, L.E.; van den Berg, B.M.; Leuning, D.G.; Lievers, E.; Koning, M.; Vanslambrouck, J.M.; Koster, A.J.; et al. Renal Subcapsular Transplantation of PSC-Derived Kidney Organoids Induces Neovasculogenesis and Significant Glomerular and Tubular Maturation In Vivo. *Stem. Cell Rep.* **2018**, *10*, 751–765. [CrossRef] [PubMed]
90. Bantounas, I.; Ranjzad, P.; Tengku, F.; Silajdžić, E.; Forster, D.; Asselin, M.C.; Lewis, P.; Lennon, R.; Plagge, A.; Wang, Q.; et al. Generation of Functioning Nephrons by Implanting Human Pluripotent Stem Cell-Derived Kidney Progenitors. *Stem. Cell Rep.* **2018**, *10*, 766–779. [CrossRef] [PubMed]
91. Schutgens, F.; Rookmaaker, M.B.; Margaritis, T.; Rios, A.; Ammerlaan, C.; Jansen, J. Tubuloids derived from human adult kidney and urine for personalized disease modeling. *Nat. Biotechnol.* **2019**, *37*, 303–313. [CrossRef] [PubMed]
92. Yousef Yengej, F.A.; Jansen, J.; Rookmaaker, M.B.; Verhaar, M.C.; Clevers, H. Kidney Organoids and Tubuloids. *Cells* **2020**, *9*, 1326. [CrossRef] [PubMed]
93. Jamalpoor, A.; van Gelder, C.A.; Yousef Yengej, F.A.; Zaal, E.A.; Berlingerio, S.P.; Veys, K.; Pou Casellas, C.; Voskuil, K.; Essa, K.; Ammerlaan, C.M.; et al. Cysteamine-bicalutamide combination therapy corrects proximal tubule phenotype in cystinosis. *EMBO Mol. Med.* **2021**, *13*, e13067. [CrossRef]
94. Cherqui, S.; Sevin, C.; Hamard, G.; Kalatzis, V.; Sich, M.; Pequignot, M.; Gogat, K.; Abitbol, M.; Broyer, M.; Gubler, M.C.; et al. Intralysosomal Cystine Accumulation in Mice Lacking Cystinosin, the Protein Defective in Cystinosis. *Mol. Cell. Biol.* **2002**, *22*, 7622–7632. [CrossRef] [PubMed]
95. Nevo, N.; Chol, M.; Bailleux, A.; Kalatzis, V.; Morisset, L.; Devuyst, O.; Gubler, M.C.; Antignac, C. Renal phenotype of the cystinosis mouse model is dependent upon genetic background. *Nephrol. Dial. Transplant.* **2010**, *25*, 1059–1066. [CrossRef]
96. Gaide Chevronnay, H.P.; Janssens, V.; Van Der Smissen, P.; N'Kuli, F.; Nevo, N.; Guiot, Y.; Levtchenko, E.; Marbaix, E.; Pierreux, C.E. Time course of pathogenic and adaptation mechanisms in cystinotic mouse kidneys. *J. Am. Soc. Nephrol.* **2014**, *25*, 1256–1269. [CrossRef]
97. Elmonem, M.A.; Khalil, R.; Khodaparast, L.; Khodaparast, L.; Arcolino, F.O.; Morgan, J.; Pastore, A.; Tylzanowski, P.; Ny, A.; Lowe, M.; et al. Cystinosis (ctns) zebrafish mutant shows pronephric glomerular and tubular dysfunction. *Sci. Rep.* **2017**, *7*, 1–17.
98. Berlingerio, S.P.; He, J.; Groef, L.; De Taeter, H.; Norton, T.; Baatsen, P.; Cairoli, S.; Goffredo, B.; de Witte, P.; van den Heuvel, L.; et al. Renal and Extra Renal Manifestations in Adult Zebrafish Model of Cystinosis. *Int. J. Mol. Sci.* **2021**, *22*, 9398. [CrossRef]
99. Festa, B.P.; Chen, Z.; Berquez, M.; Debaix, H.; Tokonami, N.; Prange, J.A.; van de Hoek, G.; Alessio, C.; Raimondi, A.; Nevo, N.; et al. Impaired autophagy bridges lysosomal storage disease and epithelial dysfunction in the kidney. *Nat. Commun.* **2018**, *9*, 1–17. [CrossRef]
100. Shimizu, Y.; Yanobu-Takanashi, R.; Nakano, K.; Hamase, K.; Shimizu, T.; Okamura, T. A deletion in the Ctns gene causes renal tubular dysfunction and cystine accumulation in LEA/Tohm rats. *Mamm. Genome* **2019**, *30*, 23–33. [CrossRef]
101. Hollywood, J.A.; Kallingappa, P.K.; Cheung, P.Y.; Martis, R.M.; Sreebhavan, S.; Chatterjee, A.; Buckels, E.J.; Mathews, B.G.; Lewis, P.M.; Davidson, A.J. Cystinosin deficient rats recapitulate the phenotype of nephropathic cystinosis. *bioRxiv* **2021**. [CrossRef]
102. Hardwick, K.G.; Pelham, H.R. ERS1 a seven transmembrane domain protein from Saccharomyces cerevisiae. *Nucleic Acids Res.* **1990**, *25*, 2177. [CrossRef]
103. Zhai, Y.; Heijne, W.H.; Smith, D.W.; Saier, M.H., Jr. Homologues of archaeal rhodopsins in plants, animals and fungi: Structural and functional predications for a putative fungal chaperone protein. *Biochim. Biophys. Acta* **2001**, *1511*, 206–223. [CrossRef]
104. Gao, X.D.; Wang, J.; Keppler-Ross, S.; Dean, N. ERS1 encodes a functional homologue of the human lysosomal cystine transporter. *FEBS J.* **2005**, *272*, 2497–2511. [CrossRef] [PubMed]
105. Simpkins, J.A.; Rickel, K.E.; Madeo, M.; Ahlers, B.A.; Carlisle, G.B.; Nelson, H.J.; Cardillo, A.L.; Weber, E.A.; Vitiello, P.F.; Pearce, D.A.; et al. Disruption of a cystine transporter downregulates expression of genes involved in sulfur regulation and cellular respiration. *Biol. Open* **2016**, *5*, 689–697. [CrossRef]
106. Kalatzis, V.; Nevo, N.; Cherqui, S.; Gasnier, B.; Antignac, C. Molecular pathogenesis of cystinosis: Effect of CTNS mutations on the transport activity and subcellular localization of cystinosin. *Hum. Mol. Genet.* **2004**, *13*, 1361–1371. [CrossRef]
107. Ratelade, J.; Lavin, T.A.; Muda, A.O.; Morisset, L.; Mollet, G.; Boyer, O.; Chen, D.S.; Henger, A.; Kretzler, M.; Hubner, N.; et al. Maternal environment interacts with modifier genes to influence progression of nephrotic syndrome. *J. Am. Soc. Nephrol.* **2008**, *19*, 1491–1499. [CrossRef]
108. Raggi, C.; Luciani, A.; Nevo, N.; Antignac, C.; Terryn, S.; Devuyst, O. Dedifferentiation and aberrations of the endolysosomal compartment characterize the early stage of nephropathic cystinosis. *Hum. Mol. Genet.* **2014**, *23*, 2266–2278. [CrossRef]
109. Sharma, A.; Gupta, R.; Sethi, S.K.; Bagga, A.; Dinda, A.K. Giant cell transformation of podocytes: A unique histological feature associated with cystinosis. *Indian J. Nephrol.* **2011**, *21*, 123–125.
110. Janssens, V.; Gaide Chevronnay, H.P.; Marie, S.; Vincent, M.F.; Van Der Smissen, P.; Nevo, N.; Vainio, S.; Nielsen, R.; Christensen, E.I.; Jouret, F.; et al. Protection of Cystinotic Mice by Kidney-Specific Megalin Ablation Supports an Endocytosis-Based Mechanism for Nephropathic Cystinosis Progression. *J. Am. Soc. Nephrol.* **2019**, *30*, 2177–2190. [CrossRef]
111. Battafarano, G.; Rossi, M.; Rega, L.R.; Di Giovamberardino, G.; Pastore, A.; D'Agostini, M.; Porzio, O.; Nebo, N.; Emma, F.; Taranta, A.; et al. Intrinsic Bone Defects in Cystinotic Mice. *Am. J. Pathol.* **2019**, *189*, 1053–1064. [CrossRef]

112. Galarreta, C.I.; Forbes, M.S.; Thornhill, B.A.; Antignac, C.; Gubler, M.C.; Nevo, N.; Murphy, M.P.; Chevalier, R.L. The swan-neck lesion: Proximal tubular adaptation to oxidative stress in nephropathic cystinosis. *Am. J. Physiol. Renal. Physiol.* **2015**, *308*, F1155–F1166. [CrossRef]
113. Yu, Y.; Kudchodkar, S.B.; Alwine, J.C. Effects of simian virus 40 large and small tumor antigens on mammalian target of rapamycin signaling: Small tumor antigen mediates hypophosphorylation of eIF4E-binding protein 1 late in infection. *J. Virol.* **2005**, *79*, 6882–6889. [CrossRef]
114. Gaide Chevronnay, H.P.; Janssens, V.; Van Der Smissen, P.; Rocca, C.J.; Liao, X.H.; Refetoff, S.; Pierreux, C.E.; Cherqui, S.; Courtoy, P.J. Hematopoietic Stem Cells Transplantation Can Normalize Thyroid Function in a Cystinosis Mouse Model. *Endocrinol.* **2016**, *157*, 1363–1371. [CrossRef]
115. Kalatzis, V.; Serratrice, N.; Hippert, C.; Payet, O.; Arndt, C.; Cazevieille, C.; Maurice, T.; Hamel, C.; Malecaze, F.; Antignac, C.; et al. The ocular anomalies in a cystinosis animal model mimic disease pathogenesis. *Pediatr. Res.* **2007**, *62*, 156–162. [CrossRef]
116. Tsilou, E.T.; Rubin, B.I.; Reed, G.; Caruso, R.C.; Iwata, F.; Balog, J.; Gahl, W.A.; Kaiser-Kupfer, M.I. Nephropathic cystinosis: Posterior segment manifestations and effects of cysteamine therapy. *Ophthalmology* **2006**, *113*, 1002–1009. [CrossRef]
117. Cheung, W.W.; Cherqui, S.; Ding, W.; Esparza, M.; Zhou, P.; Shao, J.; Lieber, R.L.; Mak, R.H. Muscle wasting and adipose tissue browning in infantile nephropathic cystinosis. *Cachexia Sarcopenia Muscle* **2016**, *7*, 152–164. [CrossRef]
118. Cheung, W.W.; Hao, S.; Wang, Z.; Ding, W.; Zheng, R.; Gonzalez, A.; Zhan, J.Y.; Zhou, P.; Li, S.; Esparza, M.C.; et al. Vitamin D repletion ameliorates adipose tissue browning and muscle wasting in infantile nephropathic cystinosis-associated cachexia. *J. Cachexia Sarcopenia Muscle.* **2020**, *11*, 120–134. [CrossRef] [PubMed]
119. Hippert, C.; Dubois, G.; Morin, C.; Disson, O.; Ibanes, S.; Jacquet, C.; Schwendener, R.; Antignac, C.; Kremer, E.J.; Kalatzis, V. Gene transfer may be preventive but not curative for a lysosomal transport disorder. *Mol. Ther.* **2008**, *16*, 1372–1381. [CrossRef] [PubMed]
120. Syres, K.; Harrison, F.; Tadlock, M.; Jester, J.V.; Simpson, J.; Roy, S.; Salomon, D.R.; Cherqui, S. Successful treatment of the murine model of cystinosis using bone marrow cell transplantation. *Blood* **2009**, *114*, 2542–2552. [CrossRef] [PubMed]
121. Yeagy, B.A.; Harrison, F.; Gubler, M.C.; Koziol, J.A.; Salomon, D.R.; Cherqui, S. Kidney preservation by bone marrow cell transplantation in hereditary nephropathy. *Kidney Int.* **2011**, *79*, 1198–1206. [CrossRef] [PubMed]
122. Harrison, F.; Yeagy, B.A.; Rocca, C.J.; Kohn, D.B.; Salomon, D.R.; Cherqui, S. Hematopoietic stem cell gene therapy for the multisystemic lysosomal storage disorder cystinosis. *Mol. Ther.* **2013**, *21*, 433–444. [CrossRef]
123. Naphade, S.; Sharma, J.; Gaide Chevronnay, H.P.; Shook, M.A.; Yeagy, B.A.; Rocca, C.J.; Ur, S.N.; Lau, A.J.; Courtoy, P.J.; Cherqui, S. Brief reports: Lysosomal cross-correction by hematopoietic stem cell-derived macrophages via tunneling nanotubes. *Stem Cells* **2015**, *33*, 301–309. [CrossRef]
124. Brasell, E.J.; Chu, L.L.; Akpa, M.M.; Eshkar-Oren, I.; Alroy, I.; Corsini, R.; Gilfix, B.M.; Yamanaka, Y.; Huertas, P.; Goodyer, P. The novel aminoglycoside, ELX-02, permits CTNSW138X translational read-through and restores lysosomal cystine efflux in cystinosis. *PLoS ONE* **2019**, *14*, e0223954. [CrossRef]
125. Schlegel, A.; Gut, P. Metabolic insights from zebrafish genetics, physiology, and chemical biology. *Cell Mol. Life Sci.* **2015**, *72*, 2249–2260. [CrossRef] [PubMed]
126. Diep, C.Q.; Ma, D.; Deo, R.C.; Holm, T.M.; Naylor, R.W.; Arora, N.; Wingert, R.A.; Bollig, F.; Djordjevic, G.; Lichman, B.; et al. Identification of adult nephron progenitors capable of kidney regeneration in zebrafish. *Nature* **2011**, *470*, 95–100. [CrossRef] [PubMed]
127. Okamura, T.; Pei, X.Y.; Miyoshi, I.; Shimizu, Y.; Takanashi-Yanobu, R.; Mototani, Y.; Kanai, T.; Satoh, J.; Kimura, N.; Kasai, N. Phenotypic Characterization of LEA Rat: A New Rat Model of Nonobese Type 2 Diabetes. *J. Diabetes Res.* **2013**, *2013*, 986462. [CrossRef]
128. Ponting, C.P.; Mott, R.; Bork, P.; Copley, R.R. Novel protein domains and repeats in Drosophila melanogaster: Insights into structure, function, and evolution. *Genome Res.* **2001**, *11*, 1996–2008. [CrossRef]
129. Jouandin, P.; Marelja, Z.; Parkhitko, A.A.; Dambowsky, M.; Asara, J.M.; Nemazanyy, I.; Simons, M.; Perrimon, N. Lysosomal cystine efflux opposes mTORC1 reactivation through the TCA cycle. *bioRxiv* **2021**. [CrossRef]

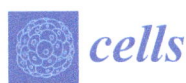

Article
Urine-Derived Kidney Progenitor Cells in Cystinosis

Koenraad Veys [1,2], Sante Princiero Berlingerio [2,†], Dries David [3,†], Tjessa Bondue [2], Katharina Held [4], Ahmed Reda [2], Martijn van den Broek [5,6], Koen Theunis [7], Mirian Janssen [8], Elisabeth Cornelissen [6], Joris Vriens [4], Francesca Diomedi-Camassei [9], Rik Gijsbers [3,10], Lambertus van den Heuvel [2,6], Fanny O. Arcolino [2,‡] and Elena Levtchenko [1,2,*,‡]

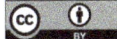

Citation: Veys, K.; Berlingerio, S.P.; David, D.; Bondue, T.; Held, K.; Reda, A.; van den Broek, M.; Theunis, K.; Janssen, M.; Cornelissen, E.; et al. Urine-Derived Kidney Progenitor Cells in Cystinosis. *Cells* **2022**, *11*, 1245. https://doi.org/10.3390/cells11071245

Academic Editor: Alfonso Eirin

Received: 31 January 2022
Accepted: 31 March 2022
Published: 6 April 2022

Publisher's Note: MDPI stays neutral with regard to jurisdictional claims in published maps and institutional affiliations.

Copyright: © 2022 by the authors. Licensee MDPI, Basel, Switzerland. This article is an open access article distributed under the terms and conditions of the Creative Commons Attribution (CC BY) license (https://creativecommons.org/licenses/by/4.0/).

1. Department of Pediatrics, University Hospitals Leuven Campus Gasthuisberg, B-3000 Leuven, Belgium; koenraad.veys@uzleuven.be
2. Laboratory of Pediatric Nephrology, Department of Development & Regeneration, KU Leuven Campus Gasthuisberg, B-3000 Leuven, Belgium; santeprinciero.berlingerio@kuleuven.be (S.P.B.); tjessa.bondue@kuleuven.be (T.B.); ahmed.reda@kuleuven.be (A.R.); bert.vandenheuvel@med.kuleuven.be (L.v.d.H.); fanny.oliveiraarcolino@kuleuven.be (F.O.A.)
3. Laboratory for Viral Vector Technology and Gene Therapy, Department of Pharmaceutical and Pharmacological Sciences, KU Leuven Campus Gasthuisberg, B-3000 Leuven, Belgium; dries.david@kuleuven.be (D.D.); rik.gijsbers@kuleuven.be (R.G.)
4. Laboratory of Endometrium, Endometriosis & Reproductive Medicine (LEERM), Department of Development & Regeneration, KU Leuven Campus Gasthuisberg, B-3000 Leuven, Belgium; kathi.held@kuleuven.be (K.H.); joris.vriens@kuleuven.be (J.V.)
5. Department of Pathology, Radboud Institute for Molecular Life Sciences, Radboud University Medical Center, 6524 Nijmegen, The Netherlands; martijn.vandenbroek@radboudumc.nl
6. Department of Pediatrics, Division of Pediatric Nephrology, Amalia Children's Hospital, Radboud University Medical Center, 6524 Nijmegen, The Netherlands; marlies.cornelissen@radboudumc.nl
7. Department of Human Genetics, KU Leuven Campus Gasthuisberg, B-3000 Leuven, Belgium; koen.theunis@kuleuven.be
8. Department of Internal Medicine, Radboud University Medical Center, 6524 Nijmegen, The Netherlands; mirian.janssen@radboudumc.nl
9. Unit of Pathology, Department of Laboratories, Bambino Gesù Children's Hospital, IRCCS, 00165 Rome, Italy; francesca.diomedi@opbg.net
10. Leuven Viral Vector Core, KU Leuven, B-3000 Leuven, Belgium
* Correspondence: elena.levtchenko@uzleuven.be; Tel.: +32-16-34-13-62
† These authors contributed equally to this work.
‡ These authors contributed equally to this work.

Abstract: Nephropathic cystinosis is an inherited lysosomal storage disorder caused by pathogenic variants in the cystinosin (*CTNS*) gene and is characterized by the excessive shedding of proximal tubular epithelial cells (PTECs) and podocytes into urine, development of the renal Fanconi syndrome and end-stage kidney disease (ESKD). We hypothesized that in compensation for epithelial cell losses, cystinosis kidneys undertake a regenerative effort, and searched for the presence of kidney progenitor cells (KPCs) in the urine of cystinosis patients. Urine was cultured in a specific progenitor medium to isolate undifferentiated cells. Of these, clones were characterized by qPCR, subjected to a differentiation protocol to PTECs and podocytes and assessed by qPCR, Western blot, immunostainings and functional assays. Cystinosis patients voided high numbers of undifferentiated cells in urine, of which various clonal cell lines showed a high capacity for self-renewal and expressed kidney progenitor markers, which therefore were assigned as cystinosis urine-derived KPCs (Cys-uKPCs). Cys-uKPC clones showed the capacity to differentiate between functional PTECs and/or podocytes. Gene addition with wild-type *CTNS* using lentiviral vector technology resulted in significant reductions in cystine levels. We conclude that KPCs present in the urine of cystinosis patients can be isolated, differentiated and complemented with *CTNS* in vitro, serving as a novel tool for disease modeling.

Keywords: cystinosis; kidney progenitors; cell model; gene therapy

1. Introduction

Cystinosis is a rare autosomal recessive lysosomal storage disorder, caused by biallelic pathogenic variants in the *CTNS* gene leading to the malfunctioning or absence of the cystine-proton cotransporter cystinosin [1]. It is a multisystem disease in which the kidney is the first and most severely affected organ [2]. In the infantile phenotype, the most common and severe form, a generalized proximal tubular dysfunction (renal Fanconi syndrome) develops in infancy, followed by progressive chronic kidney disease (CKD) leading to end-stage kidney disease (ESKD) [3]. The juvenile phenotype is characterized by a less pronounced Fanconi syndrome and slower kidney function decline. Cysteamine, a cystine-depleting amino-thiol, effectively reduces intracellular cystine accumulation and is currently the only available disease-modifying treatment [3]. Cysteamine treatment has been shown to prolong life expectancy, improve growth, postpone the onset of ESKD and reduce the number of extra-renal manifestations of cystinosis [4–6]. However, it offers no cure for renal Fanconi syndrome and does not prevent the need for renal replacement therapy [5,6].

Earlier, we demonstrated a remarkable loss of proximal tubular epithelial cells (PTECs) and podocytes in the urine of cystinosis patients [7]. Therefore, we hypothesized that in compensation for this epithelial cell loss, cystinosis kidneys might show an attempt for regeneration, which could be reflected by the presence of kidney progenitor cells in the urine. The actual existence of a stem/progenitor cell niche in the human adult kidney has been a matter of debate for more than a decade. A majority of studies have suggested the presence of a progenitor cell population by deriving them directly from kidney tissue and characterizing in vitro properties and functional potential in animal models of kidney injury, while few have investigated urine as a source for kidney progenitor cells [8–19].

In addition, current cystinosis kidney cell models show several limitations [20]. Primary cells can only be obtained by invasive means via kidney biopsies which are not required for regular clinical care and can be contaminated with several cell types. While these primary cells show a limited proliferative capacity, immortalization might affect the transcriptome, interfere with important cellular pathways and may be unreliable at high passage numbers [20–22]. The development of induced pluripotent stem cells (iPSC) is laborious and expensive and iPSC reprogramming might induce genomic side effects [23]. Therefore, alternative cystinosis cell models that demonstrate the primary phenotype of cystinosis and harbor a proliferative capacity without having the disadvantages of immortalization are desirable. These models can further improve our understanding of the cellular pathophysiology of cystinosis and help to elucidate the exclusive functions of cystinosin [20].

In this study, we describe the presence of a niche of kidney progenitor cells in cystinosis patients, which can be non-invasively isolated from urine and serve as a novel tool for disease modeling.

2. Materials and Methods

2.1. Study Participants

The ethical board of UZ/KU Leuven (Ethische Commissie Onderzoek UZ/KU Leuven) approved the study (s54695) and participants signed an informed consent form. The research was conducted in accordance with the latest version of the Declaration of Helsinki, the principles of Good Clinical Practice (GCP) and all applicable national and international legislation related to research involving human subjects [24].

Fresh urine samples were obtained from non-kidney transplanted nephropathic cystinosis patients, followed at the University Hospital Leuven (UZ Leuven), Belgium and Radboud umc Nijmegen, The Netherlands, and from healthy (not age- or gender-matched) controls. Relevant demographic and clinical data were collected from the medical records of the participants (Table 1).

Table 1. Clinical characteristics of the cystinosis patients included in the study at the moment of culturing urine samples in progenitor medium.

Patient	Age	Sex	Cystinosis Genotype	eGFR	Urine Protein/ Creatinine	WBC Cystine	# Clonal Colonies	Cys-uKPC Clones
1	10	F	57kb del + c.926dupG	78	1.97	0.5	0	
2	4	F	Hom 57kb del	>90	2.85	4.26	2	
3	16	M	Hom 57kb del	89	1.82	0.3	9	
4	13	F	c.198_218del + c.926dupG	48	3.04	0.2	16	
5	6	M	57kb del + c.926dupG	>90	4.93	0.32	5	
6 *	13	F	57kb del + c.198_218del	88	1.76	2.45	51	#1–5
7	14	F	Hom 57kb del	53	0.65	2.52	3	
8	4	M	57kb del + IVS 10-7G>A	>90	0.41	1.8	0	
9 *	16	M	Hom 57kb del	46	2.94	3.14	20	#6, #7

Age: expressed in years; eGFR: estimated glomerular filtration rate, expressed as ml/min/1.73 m^2; urine protein/creatine ratio is expressed as g/g creatinine; WBC: white blood cell; WBC cystine concentration is expressed as nmol $\frac{1}{2}$ cystine/mg protein; #: number; # clonal colonies: number of clonal colonies growing from a single fresh urine sample upon incubation in progenitor medium. *: patients that gave rise to the established Cys-uKPC clones described in this study.

2.2. Estimation of the Number of Undifferentiated Cells in Urine via Quantitative Polymerase Chain Reaction (qPCR)

Vimentin (*VIM*) is a known marker of mesenchymal cells, being expressed by undifferentiated cells of the metanephric mesenchyme in the human fetal kidney. Vimentin-expressing cells have consistently been shown to co-express CD133 and PAX2 in kidney progenitor cells. Therefore, we assessed the presence of undifferentiated cells in the urine of cystinosis patients by quantifying vimentin-positive cells [8,15,25–27]. Briefly, a calibration curve for the mRNA expression of vimentin was developed using known numbers of control human kidney stem cells, which express vimentin (kindly provided by Prof. B. Bussolati, Università degli Studi di Torino, Turin, Italy) [8,28] (Figure S1). To establish the calibration curve, cells were sorted by fluorescence activated cell sorting (FACS) using the BD FACSAria III (BD Biosciences, San Jose, CA, USA) at the VIB-KU Leuven FACS Core Facility, in a 96-well plate containing 4 µL of lysis buffer (0.2% TritonX-100 + RNase inhibitor) yielding a range of cells per well from 1 to 500 cells (Figure S1).

The Smart-Seq2 protocol allowed the preparation of cDNA from very low numbers of cells. An adaption of the protocol of Picelli et al. was applied up to PCR purification (step 26), and 18 PCR cycles were performed in step 14. qPCR was performed using the reference gene ß-Actin, and vimentin as a marker for undifferentiated cells [28] (Figure S1). The *VIM* primer used is indicated in Table S4.

After establishing the *VIM* calibration curve, urine samples were collected from cystinosis patients and healthy subjects, centrifuged (200× g, 4 °C, 5 min), and the cell pellet was resuspended in phosphate buffered saline (PBS) and diluted 100×. The cycle threshold (ct) value for *VIM* achieved in the qPCR analysis was plotted in the calibration curve for extrapolation of the number of undifferentiated cells voided in urine. Given that cystinosis patients are polyuric, urine samples of cystinosis patients showed a higher volume and were more diluted in comparison with urine samples of healthy control subjects. Therefore, results were normalized to urine volume and creatinine values, the latter to correct for the concentration of the urine sample.

2.3. Establishment of Cystinosis Urine-Derived Kidney Progenitor Cells (Cys-uKPCs)

Fresh urine samples were centrifuged (300× g, 5 min, room temperature), the supernatant was removed, and the cell pellet was washed with PBS, followed by re-centrifugation. Depending on the size of the cell pellet, cells were seeded in a single or multiple 10 cm Petri dishes and incubated in a medium containing a 1:1 ratio of keratinocyte-serum free medium (Keratinocyte-serum free medium + L-glutamine Gibco® Life Technologies reference number 17005-034, 5 ng/mL epidermal growth factor, 50 ng/mL bovine pituitary extract, 30 ng/mL cholera toxin, 100 U/mL penicillin, 1mg/ml streptomycin) and progenitor cell medium (3/4 Dulbecco's Modified Eagle's medium Lonza category number BE12-733F, ¼ Hamm's F12 Lonza category number BE12615F), 10% fetal bovine serum, 0.4 ug/mL hydrocortisone, 10^{-10} M cholera toxin, 5 ng/mL insulin, 1.8×10^{-4} M adenine, 5 ug/mL transferrin, 2×10^{-9} M 3,39,5 tri-iodo L-thyronine, 10 ng/mL epidermal growth factor, 1% penicillin-streptomycin) (1:1 mix), in the following, altogether referred to as progenitor medium, at 37 °C in 5% CO_2 [17,29].

Clonal colonies of cells could be observed after 3–5 days of culturing the fresh urine sample and were picked between 9 and 14 days. Each picked clonal colony is hereafter further named as 'clone' [30]. Each clone was seeded in a single well of a 24-well plate (passage number 1, P#1). Upon reaching 70–80% confluence, cells were trypsinized and counted using the BioRad TC20™ automated cell counter (BioRad #145-0101). In passage 2 (P#2), all cells were transferred into a 6 cm cell culture dish, while by the next passage (P#3) 2/3rd of cells were plated in a 10cm dish. From the 4th passage on, a splitting ratio of $\frac{1}{4}$ was maintained and cells were further proliferated in 10 cm Petri dishes until senescence was reached. Senescence was defined as the inability to form a subconfluent (70–80% confluence) monolayer within 14 days of culture. Mycoplasma tests were performed every 2 months and no bacterial contamination was detected in any of the culture samples.

2.4. Characterization of Cys-uKPCs

The isolated clones were characterized as Cys-uKPCs based on their proliferative capacity (doubling time), and by their gene expression profile as assessed by qPCR. The doubling times were calculated according to the following formula: doubling time = duration * log (2)/log (final concentration) − log (initial concentration) [31]. The following kidney progenitor genes were assessed by qPCR: Neural Cell Adhesion Molecule 1 (NCAM1), CBP/p300 interacting transactivators with glutamic acid (E)/aspartic acid (D)-rich C-terminal domain (CITED1), vimentin (VIM) and paired box 2 (PAX2); while β-Actin was used as the housekeeping gene. Briefly, mRNA was isolated using the RNeasy Mini or Micro Kit (Qiagen GmbH, Hilden, Germany), according to the manufacturer's protocol. RNA was synthesized to cDNA using a mix of Oligo (dT) 12–18 Primer, random primers, dNTP mix (100 mM) and SuperScript™ III Reverse Transcriptase, all from Invitrogen. qPCR was executed on a CFX96™ Real-Time PCR Detection System, using Platinum™ SYBR™ Green qPCR SuperMix-UDG w/ROX (Thermo Fisher), 10 µM of primers and 1 µL of cDNA (5 ng/µL). qPCR data were retrieved and processed using the CFX Manager™ software (Bio-Rad, Hercules, CA, USA). All antibodies and primers used are specified in Table S3 and Table S4, respectively. Clones were considered Cys-uKPCs when they (1) showed a high self-renewal capacity (mean doubling time at P#3: 35 h ± 13 h; at P#5: 56 h ± 19 h) that allowed a full characterization of these cells (including gene expression analysis in P#4 and assessment of differentiation to PTEC or podocyte in P#6), (2) cells expressed a panel of kidney progenitor genes CITED1, NCAM1, VIM and PAX2 at P#4, and (3) showed signs of differentiation to either PTEC or Podocyte as evidenced by either upregulation PTEC- or podocyte-specific genes, respectively, upon subjection to the corresponding differentiation protocol (see below) (Figure S2).

2.5. Differentiation of Cys-uKPCs to Podocytes and Proximal Tubular Epithelial Cells

All presumed Cys-uKPC clones were subjected to a differentiation protocol towards podocytes ('Cys-uKPC-Podo') in passage #6 via incubation in VRAD medium (DMEM-

F12, 10% FBS, 100nM vitamin D3, 100µM all-trans retinoic acid) for 7 days, during which the VRAD medium was refreshed 2 times (every 2–3 days). Expression of podocyte-specific markers synaptopodin (*SYNPO*), podocalyxin (*PODXL*), and Wilms' Tumor 1 (*WT1*) were assessed by qPCR, and changes in cellular morphology during differentiation were monitored by light microscopy. Depending on gene expression results, also Western blot and immunofluorescence staining were performed.

In parallel, the same Cys-uKPC clones were also subjected to a differentiation protocol towards PTECs (Cys-uKPC-PTEC) in passage #6 by incubation in PTEC medium (DMEM-F12, Insulin 5 µg/mL, Thyroxin 5 µg/mL, Selenium 5 ng/mL, Hydrocortisone 36 ng/mL, EGF 10 ng/mL, Tri-iodothyronine 40 pg/mL, 10% FBS, 1% penicillin-streptomycin) for 7 days, during which the PTEC medium was refreshed 2 times (every 2–3 days). The expression of PTEC-specific markers aquaporin 1 (*AQP1*) and P-glycoprotein (P-gp) (*ABCB1*) was demonstrated by rt-PCR and qPCR. Depending on the gene expression results, a Western blot was performed.

2.6. Western Blot

Cell pellets were lysed in RIPA lysis buffer (Thermo Fisher Scientific, Waltham, MA, USA) supplemented with protease and phosphatase inhibitors. Total protein concentrations were quantified using a Pierce BCA Protein Assay Kit (Thermo Fisher Scientific, Waltham, MA, USA). For the synaptopodin, podocalyxin and aquaporin 1 Western blot, 10 µg total protein were loaded, while for the Cystinosin-3HA Western blot, 15 µg total protein was loaded on a precast gel NuPAGE Novex 4–12% Bis–Tris (Thermo Fisher Scientific, Waltham, MA, USA) and transferred on a nitrocellulose membrane using an iBlot2 dry blotting system.

Membranes were incubated overnight at 4 °C with primary antibodies against aquaporin 1, synaptopodin, podocalyxin and β-Actin on a blocking buffer. Next, membranes were incubated with HRP-linked secondary antibodies anti-rabbit or mouse in a 1:2000 dilution in 5% milk in TBS-T. Proteins were visualized using ECL Substrate (Thermo Fisher Scientific, Waltham, MA, USA). Images were acquired using the Syngene Chemi XRQ System and quantified with ImageJ software.

The specification of all antibodies is described in Table S3.

2.7. Immunofluorescence Staining and Microscopy

Twenty to forty thousand cells were seeded, fixed, and permeabilized, followed by blocking and incubation of primary and secondary antibodies (Table S3). Microscopy was performed on the Nikon Eclipse Ci microscope (Nikon Corporation, Tokyo, Japan), while confocal microscopy images were recorded on the Zeiss® LSM 880—Airyscan (Carl Zeiss Microscopy GmbH, Jena, Germany) (Cell and Tissue Imaging cluster/Cell Imaging Core (CIC), Pieter Vanden Berghe, KU Leuven, B-3000 Leuven, Belgium). Microscopy images were processed and analyzed using the Zeiss ZEN Black and Blue imaging software and Fiji/ImageJ.

2.8. Functional Assessment of Cys-uKPC-Podo and Cys-uKPC-PTEC

2.8.1. Albumin Endocytosis Assay

The functionality of Cys-uKPC-Podo was analyzed by monitoring the capacity of endocytic uptake of albumin in an Alexa Fluor™ 555 albumin endocytosis assay in passage #7 (Figure S2). Eighty thousand Cys-uKPCs, Cys-uKPC–Podo and cystinosis conditionally immortalized podocytes (ciPodocyte$^{CTNS-/-}$) were seeded on glass coverslips. Following differentiation, cells were starved by incubation in serum- and supplement-free medium (DMEM-F12; Lonza) for 2 h. Hereafter, incubation with a complete medium supplemented with 100 µg/mL of Alexa Fluor™ 555 conjugated bovine serum albumin (BSA) (Life Technologies, Carlsbad, CA, USA) was performed for 60 minutes in parallel at 37 °C and at 4 °C, the latter for confirming the temperature dependency of specific receptor-mediated albumin endocytosis in podocytes and to rule out non-specific binding and uptake of albumin [32]. The uptake of the labeled BSA was analyzed by fluorescence microscopy using the Nikon Eclipse Ci microscope (Nikon Corporation, Tokyo, Japan). Quantification of BSA uptake was analyzed using Fiji/ImageJ software, and based on the principle of corrected total cell fluorescence (CTCF) [33]. A correct interpretation of actual BSA uptake by the individual cells was ensured by visualization of the cell border via enhancement of image brightness and contrast in Fiji/ImageJ. The experiment was performed in one Cys-uKPC clone differentiated (in triplicate) to Cys-uKPC-Podo (Cys-uKPC #1-Podo) and an average of 5 images containing on average 23 cells per image were quantified per condition.

2.8.2. Calcium Influx Assay

Given the pivotal importance of calcium dynamics in podocytes, Cys-uKPC-Podo should demonstrate a more mature system of calcium signaling as evidenced by higher responsiveness to agonists of transient receptor potential calcium channels (TRPCs) [34–36]. TRPC3 is known to be widely expressed in renal epithelial cells, while TRPC6 is of specific importance in podocytes [37,38]. Therefore, the functionality of Cys-uKPC-Podo was also analyzed by evaluating the calcium influx in a Fura calcium imaging assay in comparison to their undifferentiated Cys-uKPC counterparts in passage #7 [17,39]. Cys-uKPCs were seeded on glass coverslips and were differentiated to podocytes (Cys-uKPC-Podo). Cys-uKPC-Podo was incubated with 2 µM Fura-2 acetoxymethyl ester (Invitrogen™) for 20 min at 37 °C. Standard imaging solutions consisted of 150 mM NaCl, 2 mM $CaCl_2$, 1 mM $MgCl_2$, 10 mM HEPES (pH 7.4 by NaOH). Perfusion of the bath solutions was based on gravity via a multi-barreled pipette tip with a single outlet of 0.8 mm diameter. Intracellular Ca^{2+} concentration was determined based on the ratio of fluorescence detected upon alternating excitation at 340 and 380 nm, using a Lambda XL illuminator (Sutter Instruments, Novato, CA, USA) and an Orca Flash 4.0 camera (Hamamatsu Photonics Belgium, Mont-Saint-Guibert, Belgium) on a Nikon Eclipse Ti fluorescence microscope (Nikon Benelux, Brussels, Belgium). Data were analyzed using NIS-Elements software (Nikon) and IgorPro 6.2 (WaveMetrics, Portland, OR, USA). 1-oleoyl-2-acetyl-sn-glycerol (OAG) (Sigma-Aldrich, Burlington, MA, USA), a TRPC6 agonist, was applied (150 mM) in order to stimulate calcium influx and assess the response rate of the cell type studied. Cells showing an increase in calcium amplitude higher than 50 nM and a slope increase higher than three times the standard deviation were considered as responders to OAG stimulation. Only cells that responded to the positive control, ionomycin, at the end of the experiment were analyzed. All experiments were performed on at least 3 independent coverslips. Undifferentiated Cys-uKPCs were also assessed, while wild-type ciPodocytes (ciPodocyte^{WT}), incubated for 10–14 days at 37 °C, were used as a positive control.

2.8.3. Transferrin Endocytosis Assay

The functionality of Cys-uKPC-PTEC with regard to receptor-mediated endocytosis was assessed via a fluorescence-labeled transferrin endocytosis assay in passage #7. Cys-uKPCs were differentiated to PTEC (Cys-uKPC-PTEC), as previously described, and starved for 60 min at 37 °C in basal medium (DMEM F-12 with 1% BSA). Thereafter, Cys-uKPC-PTEC were washed with ice-cold PBS and incubated with an Alexa Fluor™ 555 conjugated transferrin (TF555, Life Technologies) (25 µg/mL) in basal medium for 30 min at 4 °C, followed by incubation at 37 °C for 15, 30, 45 and 60 min in complete medium. Immunofluorescence imaging was performed using the Eclipse CI microscope (Nikon, Tokyo, Japan). For analysis, 30 cells were studied per time point, using the ImageJ software. The fluorescence per cell was quantified and the background signal subtracted. For the analysis of endocytic uptake at different time points, data were normalized to time point zero.

2.9. Kidney Biopsy Specimen & Immunohistochemistry

A kidney tissue specimen was retrieved from the native kidney of one nephropathic cystinosis patient who had undergone nephrectomy because of ongoing renal Fanconi syndrome following kidney transplantation and assessed for the presence of the kidney progenitor cells via staining of CD133 and PAX2. Since this specimen was retrieved for clinical purposes, retrospective coverage by an ethical board for approval was not applicable. The clinical characteristics of the patient are presented in Table S3. Stainings on control biopsies are shown in Figure S5. The PAX2 control staining was performed in a developing kidney specimen, more specifically, from a healthy fetus of a gestational age of 28 weeks, of whom a biopsy was taken for regular clinical care purposes. The CD133 control staining was performed in the adult transplant kidney of a healthy 13-year-old teenager, while a kidney biopsy in the context of acute tubular injury, taken for regular clinical care purposes, was used as a positive control for CD133. The specification of the antibodies that were used for this application is indicated in Table S3.

2.10. Lentiviral Vector Design and Transduction Experiments

The Leuven Viral Vector Core (LVVC) developed several self-inactivating (SIN) lentiviral vector (LV) constructs, using a human elongation factor-1 alpha (EF-1 α) promoter to drive the expression of either *CTNS* (full-length cDNA; tagged with a 3HA tag at its C-terminus) or *eGFP* or *dATP13A2* (a deactivated version of ATP13A2, a lysosomal transmembrane protein) as a transgene, followed by an EMCV IRES-puromycin antibiotic resistance cassette, referred to as LV_CTNS-3HA, LV_eGFP and LV_dATP13A2, respectively (Figure S7, panel A) [40]. Validation of the LV constructs was performed in skin fibroblasts, that were obtained from a cystinosis patient prior to cysteamine treatment, via immunofluorescence staining and Western blot analysis (Figure S7, panel B–E) [41]. Two Cys-uKPC clonal cell lines (Cys-uKPC #1, Cys-uKPC #7) were transduced, resulting in the following cell lines: Cys-uKPC #1 LV_CTNS-3HA and Cys-uKPC #7 LV_CTNS-3HA, Cys-uKPC #1 LV_eGFP and Cys-uKPC #7 LV_eGFP, and Cys-uKPC #7 LV_dATP13A2. In order to ensure a single integrated viral vector copy per cell, viral vector transduction was conducted employing a limiting dilution series. Cells were transduced for 72 h and subsequently selected by adding puromycin (1 µg/mL) to the medium. We selected the highest dilution that still resulted in surviving cells upon puromycin selection (<20% surviving cells, which indicates a single integrated viral vector copy, corresponding to an MOI < 0.5) [42]. The corresponding non-functional p24 titers for this condition were, for Cys-uKPC #1 LV_CTNS-3HA 0.003 pg p24/mL, in Cys-uKPC #1 LV_eGFP 0.0009 pg p24/mL, while in Cys-uKPC #7 LV_CTNS-3HA the p24 titer was 0.06 pg p24/mL, 0.02 pg p24/mL for the Cys-uKPC #7 LV_eGFP and 0.04 pg p24/mL for the Cys-uKPC #7 LV_dATP13A2 transduced conditions. The resulting selected transduced Cys-uKPCs were harvested for mRNA isolation and assessment of intracellular cystine levels.

2.11. Cystine Measurements

One million cells were washed with PBS, 200 µL of ice-cold N-ethylmaleimide ('NEM') was added to block free thiol groups, followed by collecting the cells by scraping. An amount of 100 µL of 12% sulfosalicylic acid ('SSA') was added for protein precipitation, vortexed for 30 s for homogenization, and centrifuged (10 min, $10,000\times g$, 4 °C). The cystine-containing supernatants were isolated for the cystine assay and kept immediately at −80 °C, while the protein pellet was incubated with 300 µL of 0.1M NaOH (Sigma-Aldrich) overnight, and then transferred to −80 °C until the total protein concentration was determined by a BCA assay. Cystine was measured by liquid chromatography coupled to tandem mass spectrometry ('LC-MS/MS') in a kind collaboration with the Laboratory of Pathology and Metabolism of the Bambino Gesù Pediatric Hospital, Rome. Cystine concentrations were expressed as nmol cystine/mg protein.

2.12. Statistical Analysis

Graphpad Prism (version 9.3.1 (350) for Mac OS X) (GraphPad Software, La Jolla, CA, USA, www.Graphpad.com, accessed on 7 December 2021) was used for the statistical analysis. The D'Agostino & Pearson normality test was applied in order to check for normality of the distribution of the medians of the parameters of the cystinosis patients and the control subjects. Depending on this distribution, a two-tailed unpaired Student's *t*-test or Mann–Whitney U test was performed.

3. Results

3.1. Nephropathic Cystinosis Is Characterized by a Loss of Undifferentiated Cells in Urine

To test our hypothesis that a significant loss of kidney epithelial cells in cystinosis patients could be compensated with an attempt for regeneration, we first explored whether undifferentiated cells, characterized by expression of vimentin, are present in the urine of cystinosis patients [7].

Therefore, we adapted a method used for single-cell RNA extraction and amplification to quantify vimentin-expressing cells voided in urine (Figure S1). Urine samples were collected from nine cystinosis patients and nine healthy subjects (Table S1).

Cystinosis patients presented a higher number of undifferentiated cells in the urine, which were not observed in healthy subjects (Figure 1). There was no correlation between the number of undifferentiated cells with age (Spearman r -0.25, $p = 0.52$), proteinuria (Spearman r -0.62, $p = 0.09$), kidney function (eGFR; Spearman r 0.22, $p = 0.58$), the white blood cell cystine level (WBC cystine level) (Spearman r 0.15, $p = 0.71$), or the cystinosis genotype (Figure S3).

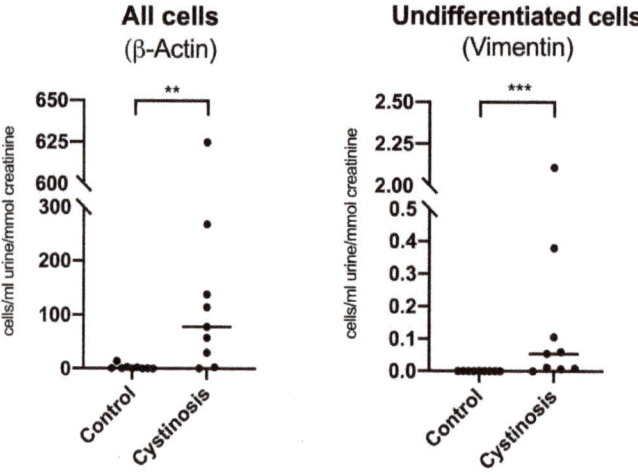

Figure 1. Quantification of undifferentiated cells in urine of cystinosis patients versus healthy controls. Total number of cells (β-Actin signal, left) and number of undifferentiated cells (vimentin signal, right) voided in urine of cystinosis patients ($n = 9$) compared to healthy controls ($n = 9$). The cycle threshold (ct) value achieved in the qPCR analysis was plotted in a calibration curve for estimation of the total number of cells and the number of undifferentiated cells voided in urine, which was normalized to urine volume and urine creatinine values. Statistical significance was evaluated using Mann–Whitney U test comparing controls versus cystinosis patients; median is indicated with the horizontal line in the midst of the individual values. $p < 0.01$: **; $p < 0.001$: ***.

3.2. Undifferentiated Cells in Urine of Cystinosis Patients Comprise Kidney Progenitor Cells (Cys-uKPCs)

In order to explore whether these undifferentiated cells comply as kidney progenitor cells, we isolated, expanded and characterized clonal cell lines following a standardized protocol in line with our method on the isolation and expansion of kidney progenitor cells from the urine of preterm born neonates (neonatal kidney stem progenitor cells, nKSPCs) (Figure S2) [17].

Therefore, urine samples of all recruited cystinosis patients were cultured in a progenitor medium (Table 1; Figure S2).

This culture yielded an average of 0.9 clonal colonies/ml urine volume (SD 1.7 clonal colonies/ml urine volume). The clonal colonies that showed the highest capacity for self-renewal were picked, expanded and further referred to as 'clones' (Figure S2). These clones showed a spindle-shaped morphology and a characteristic petal-like pattern of organization, resembling that of kidney stem progenitor cells isolated from the urine of preterm neonates (Figure 2A) [17].

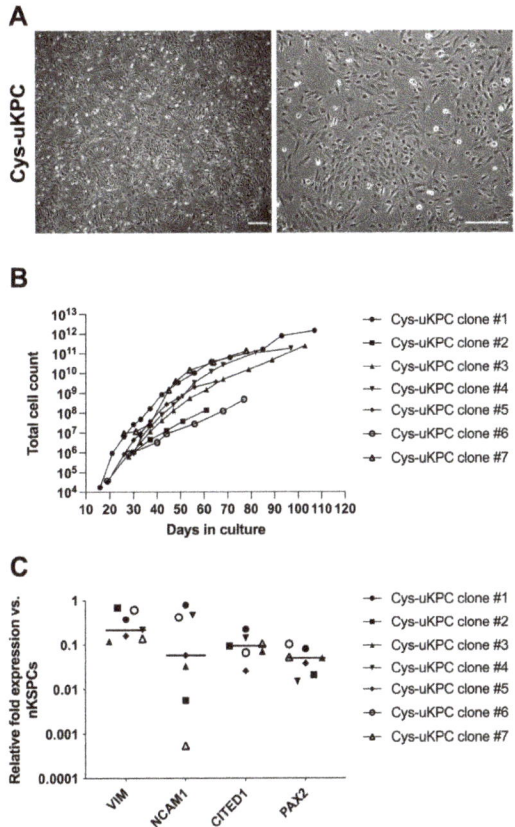

Figure 2. Characterization of cystinosis urine-derived kidney progenitor cell (Cys-uKPC) clones. (**A**) Phase contrast microscopy of a representative clone of Cys-uKPCs (Cys-uKPC #1) shows the characteristic petal-like pattern of in vitro expansion and organization (left panel) and the spindle-shaped to rhombic cellular morphology (right panel). Scale bar: 250 µm; (**B**) In vitro proliferative capacity of the seven established Cys-uKPC clones. Total number of cells grown versus days in culture before Cys-uKPC clones showed senescence and stopped proliferating. Each specific Cys-uKPC clone is represented by a symbol that is similarly used in panel (**B**,**C**) (see the legend on right in the figure). (**C**) Relative fold expression of a panel of selected nephrogenesis genes for characterizing the Cys-uKPC clones (n = 7), relative to β-actin and normalized to the expression in human neonatal kidney stem/progenitor cells (nKSPCs). In the midst of the individual values, the median of the values is represented by the horizontal line.

Since patient #6 and patient #9 showed a remarkable higher yield in a number of clonal colonies growing in the progenitor medium compared with other patients (Table 1) and both represent the full clinical spectrum of nephropathic cystinosis (patient #9: infantile phenotype, patient #6: juvenile phenotype), clonal colonies from only these two patients were selected for further experiments.

Seven clones, assigned as Cys-uKPC #1 until #7, that were isolated from these two patients (patient #6: Cys-uKPC clone #1–5; patient #9: Cys-uKPC clone #6 & #7), stayed in culture for an average 86 ± 18 days and on average 11 ± 3 passages before reaching senescence. The doubling times observed per clone in the earliest passage, in which the automated counting of cells was possible, ranged from 20.87 to 50.58 hours. The total number of cells yielded per clone before reaching senescence ranged from 1.39×10^8 to 1.46×10^{12} (Figure 2B). All seven clones showed expression of kidney progenitor genes *NCAM1*, *CITED1*, *VIM* and *PAX2* (Figure 2C) as assessed by qPCR in passage #4, in which nKSPCs were applied as a positive control.

As a result, these seven clones were used for assessing their differentiation potential into kidney epithelial cells and were presumed to be cystinosis urine-derived kidney progenitor cell (Cys-uKPC) clones.

3.3. Differentiation of Cys-uKPCs In Vitro towards Functional Podocytes and PTECs

3.3.1. Differentiation of Cys-uKPCs into Functional Podocytes

All seven Cys-uKPC clones (#1–#7) were subjected to the podocyte differentiation protocol using the VRAD medium. Following differentiation, in three of these seven Cys-uKPC clones (Cys-uKPC #1, #5, #6), the cell size increased, and cells showed multiple cellular protrusions (Figure 3A), while a proportion of cells became bi-or multi-nucleated (Figure 3C). At the mRNA level, a significant upregulation of podocyte-specific genes *SYNPO* and *PODXL* was observed (Figure 3, panel B). These differentiated Cys-uKPC clones were hereafter coined Cys-uKPC-Podo. Although Cys-uKPC-Podocytes showed a significantly lower expression of WT1 in comparison to Cys-uKPCs, kidney progenitor cells are known to show a high expression of WT1 [43]. Therefore, downregulation of WT1 following differentiation of kidney progenitors towards podocytes should not be regarded as a sign of unsuccessful differentiation [43].

We further explored protein expression of podocyte-specific genes and podocyte-related functionality in one of these three Cys-uKPC-Podo cell lines (Cys-uKPC #1-Podo), compared to its undifferentiated counterpart (Cys-uKPC #1). At the protein level, increased expression of synaptopodin and podocalyxin in Cys-uKPC-Podo compared to Cys-uKPCs was confirmed and consistent with the results of the relative increase in *SYNPO* and *PODXL* gene expression data (Figure 3C,D).

Given that the endocytic process in podocytes is fundamental to maintaining the glomerular filtration barrier, we assessed the endocytosis capacity in a fluorescence-labeled albumin endocytosis assay [44,45]. We demonstrated that, while no uptake of albumin was observed in the undifferentiated Cys-uKPC (Cys-uKPC #1), effective endocytosis of albumin was present in Cys-uKPC-Podo (Cys-uKPC #1-Podo; Figure 3E,F), comparable with a conditionally immortalized cystinosis podocyte (ciPodocyte$^{CTNS-/-}$). By comparing a 37 °C and 4 °C condition, we confirmed the temperature dependency of specific receptor-mediated albumin endocytosis in podocytes and thus were able to rule out non-specific binding and uptake of albumin. In addition, several studies demonstrated the vital role of Ca^{2+} signaling in podocytes [34–37,39,46,47]. Therefore, we evaluated the potential of calcium uptake and demonstrated that Cys-uKPC-Podo (Cys-uKPC #1-Podo) show an increased number of responders to the TRPC6 agonist OAG in a Fura-2AM calcium influx assay, compared to Cys-uKPCs (Cys-uKPC #1; Figure 3G–I). The percentage of OAG-responders from Cys-uKPC–Podo was comparable to wild-type ciPodocytes (ciPodocyte$^{CTNS\ WT}$) (Figure 3I).

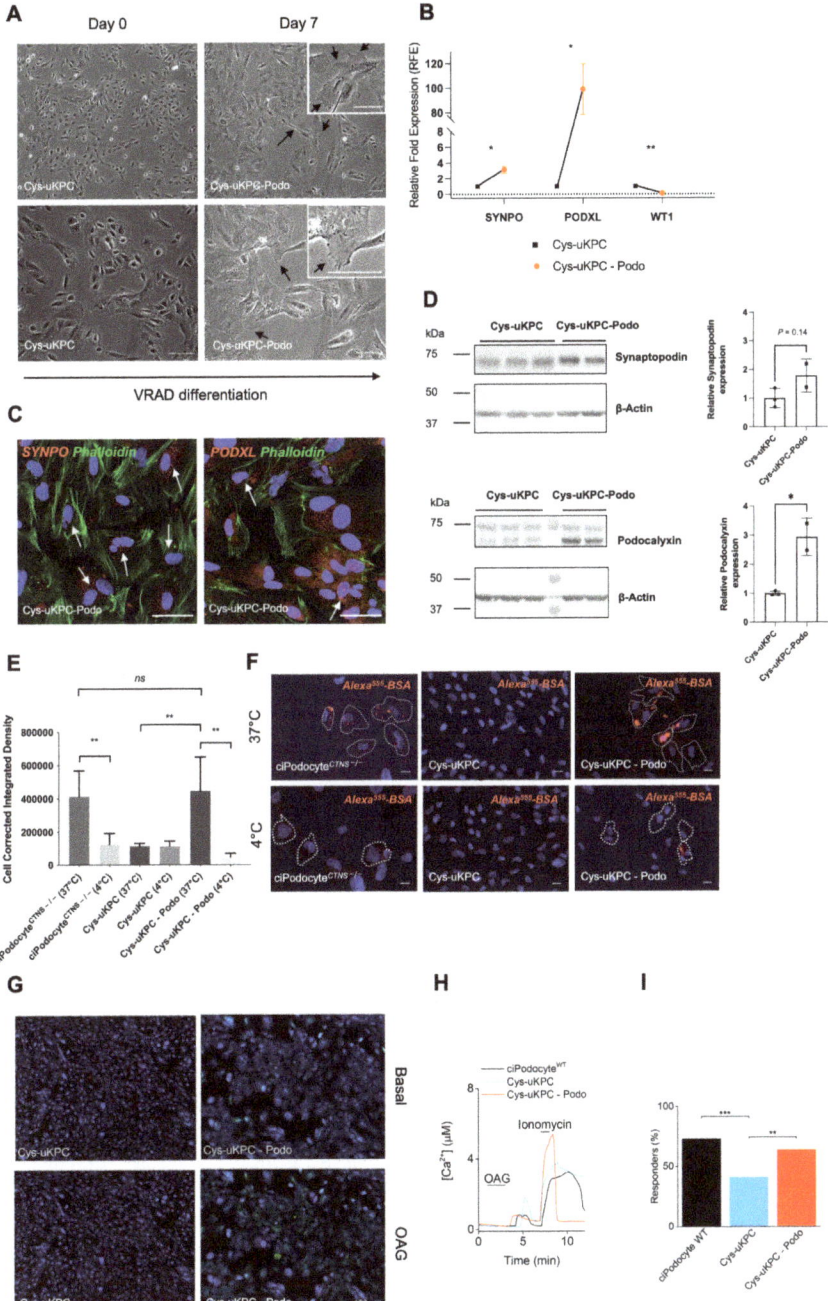

Figure 3. Differentiation of Cys-uKPC in vitro into functional podocytes. (**A**) Phase contrast microscopy of a Cys-uKPC clone with a podocyte fate (Cys-uKPC #1), demonstrating the cellular morphological

changes while undergoing differentiation from kidney progenitors (Cys-uKPC; day 0, left column) towards podocytes (Cys-uKPC-Podocyte; day 7, right column) via incubation in VRAD medium. During differentiation, cells become enlarged and show cellular protrusions (black arrows), which are specifically depicted in the zoomed subpanels in the right upper corners of the microscopy pictures in the right column. A proportion of cells became bi-or multinucleated, which can be better appreciated in panel C (white arrows). Similar results were obtained for the other clones. While the lower magnification pictures (top panels) demonstrate the growth pattern and organization of cells, the higher magnification pictures (bottom panels) illustrate better cellular morphology. Scale bar: 100 µm; (**B**) qPCR analysis of podocyte-specific gene expression in Cys-uKPC-derived podocytes relative to β-actin and normalized to Cys-uKPCs of a Cys-uKPC clone (Cys-uKPC #1) with a podocyte fate. Cys-uKPC-Podo data is indicated with an orange dot which represents the mean with bars representing the SEM of three independent experiments with three technical replicates each; Cys-uKPC data is indicated with a black square. $p < 0.05$: *; (**C**) Immunofluorescence staining for podocyte-specific proteins synaptopodin and podocalyxin (red), and F-actin filament cytoskeletal staining via phalloidin (green) in Cys-uKPC-Podo. Nuclei are stained using DAPI. Bi- or multinucleated cells are indicated with white arrows. Scale bar 50 µm. Results depicted originate from the Cys-uKPC clone #1; the individual color channels of each merged immunofluorescence picture depicted here can be appreciated in Figure S4; (**D**) Western blot and quantification for podocyte-specific proteins synaptopodin and podocalyxin in Cys-uKPC-Podo compared to their undifferentiated kidney progenitor counterparts (Cys-uKPC). Increased expression of synaptopodin and podocalyxin is observed in the Cys-uKPC-Podo condition compared to Cys-uKPC, with the corresponding quantification depicted on the right. Results depicted originate from the Cys-uKPC clone #1; (**E**) Cys-uKPC-Podo show a significantly increased capacity for albumin endocytosis that is comparable to that observed in ciPodocyte$^{CTNS-/-}$, in contrast to their undifferentiated Cys-uKPCs counterparts. Quantification of the albumin endocytosis assay using cell corrected integrated density of the signal originating from Alexa Fluor^{TM} 555 labeled albumin in the various conditions: 118,172 AU vs. 402,791 AU; actual difference: 284,619 AU; 95% CI of difference: 211,091 to 454,293; $p = 0.003$. Cell corrected integrated density ciPodocyte$^{CTNS-/-}$ vs. Cys-uKPC-Podo: 442,469 AU vs. 402,791 AU; actual difference: −39,678 AU; 95% CI of difference: −216,228 to 269,379, $p > 0.99$; (**F**) Representative immunofluorescent images of the Alexa Fluor^{TM} 555 albumin endocytosis assay for ciPodocyte$^{CTNS-/-}$, Cys-uKPC and Cys-uKPC-Podo at 37 °C and 4 °C. Results depicted originate from the Cys-uKPC clone #1. The dotted line identifies the border of the individual cells. (**G**) Cys-uKPC-Podo shows an increased number of responders to OAG in a Fura-2AM calcium influx assay compared to their undifferentiated Cys-uKPC counterparts. Cys-uKPC-Podo responders resemble the number of responders in ciPodocytes^{WT}. Results depicted originate from Cys-uKPC clone #1; microscopy fluorescence images from Cys-uKPC and Cys-uKPC-Podo during basal conditions and in presence of OAG (150 µM). Low to high calcium is indicated on a color scale that ranges from blue (low calcium) over green (medium calcium) to red (high calcium); (**H**) Example calcium traces of one cell recorded from ciPodocytes^{CTNSWT} (black), Cys-uKPC (blue) and Cys-uKPC-Podo (orange) during a standard Fura-2AM calcium imaging protocol. Percentage of responders in ciPodocytes^{WT} (total of 221 cells), Cys-uKPC (total of 440 cells) and Cys-uKPC-Podo (total of 278 cells); (**I**) Statistical significance between all groups were tested with a Chi-Square test ($p = 2.8 \times 10^{-5}$). $p < 0.05$: *; $p < 0.01$: **; $p < 0.001$: *** corrected with the Bonferroni correction for multiple-comparison of $n = 3$ groups.

3.3.2. Differentiation of Cys-uKPCs into Functional PTECs

All seven Cys-uKPC clones (#1–#7) were subjected to the PTEC differentiation protocol. Following differentiation, alterations in cellular morphology and upregulation of PTEC-specific genes were observed in six of these seven Cys-uKPC clones (Cys-uKPC #2–5 & #7), hereafter coined Cys-uKPC-PTEC. These alterations at the cellular level comprise cellular enlargement and the acquisition of an elongated, spindle- to tubular-like shape (Figure 4A), along with the significant upregulation of PTEC-specific genes *ABCB1*, and *de novo* expression of *AQP1* at the mRNA level (Figure 4B). We further explored the protein expression of PTEC-specific genes and PTEC-related functionality in one of these Cys-uKPC-PTEC cell lines (Cys-uKPC #7-PTEC), compared to its undifferentiated counterpart (Cys-uKPC #7). Protein expression of aquaporin 1 was confirmed exclusively in Cys-uKPC-PTEC in comparison with the undifferentiated Cys-uKPC (Figure 4C).

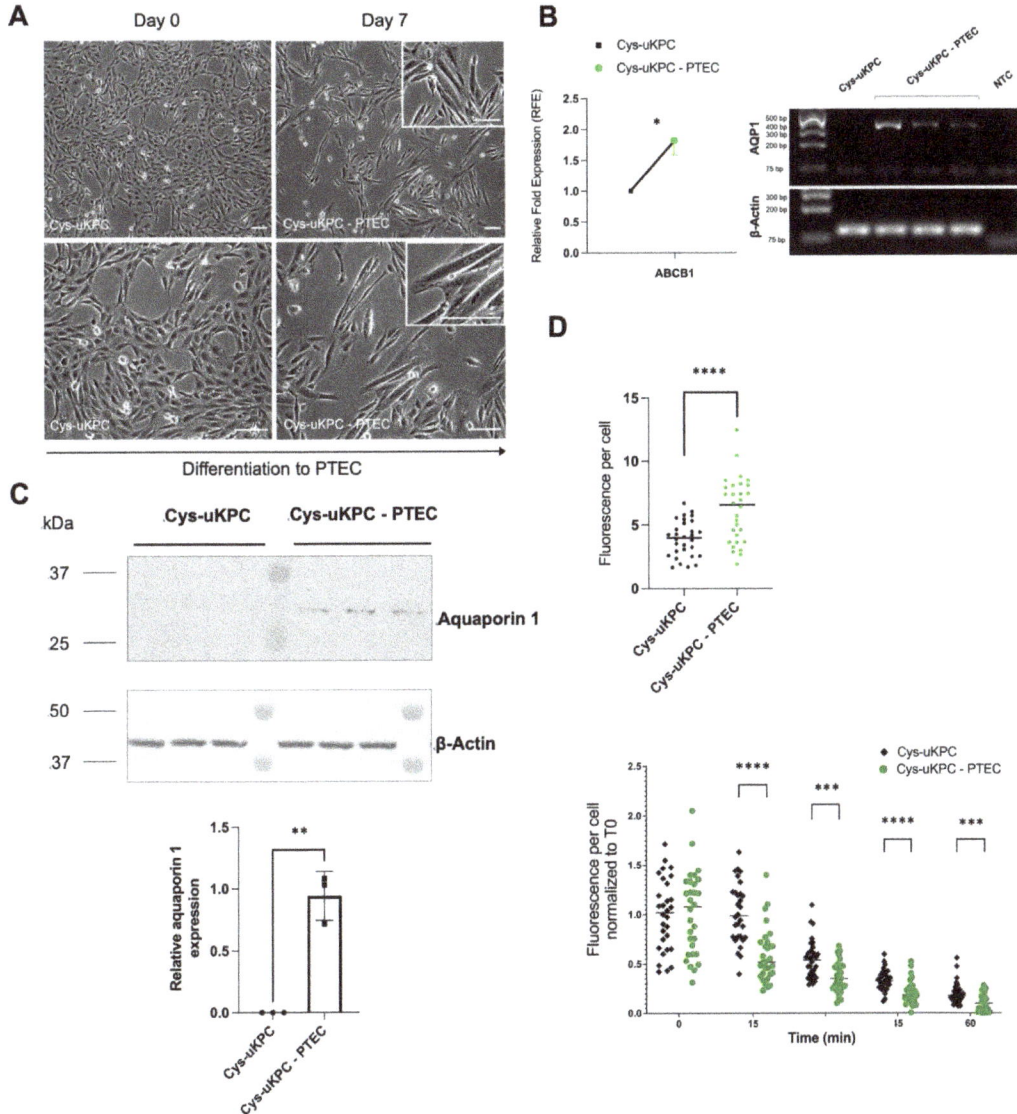

Figure 4. Cys-uKPCs can differentiate in vitro into functional proximal tubular epithelial cells. (**A**) Phase contrast microscopy of a Cys-uKPC clone with a PTEC fate, demonstrating the cellular morphological changes during differentiation (day 0, left column) towards a PTEC (day 7, right column), which is depicted more in specific in the zoomed subpanels in the right upper corner of the microscopy pictures in the right column. Scale bar: 100 μm. Results depicted originate from Cys-uKPC clone #7; (**B**) (**left**) qPCR analysis of PTEC-specific gene expression in Cys-uKPC-PTEC relative to β-actin and normalized to Cys-uKPCs of a Cys-uKPC clone (Cys-uKPC #7) with a PTEC fate. Cys-uKPC-PTEC data is indicated

with a green dot, which represents the mean with bars representing the SEM of three independent experiments with three technical replicates each; Cys-uKPC data is indicated with a black square. $p < 0.05$: *; (**right**) rt-PCR analysis of *AQP1* gene expression in Cys-uKPC-PTEC relative to β-actin, in comparison with Cys-uKPC and negative template control (NTC) showing exclusive gene expression of *AQP1* in Cys-uKPC-PTECs in contrast to Cys-uKPCs (**C**) Western blot analysis and quantification of aquaporin 1 expression in one Cys-uKPC-PTEC clone. Aquaporin 1 is undetectable in the undifferentiated Cys-uKPC, while it is clearly expressed in the Cys-uKPCs-PTEC in all three independent differentiation experiments ($p = 0.0012$: **; mean ± SD Cys-uKPC 0.00 ± 0.00; Cys-uKPC-PTEC 0.94 ± 0.2). Results depicted originate from Cys-uKPC clone #7; (**D**) Receptor-mediated endocytosis of transferrin is enhanced in Cys-uKPC-PTEC as observed in an Alexa Fluor^{TM} 555 labeled transferrin endocytosis assay. Binding of transferrin is significantly higher in Cys-uKPC-PTEC compared to Cys-uKPCs, as observed as the fluorescence per cell of Alexa Fluor^{TM} 555 labeled transferrin at time point 0 in the Alexa Fluor^{TM} 555 labeled transferrin endocytosis assay (upper part of panel, right graph). Statistical significance was reached in an unpaired *t*-test ($p < 0.0001$: ****; mean ± SD of fluorescence per cell in Cys-uKPC 3906 ± 1415, Cys-uKPC-PTEC 6178 ± 2547). Endocytic processing of transferrin is significantly enhanced in Cys-uKPC-PTECs compared to Cys-uKPCs as observed as the fluorescence per cell normalized to time point 0 at several time points (15, 30, 45 and 60 min) following internalization of transferrin via receptor-mediated endocytosis (lower part of the panel). Statistical significance was reached for time points 15, 30, 45 and 60 min via a Mann–Whitney test ($p < 0.0001$: ****, $p < 0.001$: ***; median (IQR)) of fluorescence per cell normalized to time point 0 in Cys-uKPC time point 15 min 0.99 (0.77; 1.22) compared to Cys-uKPC-PTEC time point 15 min 0.5191 (0.39; 0.72), in Cys-uKPC time point 30 min 0.54 (0.38; 0.64) compared to Cys-uKPC-PTEC time point 30 min 0.35 (0.25; 0.48), in Cys-uKPC time point 45 min 0.33 (0.26; 0.41) compared to Cys-uKPC-PTEC time point 45 min 0.19 (0.13; 0.27), and Cys-uKPC time point 60 min 0.18 (0.14; 0.23) compared to Cys-uKPC-PTEC time point 60 min 0.01 (0.03; 0.17).

We assessed the functionality of Cys-uKPC-PTEC by evaluating receptor-mediated endocytosis of transferrin and demonstrated a significant increase in the binding of fluorescent transferrin at time point 0 in the Cys-uKPC-PTEC (Cys-uKPC #7-PTEC) compared with the undifferentiated Cys-uKPC (Cys-uKPC #7), which suggests an increased expression of endocytosis receptors at the cell surface, a feature of mature PTECs (Figure 4D, upper graphs). In addition, endocytic trafficking of transferrin in Cys-uKPC-PTECs (Cys-uKPC #7-PTEC) was more enhanced in comparison to the undifferentiated Cys-uKPC (Cys-uKPC #7; Figure 4D, lower graph).

Taken together, we demonstrated that KPCs are voided in the urine of cystinosis patients, are clonogenic, can proliferate exponentially in vitro, and can be differentiated towards functional specific cells of the nephron epithelium.

3.4. A kidney Progenitor Cell Niche Is Present In Situ in the Kidneys of a Nephropathic Cystinosis Patient

The presence of Cys-uKPCs in the urine of cystinosis patients suggests an attempt at kidney regeneration. Therefore, we sought to demonstrate the presence of these cells in the native kidney of cystinosis patients. As previous studies characterized kidney progenitor cells as being PAX2$^+$/CD133$^+$, we performed immunochemistry on the kidney tissue of one nephropathic cystinosis patient by use of these markers [8,15,25–27]. The clinical characteristics of the patient are described in Table S2. PAX2 CD133 double-positive cells were present in the patient's tissue scattered throughout the parietal epithelium of the Bowman's capsule and the tubules (Figure S6, panel A, B).

3.5. Reduction in Cystine Levels in Cys-uKPCs via an Ex Vivo Gene Addition Approach

We aimed to explore the feasibility of ex vivo *CTNS* cDNA gene addition via lentiviral vector (LV) technology, in which Cys-uKPCs could be used as a tool for disease modeling.

First, we validated the LV constructs (LV_CTNS-3HA) in cystinosis fibroblasts, confirming CTNS protein expression via immunofluorescent staining and Western blot analysis (Figure S7, panel B–E).

Then, in separate transduction experiments per clone, two Cys-uKPC clonal cell lines were complemented with *CTNS* cDNA via LV transduction, followed by antibiotic selection (Cys-uKPC #1 LV_CTNS-3HA; Cys-uKPC #7 LV_CTNS-3HA). As the vehicle control, LV expressing a control protein (eGFP or dATP13A2, an inactivated lysosomal protein—LV_eGFP or LV_dATP13A2) was taken along. Protein expression of *CTNS* cDNA was confirmed by Western blot in both *CTNS* complemented clones (Cys-uKPC #1 LV_CTNS-3HA; Cys-uKPC #7 LV_CTNS-3HA) (Figure S8). In each Cys-uKPC clonal cell line, CTNS protein addition resulted in a significant, about 2.5 to 3-fold, reduction in cystine levels, compared to their vehicle controls (Figure 5; panel A: Cys-uKPC #1; panel B: Cys-uKPC #2).

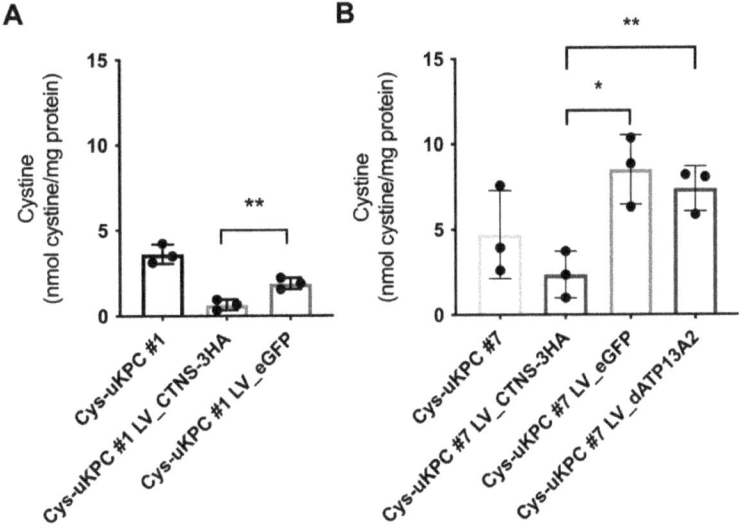

Figure 5. Complementation of *CTNS* via lentiviral vector transduction in two Cys-uKPC clonal cell lines significantly reduces intracellular cystine levels. Cystine measurement by HPLC in Cys-uKPCs (Cys-uKPC #1, #7), Cys-uKPCs transduced with LV_CTNS-3HA (Cys-uKPC #1 LV_CTNS-3HA & #7 LV_CTNS-3HA) and Cys-uKPCs transduced with LV_eGFP (Cys-uKPC #1 LV_eGFP and #7 LV_eGFP) and/or LV_dATP13A2 (Cys-uKPC #7 LV_dATP13A2) as vehicle controls. The graph shows mean ± SD of three independent measurements; $p < 0.05$: *; $p < 0.01$: **. (**A**) The cystine level of Cys-uKPC #1 LV_CTNS-3HA (0.66 ± 0.31 nmol cystine/mg protein) is significantly lower compared to the eGFP-transduced Cys-uKPC #1 as vehicle control (Cys-uKPC #1 LV_eGFP: 1.89 ± 0.34; difference between means of Cys-uKPC #1 LV_CTNS-3HA and Cys-uKPC #1 LV_eGFP cystine level: 1.23 ± 0.26; 95% CI of difference: 0.5 to 1.97; $p = 0.0097$). (**B**) Cystine levels of the Cys-uKPC #7 LV_CTNS-3HA (2.34 ± 1.36 nmol cystine/mg protein) are significantly lower compared to the eGFP (Cys-uKPC #7 LV_eGFP: 8.50 ± 2.02 nmol cystine/mg protein; difference between means: 6.16 ± 1.41; 95% CI of difference: 2.24 to 10.08; $p = 0.01$) and dATP13A2 (Cys-uKPC #7 LV_dATP13A2: 7.38 ± 1.31 nmol cystine/mg protein; difference between means: 5.04 ± 1.09; 95% CI of difference: 2.01 to 8.07; $p = 0.009$) vehicle controls.

4. Discussion

In this study, we demonstrated that, among the large number of cells voided in the urine of patients with nephropathic cystinosis, undifferentiated cells are present. These cells can be isolated and clonally expanded in vitro, amongst which specific clones express several markers reminiscent of the early stages of nephrogenesis, show a high proliferative capacity and harbor the potential to differentiate towards functional podocytes or PTECs. Therefore, the latter cells can be coined as cystinosis urine-derived kidney progenitor cells (Cys-uKPCs). In contrast with cystinosis patients, in healthy control subjects, no undifferentiated cells are present in urine. This observation can be explained by a potential attempt of cystinosis kidneys to regenerate in compensation for the epithelial cell losses. However, this attempt at regeneration obviously fails, given the progressive deterioration of the renal Fanconi syndrome and chronic kidney disease that ensues.

In our study, we established seven Cys-uKPC clones from the two cystinosis patients that showed the highest yield of clonal colonies growing from their urine in the progenitor medium. One patient had the infantile phenotype and another the juvenile phenotype; these two patients represented the full spectrum of nephropathic cystinosis. Confirming their nature as nephron progenitors, Cys-uKPC expressed *CITED1*, which is a specific marker of the cap mesenchyme cells [48], and *NCAM1*, which has shown to define a population of kidney epithelial cells with clonogenic and stem/progenitor cell properties [14,15]. Not surprisingly, the shortest doubling times and highest proliferative potential were observed in the Cys-uKPC clone with the highest level of co-expression of *NCAM1*, *CITED1*, *VIM* and *PAX2*. However, mRNA expression levels of *CITED1*, *NCAM1*, *VIM* and *PAX2*, were lower in Cys-uKPCs compared to nKSPCs, which show a higher potency as kidney progenitor cells as demonstrated by their higher proliferative potential [17]. Cys-uKPCs showed the potential to differentiate between functional podocytes and/or proximal tubular epithelial cells, as demonstrated by the results of gene and protein expression experiments of specific markers and functional assays.

In contrast to previous studies, the kidney progenitor cells of cystinosis patients that we describe here are derived from urine, and the group of undifferentiated cells of which they have been derived has been quantified via a novel accurate method [15,17]. The factors determining the yield of Cys-uKPC that can be isolated from a random urine sample, remain however unclear since no correlation has been observed between the number of undifferentiated cells in the urine and some clinical features of the patients, including the age, cystinosis genotype, the WBC cystine level, eGFR and proteinuria (Figure S3). Nevertheless, Cys-uKPCs show the advantage of a high potential for self-renewal and our approach eliminates the need for laborious isolation and immortalization procedures, while it avoids the complex differentiation protocols from iPSCs, side effects of iPSC reprogramming and the limitations of application of iPSC-derived cell lines [23].

Various hypotheses have been proposed to determine the in vivo origin of regenerating cells of the kidney, depending on their potency and fate [8,9,12,13,15,26]. While an attempt was made to delineate this niche of progenitor cells in vivo, detailed localization of cells in cystinosis kidneys was hampered by a very limited amount of available kidney tissue, as a biopsy is not required for the diagnosis or the clinical follow-up of cystinosis patients. Being able to examine only a single historic cystinosis kidney specimen, we demonstrated cells co-expressing $CD133^+/PAX2^+$ scattered through the tubular epithelium and the parietal epithelium of the Bowman's capsule. However, no sufficient material was available to perform co-localization studies with specific nephron segment markers. Although we have no direct proof that Cys-uKPCs and $CD133^+/PAX2^+$ cells found in this single cystinosis kidney represent the same cell population, both findings are in line with our hypothesis that epithelial cell loss in the urine of cystinosis patients is accompanied by the presence of cells with nephron progenitor characteristics.

The most intriguing question launched by this study is whether the niche of KPCs found in cystinosis is the response to kidney damage or the reflection of regeneration, which limits the disease progression. Gaide Chevronnay et al. showed in kidney tissue of the cystinosis mouse model that the development of progressive proximal tubular atrophy close to glomerular junctions caused by increased apoptosis, was compensated by a proliferation of PTECs, which was interpreted as an adaptive mechanism of ongoing tissue repair [49,50]. On the other hand, Festa et al. found that abnormal proximal tubule dedifferentiation is part of the pathologic process, resulting in a reduced expression of the PTEC transporters in the apical membrane, resulting in renal Fanconi syndrome [51]. Hence, Cys-KPCs might present the yin-yang endeavor of the cystinosis kidney to regenerate at the expense of proper proximal tubular function.

Another question that has been addressed in our study is whether the pathologic phenotype of Cys-uKPCs can be corrected using a gene addition strategy. Upon complementation of *CTNS*-depleted Cys-uKPCs via LV vector technology, we demonstrated a significant reduction in cystine levels in Cys-uKPCs, indicating that our approach results in a substantial improvement of lysosomal cystine-transporting functions in the *CTNS* complemented cells.

The most practical future application of the Cys-uKPCs described in this study is a novel platform for disease modeling, including the development of organoids and tubuloids. Indeed, urine can serve as a non-invasive, cost-effective and virtually unlimited source for cell lines in cystinosis patients [52–54].

Investigating the therapeutic application of gene-corrected Cys-KPCs was beyond the scope of this study. Nevertheless, we might speculate that in vivo complementation of *CTNS* cDNA in the kidney progenitor cell niche in situ, using directly in vivo gene addition with, for example, AAV based viral vectors, could yield promising results [55,56]. For example, in C57BL/6 mice, nephron segment-specific gene expression was shown to be feasible by administration of an AAV9 vector with segment-specific promotors via retrograde ureteric infusion [55]. In another study, specific and highly efficient transduction of kidney stromal and mesangial cells with a synthetic AAV allowing inducible knockout of genes was demonstrated in mice, resulting in a reduction in interstitial fibrosis [56]. These studies might be particularly useful for cystinosis since they highlight a potential route for administration and show the feasibility of targeting renal cells of interest. On the other hand, gene-corrected cystinosis progenitor cells can represent an interesting source of cells for autologous cell therapy. Recently, ex vivo hematopoietic stem cell gene therapy using autologous hematopoietic stem and progenitor cells (HSPCs) transduced with lentiviral vector technology was reported to be successful in Hurler disease, another rare lysosomal storage disorder, yielding extensive metabolic correction in peripheral tissues and the central nervous system [57]. Further studies investigating the potential of Cys-uKPCs to integrate into cystinosis structures in vitro (e.g., organoids) or in (damaged) kidneys in cystinosis animal models, are required to explore these exciting possibilities.

Taken together, we demonstrate that cystinosis patients shed KPCs in urine. These cells can be readily isolated and carry the potential to differentiate between functional podocytes or proximal tubular cells in vitro. We showed that the improvement of the cellular cystine accumulation in cystinosis KPCs can be achieved by ex vivo gene addition, making them a valuable novel in vitro model, and a potential tool for gene therapeutic applications.

Supplementary Materials: The following supporting information can be downloaded at: https://www.mdpi.com/article/10.3390/cells11071245/s1, Table S1: Control healthy subjects recruited in the study; Table S2: Clinical characteristics of the cystinosis patients whose native kidney specimen was analyzed; Table S3: Antibodies used in Western blot, IF & ICH stainings; Table S4: Primers used to test steady-state mRNA level via qPCR; Figure S1: Protocol of the quantification of undifferentiated cells in urine of cystinosis patients compared with healthy control subjects. Panel A: Establishment of a calibration curve of known numbers of vimentin-positive renal papilla cells. Known numbers of renal papilla cells (1, 5, 10, 50, 100, 300, 500, 1000 cells per well) were seeded using fluorescence activated cell sorting (FACS) in a 96-well plate. cDNA was synthesized and pre-amplified according to the protocol of Picelli et al. qPCR was performed and the resulting Ct value for Beta-actin and vimentin for each known number of renal papilla cells, was used to establish a calibration curve for the total number of cells voided in urine (Ct value for Beta-actin), and the number of undifferentiated cells voided in urine, respectively (Ct value for vimentin). Panel B: Quantification of number of undifferentiated cells in urine of a cystinosis patient or healthy control subject (progenituria). A freshly voided urine sample was collected and a cell pellet was acquired via centrifugation. cDNA was synthesized and pre-amplified according to the protocol of Picelli et al. qPCR was performed and the resulting Ct value for Beta-actin and vimentin for each urine sample was plotted against the established calibration curve for defining the total number of cells voided in urine and the number of undifferentiated cells; Figure S2: Protocol of the isolation, characterization and establishment of Cys-uKPC clones, Cys-uKPC-PTEC and Cys-uKPC-Podo from urine of cystinosis patients; Figure S3: Correlation between the number of undifferentiated cells voided in urine of cystinosis patients, and age, proteinuria (protein/creatinine ratio; g/g creatinine), kidney function (eGFR; mL/min/1.73 m^2), white blood cell cystine level (WBC cystine level; nmol $\frac{1}{2}$ cystine/mg protein) and cystinosis genotype at the moment of quantification; Figure S4: Immunofluorescence staining for synaptopodin (SYNPO) and podocalyxin (PODXL) in Cys-uKPC-Podocytes. Immunofluorescence pictures of individual color channels (Synaptopodin or Podocalyxin: red; phalloidin: green; DAPI: blue) are provided in order to better discriminate the individual signals. Figure S5: Control stainings for CD133 and PAX2 as markers of kidney progenitor cells; Figure S6: A kidney progenitor cell niche expressing CD133$^+$/PAX2$^+$ is present in situ in cystinosis kidney; Figure S7: Graphical representation and validation of the SIN lentiviral vector (LV) constructs used in the transduction experiments for complementation of *CTNS* cDNA. Figure S8: Confirmation of protein expression of CTNS-3HA in Cys-uKPC #1 LV_CTNS-3HA and Cys-uKPC #7 LV_CTNS-3HA.

Author Contributions: Conceptualization: K.V., F.O.A., R.G., L.v.d.H. and E.L.; methodology: K.V., F.O.A., K.H., J.V., K.T., D.D., A.R., M.v.d.B., R.G., L.v.d.H. and E.L.; software: K.V., F.O.A., K.H. and M.v.d.B.; validation: K.V., F.O.A., D.D. and R.G.; formal analysis: K.V., F.O.A., A.R., D.D., K.H., S.P.B., T.B., M.v.d.B. and E.L.; investigation: K.V., F.O.A., K.H., K.T., A.R., D.D., F.D.-C., R.G., S.P.B., T.B. and M.v.d.B.; resources: K.V., F.O.A., M.v.d.B., M.J., E.C., L.v.d.H., D.D., R.G., F.D.-C. and E.L.; data curation: K.V.; writing—original draft preparation: K.V.; writing—review and editing: K.V., F.O.A., M.v.d.B., M.J., E.C., K.T., E.C., A.R., J.V., D.D., L.v.d.H., F.D.-C., R.G., E.L., S.P.B. and T.B.; visualization: K.V. and F.O.A.; supervision: F.O.A., L.v.d.H. and E.L.; project administration: K.V., F.O.A. and E.L.; funding acquisition: K.V., F.O.A., L.v.d.H., R.G. and E.L. All authors have read and agreed to the published version of the manuscript.

Funding: This research was funded by the Research Foundation—Flanders (F.W.O. Vlaanderen), grant number 1801110N, the Cystinosis Research Network (CRN), Cystinosis Ireland and KU Leuven (C1 Internal Funding grant 3M170322). KV, FOA and DD are funded by the Research Foundation—Flanders (F.W.O Vlaanderen), grants 11Y5216N, 12Q99171N and 1S22919N, respectively.

Institutional Review Board Statement: The study was conducted in accordance with the Declaration of Helsinki, and approved by the Institutional Review Board (or Ethics Committee) of UZ/KU Leuven (Ethische Commissie Onderzoek UZ/KU Leuven) (protocol code s54695; date of approval: 14 December 2012).

Informed Consent Statement: Informed consent was obtained from all subjects involved in the study.

Data Availability Statement: Not applicable.

Acknowledgments: We thank Louise Medaer and Maxime Smits for their assistance with experiments while replacing Dries David. We also thank Inge Bongaers, Sandra van Aerschot, Irina Thiry, Christiana Adebayo, Sem Tuerlings and Antonina Mikorska for their technical assistance. We acknowledge M. van Dyck (UZ Leuven) for the collection of urine samples and care for our cystinosis patients; P. Van den Berghe (KU Leuven) of the Cell and Tissue Imaging cluster/Cell Imaging Core (CIC), supported by Hercules AKUL/15/37_GOH1816N and FWO G.0929.15 for support with confocal microscopy; B. Bussolatti (University of Turin, Italy) for sharing human papilla kidney stem cells; R. Masereeuw (University of Utrecht, Utrecht, The Netherlands) and F Emma (Laboratory of Pathology and Metabolism, Università Bambino Gesù, Rome, Italy) for cystine measurements. Library preparation, sequencing and statistical data analysis were performed by VIB Nucleomics Core (www.nucleomics.be; accessed date 13 March 2022). The authors acknowledge the internal fund from KU Leuven (C1 grant 3M170322). E.L. is supported by the Research Foundation—Flanders (F.W.O Vlaanderen), grant 1801110N, the Cystinosis Research Network (CRN) and Cystinosis Ireland. K.V, F.O.A and D.D are funded by the Research Foundation—Flanders (F.W.O Vlaanderen), grants 11Y5216N, 12Q9917N and 1S22919N, respectively.

Conflicts of Interest: E.L. performs consultancy for Recordati, Chiesi, Kyowa Kirin, Advicenne, and was supported by a research grant from Horizon Pharma. The funders of this study had no role in the design of the study; in the collection, analyses, or interpretation of data; in the writing of the manuscript, or in the decision to publish the results.

References

1. Town, M.; Jean, G.; Cherqui, S.; Attard, M.; Forestier, L.; Whitmore, S.A.; Callen, D.F.; Gribouval, O.; Broyer, M.; Bates, G.P.; et al. A novel gene encoding an integral membrane protein is mutated in nephropathic cystinosis. *Nat. Genet.* **1998**, *18*, 319–324. [CrossRef] [PubMed]
2. Gahl, W.A.; Thoene, J.G.; Schneider, J.A. Cystinosis. *N. Engl. J. Med.* **2002**, *347*, 111–121. [CrossRef] [PubMed]
3. Elmonem, M.A.; Veys, K.R.; Soliman, N.A.; Van Dyck, M.; Van Den Heuvel, L.P.; Levtchenko, E. Cystinosis: A review. *Orphanet J. Rare Dis.* **2016**, *11*, 47. [CrossRef] [PubMed]
4. Markello, T.C.; Bernardini, I.M.; Gahl, W.A. Improved renal function in children with cystinosis treated with cysteamine. *N. Engl. J. Med.* **1993**, *328*, 1157–1162. [CrossRef]
5. Gahl, W.A.; Balog, J.Z.; Kleta, R. Nephropathic cystinosis in adults: Natural history and effects of oral cysteamine therapy. *Ann. Intern. Med.* **2007**, *147*, 242–250. [CrossRef]
6. Brodin-Sartorius, A.; Tête, M.J.; Niaudet, P.; Antignac, C.; Guest, G.; Ottolenghi, C.; Charbit, M.; Moyse, D.; Legendre, C.; Lesavre, P.; et al. Cysteamine therapy delays the progression of nephropathic cystinosis in late adolescents and adults. *Kidney Int.* **2012**, *81*, 179–189. [CrossRef]
7. Ivanova, E.A.; Arcolino, F.O.; Elmonem, M.A.; Rastaldi, M.P.; Giardino, L.; Cornelissen, E.M.; Van Den Heuvel, L.P.; Levtchenko, E.N. Cystinosin deficiency causes podocyte damage and loss associated with increased cell motility. *Kidney Int.* **2016**, *89*, 1037–1048. [CrossRef]
8. Bussolati, B.; Bruno, S.; Grange, C.; Buttiglieri, S.; Deregibus, M.C.; Cantino, D.; Camussi, G. Isolation of renal progenitor cells from adult human kidney. *Am. J. Pathol.* **2005**, *166*, 545–555. [CrossRef]
9. Sagrinati, C.; Netti, G.S.; Mazzinghi, B.; Lazzeri, E.; Liotta, F.; Frosali, F.; Ronconi, E.; Meini, C.; Gacci, M.; Squecco, R.; et al. Isolation and characterization of multipotent progenitor cells from the Bowman's capsule of adult human kidneys. *J. Am. Soc. Nephrol.* **2006**, *17*, 2443–2456. [CrossRef]
10. Huling, J.; Yoo, J.J. Comparing adult renal stem cell identification, characterization and applications. *J. Biomed. Sci.* **2017**, *24*, 32. [CrossRef]
11. Marcheque, J.; Bussolati, B.; Csete, M.; Perin, L. Concise reviews: Stem cells and kidney regeneration: An update. *Stem Cells Transl. Med.* **2019**, *8*, 82–92. [CrossRef] [PubMed]
12. Ronconi, E.; Sagrinati, C.; Angelotti, M.L.; Lazzeri, E.; Mazzinghi, B.; Ballerini, L.; Parente, E.; Becherucci, F.; Gacci, M.; Carini, M.; et al. Regeneration of glomerular podocytes by human renal progenitors. *J. Am. Soc. Nephrol.* **2009**, *20*, 322–332. [CrossRef] [PubMed]
13. Angelotti, M.L.; Ronconi, E.; Ballerini, L.; Peired, A.; Mazzinghi, B.; Sagrinati, C.; Parente, E.; Gacci, M.; Carini, M.; Rotondi, M.; et al. Characterization of renal progenitors committed toward tubular lineage and their regenerative potential in renal tubular injury. *Stem Cells* **2012**, *30*, 1714–1725. [CrossRef] [PubMed]
14. Harari-Steinberg, O.; Metsuyanim, S.; Omer, D.; Gnatek, Y.; Gershon, R.; Pri-Chen, S.; Ozdemir, D.D.; Lerenthal, Y.; Noiman, T.; Ben-Hur, H.; et al. Identification of human nephron progenitors capable of generation of kidney structures and functional repair of chronic renal disease. *EMBO Mol. Med.* **2013**, *5*, 1556–1568. [CrossRef] [PubMed]
15. Buzhor, E.; Omer, D.; Harari-Steinberg, O.; Dotan, Z.; Vax, E.; Pri-Chen, S.; Metsuyanim, S.; Pleniceanu, O.; Goldstein, R.S.; Dekel, B. Reactivation of NCAM1 defines a subpopulation of human adult kidney epithelial cells with clonogenic and stem/progenitor properties. *Am. J. Pathol.* **2013**, *183*, 1621–1633. [CrossRef]
16. Lazzeri, E.; Ronconi, E.; Angelotti, M.L.; Peired, A.; Mazzinghi, B.; Becherucci, F.; Conti, S.; Sansavini, G.; Sisti, A.; Ravaglia, F.; et al. Human urine-derived renal progenitors for personalized modeling of genetic kidney disorders. *J. Am. Soc. Nephrol.* **2015**, *26*, 1961–1974. [CrossRef]
17. Arcolino, F.O.; Zia, S.; Held, K.; Papadimitriou, E.; Theunis, K.; Bussolati, B.; Raaijmakers, A.; Allegaert, K.; Voet, T.; Deprest, J.; et al. Urine of preterm neonates as a novel source of kidney progenitor cells. *J. Am. Soc. Nephrol.* **2016**, *27*, 2762–2770. [CrossRef]
18. Leuning, D.G.; Reinders, M.E.J.; Li, J.; Peired, A.J.; Lievers, E.; de Boer, H.C.; Fibbe, W.E.; Romagnani, P.; van Kooten, C.; Little, M.H.; et al. Clinical-grade isolated human kidney perivascular stromal cells as an organotypic cell source for kidney regenerative medicine. *Stem Cells Transl. Med.* **2017**, *6*, 405–418. [CrossRef]
19. Eymael, J.; Smeets, B. Origin and fate of the regenerating cells of the kidney. *Eur. J. Pharmacol.* **2016**, *790*, 62–73. [CrossRef]
20. Cheung, P.Y.; Harrison, P.T.; Davidson, A.J.; Hollywood, J.A. In Vitro and In Vivo Models to Study Nephropathic Cystinosis. *Cells* **2021**, *11*, 6. [CrossRef]
21. Racusen, L.C.; Fivush, B.A.; Andersson, H.; Gahl, W.A. Culture of renal tubular cells from the urine of patients with nephropathic cystinosis. *J. Am. Soc. Nephrol.* **1991**, *1*, 1028–1033. [CrossRef] [PubMed]
22. Hollywood, J.A.; Przepiorski, A.; D'Souza, R.F.; Sreebhavan, S.; Wolvetang, E.J.; Harrison, P.T.; Davidson, A.J.; Holm, T.M. Use of human induced pluripotent stem cells and kidney organoids to develop a cysteamine/mtor inhibition combination therapy for cystinosis. *J. Am. Soc. Nephrol.* **2020**, *31*, 962–982. [CrossRef] [PubMed]

23. Ruiz, S.; Diep, D.; Gore, A.; Panopoulos, A.D.; Montserrat, N.; Plongthongkum, N.; Kumar, S.; Fung, H.-L.; Giorgetti, A.; Bilic, J.; et al. Identification of a specific reprogramming-associated epigenetic signature in human induced pluripotent stem cells. *Proc. Natl. Acad. Sci. USA* **2012**, *109*, 16196–16201. [CrossRef] [PubMed]
24. The World Medical Association. Declaration of Helsinki. Available online: http://www.wma.net/e/policy/b3.htm (accessed on 13 March 2022).
25. Ye, Y.; Wang, B.; Jiang, X.; Hu, W.; Feng, J.; Li, H.; Jin, M.; Ying, Y.; Wang, W.; Mao, X.; et al. Proliferative capacity of stem/progenitor-like cells in the kidney may associate with the outcome of patients with acute tubular necrosis. *Hum. Pathol.* **2011**, *42*, 1132–1141. [CrossRef] [PubMed]
26. Lindgren, D.; Boström, A.K.; Nilsson, K.; Hansson, J.; Sjölund, J.; Möller, C.; Jirström, K.; Nilsson, E.; Landberg, G.; Axelson, H.; et al. Isolation and characterization of progenitor-like cells from human renal proximal tubules. *Am. J. Pathol.* **2011**, *178*, 828–837. [CrossRef]
27. Smeets, B.; Boor, P.; Dijkman, H.; Sharma, S.; Jirak, P.; Mooren, F.; Berger, K.; Borneman, J.; Gelman, H.; Floege, J.; et al. Proximal tubular cells contain a phenotypically distinct, scattered cell population involved in tubular regeneration. *J. Pathol.* **2013**, *229*, 645–659. [CrossRef]
28. Picelli, S.; Faridani, O.R.; Björklund, Å.K.; Winberg, G.; Sagasser, S.; Sandberg, R. Full-length RNA-seq from single cells using Smart-seq2. *Nat. Protoc.* **2014**, *9*, 171. [CrossRef]
29. Zhang, Y.; McNeill, E.; Tian, H.; Soker, S.; Andersson, K.E.; Yoo, J.J.; Atala, A. Urine derived cells are a potential source for urological tissue reconstruction. *J. Urol.* **2008**, *180*, 2226–2233. [CrossRef]
30. DeKoninck, P.; Toelen, J.; Zia, S.; Albersen, M.; Lories, R.; De Coppi, P.; Deprest, J. Routine isolation and expansion late mid trimester amniotic fluid derived mesenchymal stem cells in a cohort of fetuses with congenital diaphragmatic hernia. *Eur. J. Obs. Gynecol. Reprod. Biol.* **2014**, *178*, 157–162. [CrossRef]
31. V, R. Doubling Time Computing. Available online: https://www.doubling-time.com/compute.php (accessed on 14 March 2022).
32. Gianesello, L.; Priante, G.; Ceol, M.; Radu, C.M.; Saleem, M.A.; Simioni, P.; Terrin, L.; Anglani, F.; Prete, D. Del Albumin uptake in human podocytes: A possible role for the cubilin-amnionless (CUBAM) complex. *Sci. Rep.* **2017**, *7*, 13705. [CrossRef]
33. Chan, P.M.; Tan, Y.S.; Chua, K.H.; Sabaratnam, V.; Kuppusamy, U.R. Attenuation of Inflammatory Mediators (TNF-α and Nitric Oxide) and Up-Regulation of IL-10 by Wild and Domesticated Basidiocarps of Amauroderma rugosum (Blume & T. Nees) Torrend in LPS-Stimulated RAW264.7 Cells. *PLoS ONE* **2015**, *10*, e0139593. [CrossRef]
34. Greka, A.; Mundel, P. Regulation of podocyte actin dynamics by calium. *Semin. Nephrol.* **2012**, *32*, 319–326. [CrossRef] [PubMed]
35. Wieder, N.; Greka, A. Calcium, TRPC channels, and regulation of the actin cytoskeleton in podocytes: Towards a future of targeted therapies. *Pediatr. Nephrol.* **2016**, *31*, 1047–1054. [CrossRef] [PubMed]
36. Piwkowska, A.; Rogacka, D.; Audzeyenka, I.; Kasztan, M.; Angielski, S.; Jankowski, M. Intracellular calcium signaling regulates glomerular filtration barrier permeability: The role of the PKGIα-dependent pathway. *FEBS Lett.* **2016**, *590*, 1739–1748. [CrossRef]
37. Khayyat, N.H.; Tomilin, V.N.; Zaika, O.; Pochynyuk, O. Polymodal roles of TRPC3 channel in the kidney. *Channels* **2020**, *14*, 257–267. [CrossRef]
38. Ilatovskaya, D.V.; Staruschenko, A. TRPC6 channel as an emerging determinant of the podocyte injury susceptibility in kidney diseases. *Am. J. Physiol. Physiol.* **2015**, *309*, F393–F397. [CrossRef]
39. Reiser, J.; Polu, K.R.; Möller, C.C.; Kenlan, P.; Altintas, M.M.; Wei, C.; Faul, C.; Herbert, S.; Villegas, I.; Avila-casado, C.; et al. TRPC6 is a glomerular slit diaphragm-associated channel required for normal renal function. *Nat. Genet.* **2005**, *37*, 739–744. [CrossRef]
40. van Veen, S.; Martin, S.; Van den Haute, C.; Benoy, V.; Lyons, J.; Vanhoutte, R.; Kahler, J.P.; Decuypere, J.P.; Gelders, G.; Lambie, E.; et al. ATP13A2 deficiency disrupts lysosomal polyamine export. *Nature* **2020**, *578*, 419–424. [CrossRef]
41. Levtchenko, E.N.; de Graaf-Hess, A.; Wilmer, M.; van den Heuvel, L.; Monnens, L.; Blom, H. Altered status of glutathione and its metabolites in cystinotic cells. *Nephrol. Dial. Transplant.* **2005**, *20*, 1828–1832. [CrossRef]
42. Fehse, B.; Kustikova, O.S.; Bubenheim, M.; Baum, C. Pois(s)on—It's a question of dose. *Gene Ther.* **2004**, *11*, 879–881. [CrossRef]
43. Fanni, D.; Fanos, V.; Monga, G.; Gerosa, C.; Locci, A.; Nemolato, S.; Van Eyken, P.; Faa, G. Expression of WT1 during normal human kidney development. *J. Matern. Neonatal Med.* **2011**, *24*, 45–48. [CrossRef] [PubMed]
44. Inoue, K.; Ishibe, S. Podocyte endocytosis in the regulation of the glomerular filtration barrier. *Am. J. Physiol. Physiol.* **2015**, *309*, F398–F405. [CrossRef] [PubMed]
45. Perico, L.; Conti, S.; Benigni, A.; Remuzzi, G. Podocyte-actin dynamics in health and disease. *Nat. Rev. Nephrol.* **2016**, *12*, 692–710. [CrossRef]
46. Huber, T.B.; Köttgen, M.; Schilling, B.; Walz, G.; Benzing, T. Interaction with podocin facilitates nephrin signaling. *J. Biol. Chem.* **2001**, *276*, 41543–41546. [CrossRef] [PubMed]
47. Huber, T.B.; Schermer, B.; Muller, R.U.; Hohne, M.; Bartram, M.; Calixto, A.; Hagmann, H.; Reinhardt, C.; Koos, F.; Kunzelmann, K.; et al. Podocin and MEC-2 bind cholesterol to regulate the activity of associated ion channels. *Proc. Natl. Acad. Sci. USA* **2006**, *103*, 17079–17086. [CrossRef] [PubMed]
48. Plisov, S.; Tsang, M.; Shi, G.; Boyle, S.; Yoshino, K.; Dunwoodie, S.L.; Dawid, I.B.; Shioda, T.; Perantoni, A.O.; de Caestecker, M.P. Cited1 Is a bifunctional transcriptional cofactor that regulates early nephronic patterning. *J. Am. Soc. Nephrol.* **2005**, *16*, 1632–1644. [CrossRef]

49. Gaide Chevronnay, H.P.; Janssens, V.; Van Der Smissen, P.; Rocca, C.J.; Liao, X.H.; Refetoff, S.; Pierreux, C.E.; Cherqui, S.; Courtoy, P.J. Hematopoietic stem cells transplantation can normalize thyroid function in a cystinosis mouse model. *Endocrinology* **2016**, *157*, 1363–1371. [CrossRef]
50. Gaide Chevronnay, H.P.; Janssens, V.; Van Der Smissen, P.; N'Kuli, F.; Nevo, N.; Guiot, Y.; Levtchenko, E.; Marbaix, E.; Pierreux, C.E.; Cherqui, S.; et al. Time course of pathogenic and adaptation mechanisms in cystinotic mouse kidneys. *J. Am. Soc. Nephrol.* **2014**, *25*, 1256–1269. [CrossRef]
51. Festa, B.P.; Chen, Z.; Berquez, M.; Debaix, H.; Tokonami, N.; Prange, J.A.; Van De Hoek, G.; Alessio, C.; Raimondi, A.; Nevo, N.; et al. Impaired autophagy bridges lysosomal storage disease and epithelial dysfunction in the kidney. *Nat. Commun.* **2018**, *9*, 191. [CrossRef]
52. Pavathuparambil Abdul Manaph, N.; Al-Hawaas, M.; Bobrovskaya, L.; Coates, P.T.; Zhou, X.F. Urine-derived cells for human cell therapy. *Stem Cell Res. Ther.* **2018**, *9*, 189. [CrossRef]
53. Oliveira Arcolino, F.; Tort Piella, A.; Papadimitriou, E.; Bussolati, B.; Antonie, D.J.; Murray, P.; van den Heuvel, L.; Levtchenko, E. Human Urine as a Noninvasive Source of Kidney Cells. *Stem Cells Int.* **2015**, *2015*, 362562. [CrossRef] [PubMed]
54. Janssen, M.J.; Arcolino, F.O.; Schoor, P.; Kok, R.J.; Mastrobattista, E. Gene Based Therapies for Kidney Regeneration. *Eur. J. Pharmacol.* **2016**, *790*, 99–108. [CrossRef] [PubMed]
55. Asico, L.D.; Cuevas, S.; Ma, X.; Jose, P.A.; Armando, I.; Konkalmatt, P.R. Nephron segment-specific gene expression using AAV vectors. *Biochem. Biophys. Res. Commun.* **2018**, *497*, 19–24. [CrossRef] [PubMed]
56. Ikeda, Y.; Sun, Z.; Humphreys, B.D.; Ru, X.; Vandenberghe, L.H. Efficient gene transfer to kidney mesenchymal cells using a synthetic adeno-associated viral vector. *J. Am. Soc. Nephrol.* **2018**, *29*, 2287–2297. [CrossRef]
57. Gentner, B.; Tucci, F.; Galimberti, S.; Fumagalli, F.; De Pellegrin, M.; Silvani, P.; Camesasca, C.; Pontesilli, S.; Darin, S.; Ciotti, F.; et al. Hematopoietic Stem- and Progenitor-Cell Gene Therapy for Hurler Syndrome. *N. Engl. J. Med.* **2021**, *385*, 1929–1940. [CrossRef]

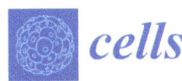

Article

Bioengineered Cystinotic Kidney Tubules Recapitulate a Nephropathic Phenotype

Elena Sendino Garví, Rosalinde Masereeuw and Manoe J. Janssen *

Division Pharmacology, Utrecht Institute for Pharmaceutical Sciences, Utrecht University, Universiteitsweg 99, 3584 CG Utrecht, The Netherlands; e.sendinogarvi@uu.nl (E.S.G.); r.masereeuw@uu.nl (R.M.)
* Correspondence: m.j.janssen1@uu.nl

Abstract: Nephropathic cystinosis is a rare and severe disease caused by disruptions in the *CTNS* gene. Cystinosis is characterized by lysosomal cystine accumulation, vesicle trafficking impairment, oxidative stress, and apoptosis. Additionally, cystinotic patients exhibit weakening and leakage of the proximal tubular segment of the nephrons, leading to renal Fanconi syndrome and kidney failure early in life. Current in vitro cystinotic models cannot recapitulate all clinical features of the disease which limits their translational value. Therefore, the development of novel, complex in vitro models that better mimic the disease and exhibit characteristics not compatible with 2-dimensional cell culture is of crucial importance for novel therapies development. In this study, we developed a 3-dimensional bioengineered model of nephropathic cystinosis by culturing conditionally immortalized proximal tubule epithelial cells (ciPTECs) on hollow fiber membranes (HFM). Cystinotic kidney tubules showed lysosomal cystine accumulation, increased autophagy and vesicle trafficking deterioration, the impairment of several metabolic pathways, and the disruption of the epithelial monolayer tightness as compared to control kidney tubules. In particular, the loss of monolayer organization and leakage could be mimicked with the use of the cystinotic kidney tubules, which has not been possible before, using the standard 2-dimensional cell culture. Overall, bioengineered cystinotic kidney tubules recapitulate better the nephropathic phenotype at a molecular, structural, and functional proximal tubule level compared to 2-dimensional cell cultures.

Keywords: nephropathic cystinosis; lysosomal storage disease; hollow fiber membrane; 3-dimensional models; autophagy

Citation: Sendino Garví, E.; Masereeuw, R.; Janssen, M.J. Bioengineered Cystinotic Kidney Tubules Recapitulate a Nephropathic Phenotype. *Cells* 2022, 11, 177. https://doi.org/10.3390/cells 11010177

Academic Editor: Alfonso Eirin

Received: 25 November 2021
Accepted: 25 December 2021
Published: 5 January 2022

Publisher's Note: MDPI stays neutral with regard to jurisdictional claims in published maps and institutional affiliations.

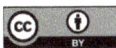

Copyright: © 2022 by the authors. Licensee MDPI, Basel, Switzerland. This article is an open access article distributed under the terms and conditions of the Creative Commons Attribution (CC BY) license (https://creativecommons.org/licenses/by/4.0/).

1. Introduction

Nephropathic cystinosis is an autosomal recessive chronic kidney disease condition caused by mutations in the *CTNS* gene [1,2]. Several mutations have been associated with this disease, but the most recurrent in Europe is a 57kb deletion including the first 10 exons of the *CTNS* gene [3]. This gene encodes for a cystine/proton symporter located in the lysosomal membrane. The impairment or loss of cystinosin leads to the accumulation of cystine inside the lysosomes in all the cells of the body [4–6], which causes severe and chronic damage to several organs, particularly the kidneys. One of the first manifestations of cystinosis is the clinical presentation of renal Fanconi syndrome, characterized by a severe proximal tubule cell dysfunction at early stages of the disease, which results in a total loss of integrity of the proximal tubule [7]. Great efforts have been made to elucidate further the underlying pathological mechanisms of nephropathic cystinosis that revealed several hallmarks beyond cystine accumulation, including impaired autophagy, mTOR activation, disrupted vesicle dynamics (lysosomes-autophagosomes interactions), mitochondrial impairment, reactive oxygen species (ROS), and increased cell stress [8–13]. Despite clinical improvements in prognosis, there is, as of yet, no curative therapy available for cystinosis. Therapy with cysteamine, the only treatment available, is symptomatic and its regime comprises of life-long drug intake with multiple reported side effects [14].

Most knowledge on the pathology of cystinosis results from in vitro models. Human fibroblast, obtained from cystinotic patients and widely available, are a common in vitro model which have been used for many years [15,16]. However, these cells lack the kidney phenotype and, therefore, their use for studying nephropathic cystinosis is limited. In vitro human proximal tubule models can be generated from fresh urine samples [17–20] and kidney tissue (biopsies) [21–23] from cystinotic patients. While valuable, their restricted availability and lack of capacity to stay in culture for more than a few passages urged researchers to immortalize primary cultures following different strategies. An example forms the ciPTEC (conditionally immortalized proximal tubule epithelial cells) [24], a model that has been shown to be particularly useful for investigating the molecular mechanisms affected in nephropathic cystinosis [9]. However, individual variability and the lack of a healthy control with the same genetic background as the cystinotic donor are major hurdles in pinpointing the molecular mechanism associated with the disease. To overcome this issue, recent studies have created isogenic cell lines using CRISPR-Cas by knocking out the *CTNS* gene [9,10]. In addition, advancements in the culture of primary cells obtained from patients' urine now allow prolonged in vitro expansion in the form of adult organoids. This system also offers a 3-dimensional structure and a heterogeneous cell population that better recapitulate native kidney tissue and can be useful for disease modeling and personalized medicine [25]. Furthermore, the use of human induced pluripotent stem cells (hiPSC) has been presented as an unlimited source of patient specific material. Using this approach pluripotent stem cells can be obtained from any human tissue after de-differentiation and re-programming into kidney-like cells and organoids [26,27]. Coupling hiPSC and genome-editing tools such as CRISPR/Cas, can be used to create isogenic knock-out diseased cell lines from healthy hiPSC and, therefore, eliminate the variations that the differential genetic background between donors could carry [28].

Despite the advantages in human disease models for the proximal tubule, it remains challenging to replicate some of the features that the proximal tubule exhibits in nephropathic cystinosis, such as the total integrity loss of the nephron segment in renal Fanconi syndrome. We, therefore, aimed in this study to develop a cystinotic in vitro model that allows for perfusion and flow. The use of hollow fiber membranes (HFM) for the generation of microphysiological in vitro models has recently been described and has proven to be a promising in vitro platform for multiple organs that form tube-like structures, including kidney tubules and intestines [29–31]. The bioengineered kidney tubules consist of conditionally immortalized proximal tubule epithelial cells (ciPTEC) grown on stable and inexpensive biocompatible, poly-ether sulfone (PES) fibers [32]. The connection of the fibers to tubing and the application of flow allows for studying tubular epithelial integrity and transporter activity [32,33]. The ciPTEC line used for this work has been shown to stably express the proximal tubule phenotype over a very high number of passages, and when grown as kidney tubules on a fiber, these cells are capable of organic cation transporter (OCT)-mediated ASP+ transport, albumin reabsorption, organic anion secretion, and the secretion of immune modulators upon an inflammatory response [24,29,32,33].

In this study, we aimed to generate and characterize two cystinotic 3-dimensional models and to establish the added benefit of culturing cystinotic cells on HFM. We focused on the characterization of the cystinotic phenotype when cultured in these advanced in vitro platforms including epithelial monolayer organization and functional integrity. We hypothesize that the generation of advanced in vitro models that better reflect the pathophysiology of cystinosis in the proximal tubule is crucial to gain further knowledge about the molecular mechanisms underlying the tubular epithelium and functional disruption. This would also allow investigating novel treatment and potential curative options.

2. Materials and Methods

2.1. Reagents and Antibodies

All reagents used were obtained from Sigma-Aldrich (Zwijndrecht, The Netherlands) unless specified otherwise. The primary antibodies and probes used for monolayer assessment were Phalloidin-AF488 (Invitrogen, Carlsbad, CA, USA) diluted 1:100, Mouse anti-α-tubulin (#EP1332Y; Invitrogen, Carlsbad, CA, USA) diluted 1:500 and rabbit anti-Na+/K+ATP-ase (a kind gift from Dr. Jan Koenderink, Radboudumc, The Netherlands) diluted 1:500. The primary antibodies used for autophagy and vesicle trafficking assessment were rabbit anti-LC3 (Novus Biologicals, Abingdon, UK #NB600-1384SS) diluted 1:1000, mouse anti-P62 (SQSTM1) (#610832; BD Biosciences, Mississauga, ON, Canada) diluted 1:1000, mouse anti-LAMP1 (#sc-18821; Santa Cruz Biotechnology, Dallas, TX, USA) diluted 1:200, and rabbit anti-mTOR (#2983; Cell Signaling Technology, Leiden, The Netherlands) diluted 1:400. The secondary antibodies used for detection were Polyclonal goat anti-rabbit (#P0448, Dako products, Carpinteria, CA, USA) diluted 1:5000, and polyclonal goat anti-mouse (#P0447, Dako products, Carpinteria, CA, USA) diluted 1:5000. Additionally, Alexa-488 goat anti- mouse (#ab150113; diluted 1:500), Alexa-647 goat anti-rabbit (#ab150083; diluted 1:200), donkey anti-rabbit (#AF647; diluted 1:300), and donkey anti-mouse (#AF568; diluted 1:200) secondary antibodies were all from Abcam (Amsterdam, The Netherlands).

2.2. Cell Culture

Three ciPTECs lines were used for this study: the healthy control ciPTEC, $CTNS^{WT}$ (also referred to as ciPTEC14.4 in previous literature) [24], and two cystinotic models ciPTEC $CTNS^{Patient}$ (ciPTEC46.2) [34] and ciPTEC $CTNS^{-/-}$. $CTNS^{-/-}$ is an isogenic immortalized cell line derived from ciPTEC14.4 and generated in-house previously [9], which harbors a biallelic mutation in the exon 4 of the *CTNS* gene. The ciPTEC46.6 (referred to as "Patient") is an immortalized cell line derived from a urine sample of a cystinotic patient harboring a 57 kb deletion which includes the first 10 exons of the *CTNS* gene. All ciPTEC were cultured as described previously [24]. Cells were seeded at a density of 48,400 cells/cm^2 and allowed to grow at 33 °C for 24 h to enable proliferation and subsequently cultured at 37 °C for 7 days to mature them into fully differentiated PTECs. The culture medium used was Dulbecco's modified Eagle medium DMEM/F-12 (GIBCO, Life Technologies, Paisley, UK) supplemented with fetal calf serum 10% (v/v), insulin 5 µg/mL, transferrin 5 µg/mL, selenium 5 µg/mL, hydrocortisone 35 ng/mL, epidermal growth factor 10 ng/mL, and triiodothyronine 40 pg/mL.

2.3. Hollow Fiber Membrane Culture

All cells were passaged and seeded on the HFM after reaching 80–90% confluency, as described previously [35,36]. MicroPES type TF10 hollow fiber capillary membranes (Membrana GmbH, Wuppertal, Germany) were cut into 175 cm pieces and sterilized in EtOH (70%, v/v) for 45 min. After sterilization, HFM were washed once with HBSS (Hanks' Balanced Salt Solution, Gibco, Life Technologies, Paisley, UK) and put into sterile L-3,4-di-hydroxy-phenylalanine (L-Dopa, 2 mg/mL in 10 mM Tris buffer, pH 8.5) and incubated at 37 °C for 5 h. Next, HFM were washed with HBSS and incubated in a human collagen IV solution (25 µg/mL in HBBS) for 1 h at 37 °C. Unbound collagen IV was washed three times with HBSS. For cell seeding on the HFM, ciPTEC cells were washed and detached with accutase solution (Invitrogen, Carlsbad, CA, USA) and added to 1.5 mL Eppendorf tubes containing individual HFM at a density of 1 million cells/mL and incubated for 6 h at 37 °C, rotating the Eppendorf tubes 90° every 30 min. Lastly, seeded HFM were carefully placed into 6-well plates containing 3 mL of warm culture medium and allowed to grow for 3 days at 33 °C to facilitate the full coverage of the HFM by a cell monolayer, before transferring them to 37 °C for 7–10 days to obtained fully mature bioengineered kidney tubules. Medium was replaced every 3 days.

2.4. Immunostainings

Cells and kidney tubules were fixed using 4% PFA solution (Pierce™ 16% formaldehyde (w/v), methanol-free, ThermoFisher, Waltham, MA, USA) and subsequently permeabilized in 0.3% (v/v) Triton X-100 in HBSS. Kidney tubules were incubated with a blocking solution (2% (w/v) bovine serum albumin (BSA) fraction V and 0.1% (v/v) Tween-20 in HBSS) to prevent the non-specific binding of antibodies. Next, kidney tubules were incubated with the corresponding primary antibodies diluted in blocking solution overnight at 4 °C on a rocking platform. After washing off the primary antibodies, incubation with the secondary antibodies at RT for 2h was followed. Lastly, cells were incubated with Hoechst 33342 (dilution 1:10,000) and kidney tubules were mounted using Prolong gold containing DAPI (Cell Signaling Technology, Leiden, The Netherlands) for nuclei staining. Images were acquired using the confocal microscope Leica TCS SP8 X (Leica Biosystems, Amsterdam, The Netherlands).

2.5. FITC-Inulin Leakage Assay

To quantify the tightness of the kidney tubules cell monolayer, a FITC-inulin solution (0.1 mg/mL in HBSS) was prepared. The kidney tubules were connected to a custom-made 3D-printer chamber [31] made of cytocompatible polyester after washing once with HBSS and sterilizing the chambers with EtOH 70%. The HFM were subsequently connected to a cannula (inner diameter 120–150 μm) DMT Trading, Aarhus, Denmark) using microsuture silk (Pearsalls Limited, Taunton, UK). The apical compartment of the chamber was filled with 1 mL of HBSS, and the kidney tubules were perfused with HBSS. Once leakage of the chamber was resolved, the kidney tubules were perfused with FITC-inulin solution at a rate speed of 0.1 mL/min for 10 min using a Terumo Syringe Pump TE-311 (Terumo, Leuven, Belgium). After completing the perfusion, three technical replicate samples of 100 uL were taken from the apical chamber and transferred to a 96 well-plate. Fluorescence was measured using a Tecan infinite M200PRO plate reader (Tecan Austria GmbH, Grödig, Austria) at an excitation and emission wavelength of 492 nm and 518 nm, resp.

2.6. Isolation of mRNA and Quantification by Real-Time PCR

To be able to obtain enough mRNA for a reliable gene expression measurement, three kidney tubules were pooled together in a 1.5 mL Eppendorf tube. Cell pellets were collected by detaching the cells from the HFM using accutase solution (Invitrogen, Carlsbad, CA, USA) neutralized with culture medium and centrifuged for 10 min at 300× g. The mRNAs were extracted using the RNeasy mini kit (Qiagen, Venlo, The Netherlands) following the manufacturer's instructions. A total of 600 ng of mRNA was reverse transcribed using iScript Reverse Transcriptase Supermix (Bio-Rad Laboratories, Hercules, CA, USA). Lastly, quantitative real-time PCR was performed using iQ Universal SYBR Green Supermix (Bio-Rad Laboratories, Hercules, CA, USA) using RPS-13 (ribosomal protein subunit 13) as a reference gene for normalization. Relative gene expression levels were calculated as fold changes using the $2^{-\Delta\Delta Ct}$ method. Primers were designed using the free access online tool: https://ncbi.nlm.nih.gov/ (accessed on 1 February 2021) and ordered from ThermoFisher (Waltham, MA, USA). The primers used are shown in Table 1.

Table 1. Primer sets used for quantification by Real-time PCR.

Gene	Forward Primer (5'-3')	Reverse Primer (5'-3')
CTNS	AGCTCCCCGATGAAGTTGTG	GTCAGGTTCAGAGCCACGAA
TFEB	GCAGTCCTACCTGGAGAATC	GTGGGCAGCAAACTTGTTCC
SQSTM1 (p62)	CTGAGCTCTGCCTCTTCCAG	GACAGGAGGAACAGTGAGGC
AKGDH	GATCTGGACTCCTCCGTGCC	ATCTCCCGCAGAGGAAGTGC
RPS-13	GCTCTCCTTTCGTTGCCTGA	ACTTCAACCAAGTGGGGACG

2.7. Lysosomal Cystine Measurement

Lysosomal cystine was quantified using HPLC-MS following an optimized assay previously developed in-house [37]. In short, six kidney tubules were pooled together in 1.5 mL. Eppendorf tubes and washed with ice-cold HBSS. Cells were then detached with accutase solution (Invitrogen, Carlsbad, CA, USA) and resuspended in HBSS before centrifugation at 300× g for 10 min. Cell pellets were neutralized with N-Ethylmaleimide

(NEM) solution (5 mM NEM in 0.1 mM sodium phosphate buffer pH 7.4) to avoid the unwanted measurement of cytosolic cystine. Cell suspension was precipitated, and protein was extracted by adding sulfosalicylic acid 15% (w/v) and centrifuging at 20,000× g for 10 min at 4 °C. In parallel, the total protein quantification was assessed by the PierceTM BCA protein assay kit (Thermo Fischer, Waltham, MA, USA) following the manufacturer's instructions. Lysosomal cystine measurement was performed using HPLC-MS/MS. Data is expressed as the lysosomal cystine normalized by total protein content.

2.8. Metabolomics Profiling

To be able to obtain enough metabolites for a reliable measurement, six kidney tubules were pooled in a 1.5 mL Eppendorf tube and washed with ice-cold HBSS. Next, cells pellets were collected by detaching the cells from the HFM using accutase solution (Invitrogen, Carlsbad, CA, USA), neutralized with culture medium, and centrifuged for 10 min at 300× g. Cell pellets were then incubated for 1 min with 1 mL of lysis buffer (methanol/acetonitrile/dH2O at a 2:2:1 ratio), vortexed for 30 s with intervals of 30 s in ice for 5 min, and put in a shaker platform at 4 °C for 20 min. The suspension was centrifuged at 16,000× g for 20 min at 4 °C and, lastly, supernatants containing the metabolite suspension were collected and stored at −80 °C until LC-MS measurement was performed. In parallel, six coated but unseeded HFM were pooled and identically processed as the seeded HFM, as the negative control. Additionally, medium samples of each well with unseeded HFM were cultured and identically processed as the other samples, as additional controls. All samples were sent to the Metabolism Expertise Center (Utrecht University, Utrecht, The Netherlands) and analyzed as described before [9]. In short, LC-MS analysis was performed on an Exactive mass spectrometer (ThermoFisher Scientific, Waltham, MA, USA) coupled to a Dionex Ultimate 3000 autosampler and pump (ThermoFisher Scientific, Waltham, MA, USA). Metabolites were separated using a Sequant ZIC-pHILIC column (2.1 cm × 150 mm, 5 µm, guard column 2.1 cm × 20 mm, 5 µm; Merck) with elution buffers acetonitrile (A) and eluent B (20 mM $(NH_4)_2CO_3$, 0.1% NH_4OH in ULC/MS-grade water (Biosolve, Valkenswaard, The Netherlands)). Gradient ran from 20% eluent B to 60% eluent B in 20 min, followed by a wash step at 80% and equilibration at 20%. Flow rate was set at 150 µL/min. Analysis was performed using the TraceFinder software (ThermoFisher Scientific, Waltham, MA, USA). Metabolites were identified and quantified based on exact mass within 5 ppm and further validated by concordance with retention times of standards. Data was further analyzed with R studio using the publicly available code from MetaboAnalyst.

2.9. Statistical Analysis

Every experiment was performed in at least three biological replicates, including at least 3 technical replicates each, unless specified otherwise. Results are shown as the mean ± standard error of the mean (SEM). All statistical analyses, except for metabolomics and image analysis, were performed in GraphPad version 8 (GraphPad software, La Jolla, CA, USA), using one-way ANOVA followed by a Tukey's post-hoc test, and two-way ANOVA for multiple comparison analyses. Metabolomics analysis was performed using R-studio (version 1.4.1103-3), using the publicly available code from MetaboAnalyst online tool. Image analysis was performed using Fiji (ImageJ software version 1.49, National Institutes of Health, Bethesda, MD, USA). For the actin filament orientation analysis, the plug-in "directionality" was used. For the puncta analysis, single channel images were first converted to binary and corrected for background. The puncta were counted by setting the same the threshold for all samples (between 30–255 and 3–255 for LC3/p62 and LAMP1/mTOR, respectively). Lastly, the plug-in "analyze particles" was used to count the particles. A p-value of <0.05 was considered as statistically significant.

3. Results

3.1. Healthy and Cystinotic ciPTECs Form Mature Kidney Tubules When Cultured on HFM

To develop a 3-dimensional bioengineered model of nephropathic cystinosis, we cultured different ciPTEC lines on HFM. We used the ciPTEC $CTNS^{WT}$ cells as our healthy control line; these cells have been well characterized in the past and are known to maintain many proximal tubules cell functions in culture [24]. The ciPTEC $CTNS^{-/-}$ cell line has been obtained by knocking out CTNS from the $CTNS^{WT}$ parent cell line [9]. These cell lines are isogenic and therefore any differences seen between these lines then can be directly attributed to CTNS loss. In addition, we include the $CTNS^{Patient}$ ciPTEC line, which was derived from cystinotic patient harboring a 57kb deletion and presents a strong cystinotic phenotype.

To determine whether all three ciPTEC lines can grow into a functional monolayer on the HFM, the polarization of the barrier was evaluated by immunofluorescent staining of the apically expressed cilia and the basolaterally located Na^+/K^+-ATPase. Imaging results confirmed that all three cell lines were able to attach and grow for at least 15 days on the double-coated HFM and exhibit one cilium at the apical side, and express Na^+/K^+-ATPase at the basolateral side of each cell (Figure 1A–C)

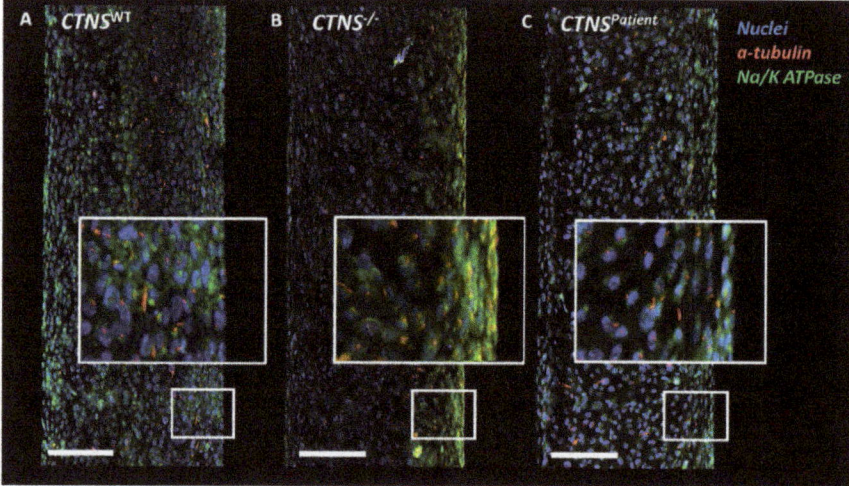

Figure 1. Confocal images of healthy and cystinotic ciPTECs kidney tubules. After maturation of 7 days, the control ciPTEC (**A**) form an organized 3-dimensional structure including primary cilia. Both cystinotic kidney tubule models (**B**,**C**) show visible holes in the monolayer when compared to the healthy proximal tubule model (**A**). The close-up images represent a 3-fold zoom increase. In blue: DAPI (nuclei staining), in red: α-tubulin staining, in green: Na^+/K^+-ATPase. Scale bar: 100 µm.

3.2. Bioengineered Cystinotic Kidney Tubules Present Disrupted Epithelial Monolayer

To assess the organization of the cell monolayer, kidney tubules were evaluated by immunofluorescent stainings and quantification of the intracellular actin filaments using the fluorescently labeled phalloidin probe. Imaging results revealed a loss of organization of the actin filaments in both cystinotic models when compared to the healthy proximal tubule model (Figure 2A–C). Moreover, directionality image analysis revealed that actin filaments were mostly oriented in a 90° angle (relative to the length of the tubule) in the healthy kidney tubules, an organization that was lost in the cystinotic models (Figure 2D–F). Besides, both cystinotic models exhibited holes along the monolayer where cells detached from the fiber membrane, consistent with a weaker and leakier monolayer.

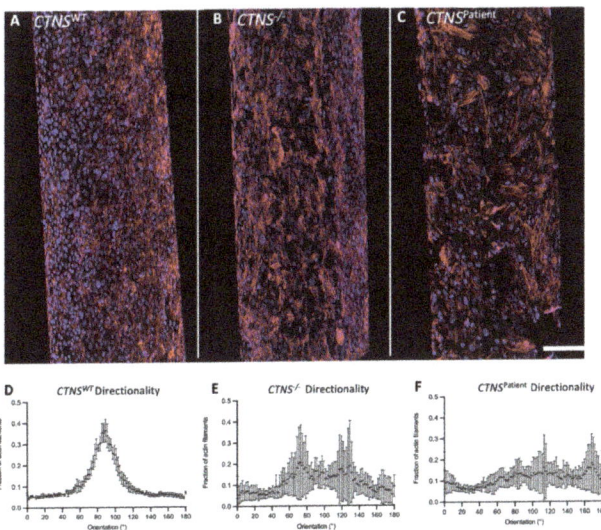

Figure 2. Cellular organization of kidney tubules. Kidney tubules were stained using phalloidin to show the organization of actin filaments in ciPTEC $CTNS^{WT}$ (**A**), $CTNS^{-/-}$ (**B**), and $CTNS^{Patient}$ (**C**). Both cystinotic models (**B**,**C**) present a disrupted cell monolayer with visible holes along the membrane when compared to the control cells (**A**), which is also seen in the image directionality quantification (**D**–**F**). In blue: DAPI (nuclei staining), in red: Phalloidin (binds to actin filaments). Directionality analysis was performed in three biological replicates. Scale bar: 100 μm.

Next, we compared the phenotype of the 3D bioengineered kidney tubules to a 2D environment. The same cell lines used for the kidney tubules were seeded under the same conditions as in the HFM, on top of a layer of L-dopa and a layer of collagen IV to ensure that the results are not dependent on the extracellular matrix provided (Figure 3). Quantification of the phalloidin staining showed no organization of the actin filaments in either of the models (Figure 3), including the healthy control, indicating that the directional cell monolayer organization is due to the 3-dimensional architecture of the HFM.

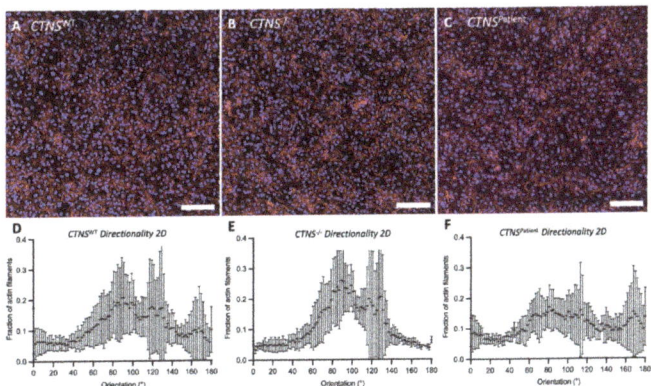

Figure 3. Cellular organization in 2D cell culture. Cells were stained using phalloidin to show the organization of actin filaments in ciPTEC $CTNS^{WT}$ (**A**), $CTNS^{-/-}$ (**B**), and $CTNS^{Patient}$ (**C**). Image directionality analysis revealed loss of organization in all the cell lines when cultured in 2D (**D**–**F**). In blue: DAPI (nuclei staining), in red: Phalloidin (binds to actin filaments). Directionality analysis was performed in two biological replicates Scale bar: 100 μm.

To further assess the integrity and the tightness of the kidney tubules monolayer, a FITC-inulin leakage assay was performed (Figure 4A). The results confirmed that the monolayer of both cystinotic kidney tubule models is less tight in comparison to the healthy control, with the cystinotic models 2.5- ($CTNS^{-/-}$) and 3.7-fold ($CTNS^{Patient}$) leakier than the healthy control (Figure 4B).

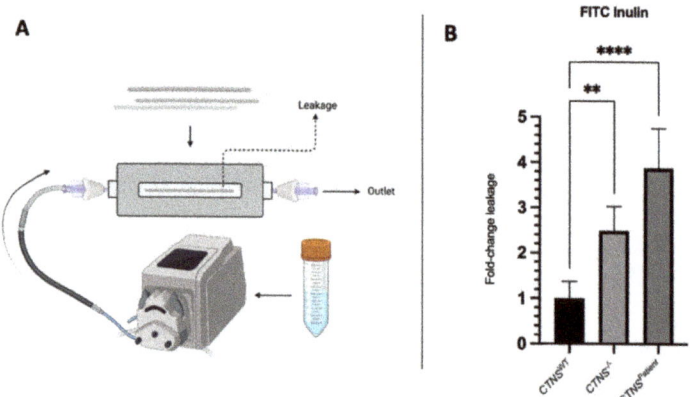

Figure 4. FITC inulin leakage assay in kidney. (**A**) Graphical presentation of the experimental set-up for the assessment of the monolayer leakage. The kidney tubules were secured into a 3-D printed chamber and connected to a pump with an in-let and out-let needle. Fluorescent FITC-inulin solution was perfused through the inside of the fiber and after 10 min, the solution that leaked through the kidney tubules to the extraluminal compartment was collected and measured. (**B**) Leakage of the healthy and cystinotic kidney tubules is expressed in fold change compared to the healthy control and normalized to a double-coated but unseeded HFM. One-way ANOVA statistical analysis was performed (N = 3; ** p-value < 0.01; **** p-value < 0.0001).

3.3. Cystinotic Kidney Tubules Accumulate Cystine Due to Cystinosin Absence

To evaluate the key phenotypical features of renal cystinosis, the expression of the *CTNS* gene and the accumulation of cystine in the lysosomes of the kidney tubules were measured. Real-time PCR results show that the *CTNS* gene expression was reduced by 60% in the $CTNS^{-/-}$ kidney tubules and a total loss of *CTNS* expression in the $CTNS^{Patient}$ tubules compared to the healthy kidney tubules (Figure 5A). The loss of *CTNS* expression led to a 100- and 360-fold increase in cystine accumulation in the $CTNS^{-/-}$ and $CTNS^{Patient}$ kidney tubules, respectively (Figure 5B).

3.4. Intracellular Vesicle Trafficking Is Impaired in Cystinotic Kidney Tubules

We evaluated further the downstream effects of lysosomal cystine accumulation by assessing autophagy using LC3 and p62 protein levels, which are part of the autophagosomal membrane and autophagosome cargo, respectively. Image analyses revealed a significant accumulation of both LC3 (5-fold in $CTNS^{-/-}$ and 8-fold in $CTNS^{Patient}$ kidney tubules) and p62 (2-fold in $CTNS^{-/-}$ and 2.6-fold in $CTNS^{Patient}$ kidney tubules) in the cytosol of the cystinotic models (Figure 6A–D), indicating increased levels of autophagy in the cystinotic kidney tubules. Real-time PCR quantification show the dysregulation of *TFEB* and *SQSTM1* (the gene coding for p62) in both cystinotic kidney tubules when compared to baseline healthy kidney tubules expression levels. *TFEB* is a transcriptional regulator of autophagy which is known to downregulate its own expression after autophagy activation. Indeed, its expression appeared significantly reduced by 40% to 80% in $CTNS^{-/-}$ and $CTNS^{Patient}$ kidney tubules, respectively (Figure 6E). Interestingly, mRNA expression of p62 was 2-fold higher in $CTNS^{-/-}$ kidney tubules than the healthy control, while in the $CTNS^{Patient}$ kidney tubules, a 44% reduction in p62 gene expression was found (Figure 6E).

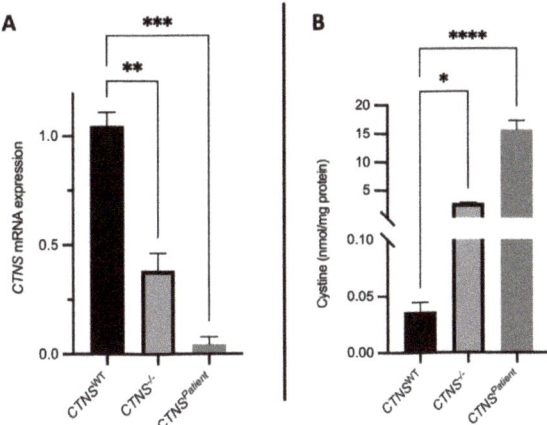

Figure 5. Cystine accumulation and *CTNS* expression in kidney tubules. Real-time PCR quantification showed significant reduction of *CTNS* gene expression in both cystinotic tubule models when compared to the healthy control (**A**), which led to an increase in cystine accumulation in the cystinotic kidney tubules (**B**). One-way ANOVA statistical analysis was performed (N = 3; * p-value < 0.05; ** p-value < 0.01; *** p-value < 0.001; **** p-value < 0.0001).

To confirm the activation of autophagy, we evaluated the subcellular localization of the mammalian target of rapamycin (mTOR). Under normal conditions the active mTOR complex 1 (mTORC1) is located at the lysosomal membrane and colocalizes with lysosomal membrane protein LAMP1. Imaging analysis showcased a 5-fold loss of co-localization of the LAMP1-mTOR complex in both $CTNS^{-/-}$ and $CTNS^{Patient}$ kidney tubules (Figure 7), when compared to the healthy kidney tubules. These results indeed suggest the inactivation of mTOR, which will in turn activate autophagy.

3.5. Cystinotic Kidney Tubules Present Metabolic Impairment

To gain in-depth knowledge on the intracellular molecular pathways affected in the cystinotic kidney tubules, we evaluated the metabolomic profile of 100 key metabolites in all three models. Principal component analysis (PCA) of the metabolites measured show that $CTNS^{-/-}$ and $CTNS^{Patient}$ kidney tubules account for most of the variability of the dataset (74.2%); Figure 8A). To explore which metabolites and pathways are directly linked to a cystinotic phenotype, the top 60 most differentially expressed metabolites in cystinotic *vs* healthy kidney tubules were plotted together in a heatmap (Figure 8B). Significantly altered metabolites are either up or downregulated, such as the accumulation of alanine and glucose, and the loss of threonine and glutamine in the cystinotic models when compared to the healthy kidney tubules. Interestingly, despite the uniqueness of the genetic background of the $CTNS^{-/-}$ and the $CTNS^{Patient}$ models, the metabolic profiling appears to be similar when compared to the healthy kidney tubules, indicating that these metabolites are directly linked to *CTNS* loss rather than to differences in the genetic background of the cells.

To elucidate the molecular pathways altered in cystinosis due to complete *CTNS* loss, we performed a pathway analysis that revealed the pathways significantly correlated ($p < 0.05$) with *CTNS* loss: ubiquinone biosynthesis, phenylalanine, tyrosine and tryptophan biosynthesis, arginine biosynthesis, cystine and methionine metabolism, D-Glutamine and D-glutamate metabolism, alanine, aspartate and glutamate metabolism, and the TCA cycle (tricarboxylic acid cycle), in decreasing order of impact. In line with previous studies, we found α-ketoglutarate (α-KG) to be among the key metabolites altered when comparing cystinotic to healthy kidney tubules (Figure 9B). Alpha-Ketoglutarate dehydrogenase is the enzyme encoded by the *AKGDH* gene and is responsible for the degradation of α-KG in the cytosol. We found a significant reduction in *AKGDH* expression in both cystinotic models (Figure 9A), which correlates directly with the cytosolic accumulation of a-KG (Figure 9B).

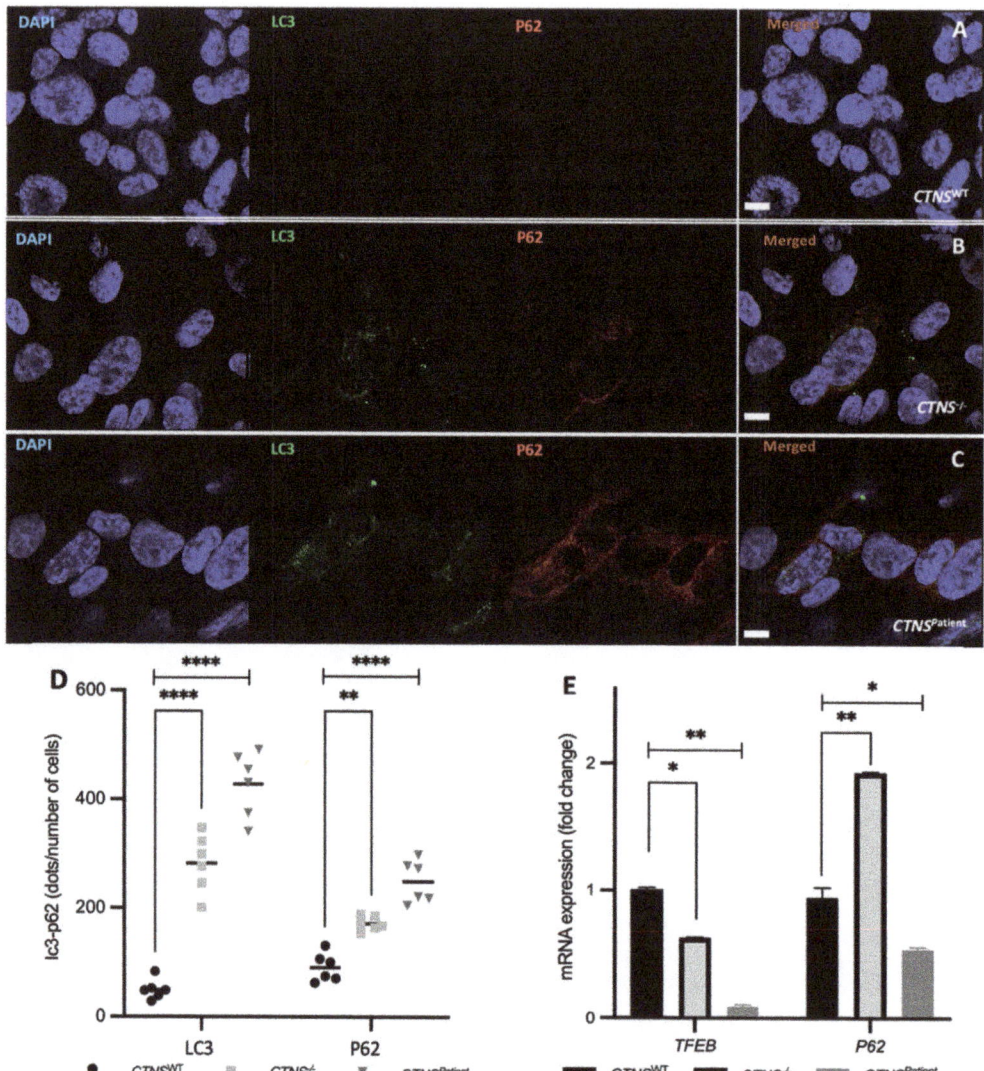

Figure 6. Autophagic markers in kidney tubules. Images obtained with a confocal microscope at 63X of the ciPTEC *CTNS^{WT}* (**A**), *CTNS$^{-/-}$* (**B**), and *CTNS^{Patient}* (**C**) kidney tubules. Image quantification analysis showed a significant increase of the autophagy markers LC3 and p62 in the cystinotic 3D models when compared to the healthy control (**D**). Real-time PCR quantification also showed a significant impairment of the autophagy-related genes TFEB and p62 in the cystinotic models when compared to the healthy control (**E**). In blue: nuclei, in green: LC3 protein, in red: p62 protein. Scale bar: 10 μm. One-way ANOVA statistical analysis was performed (N = 3; * p-value < 0.05; ** p-value < 0.01; **** p-value < 0.0001).

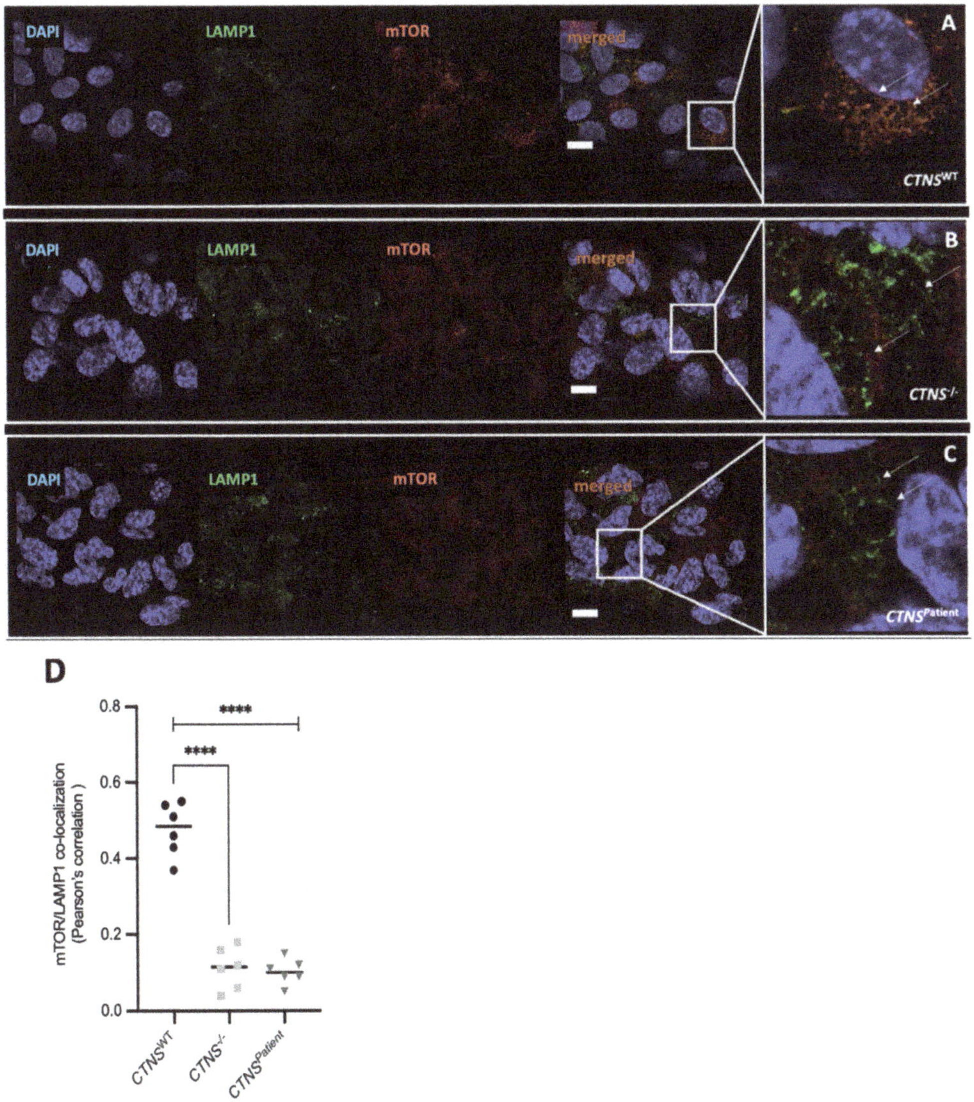

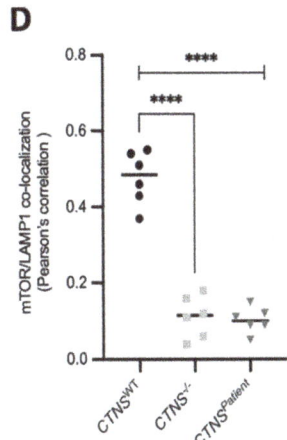

Figure 7. mTOR and LAMP1 staining and colocalization in kidney tubules. Confocal microscopy images taken at 63X of the ciPTEC $CTNS^{WT}$ (**A**), $CTNS^{-/-}$ (**B**), and $CTNS^{Patient}$ (**C**) kidney tubules. Image analysis quantification showed co-localization of the mTOR/LAMP1 complex in the healthy control and loss of co-localization in both cystinotic models (**D**), suggesting an impaired autophagosome-lysosome trafficking. In blue: DAPI (nuclei), in green: LAMP1 protein, in red: mTOR protein. Scale bar: 10 µm. One-way ANOVA statistical analysis was performed (N = 3; **** p-value < 0.0001).

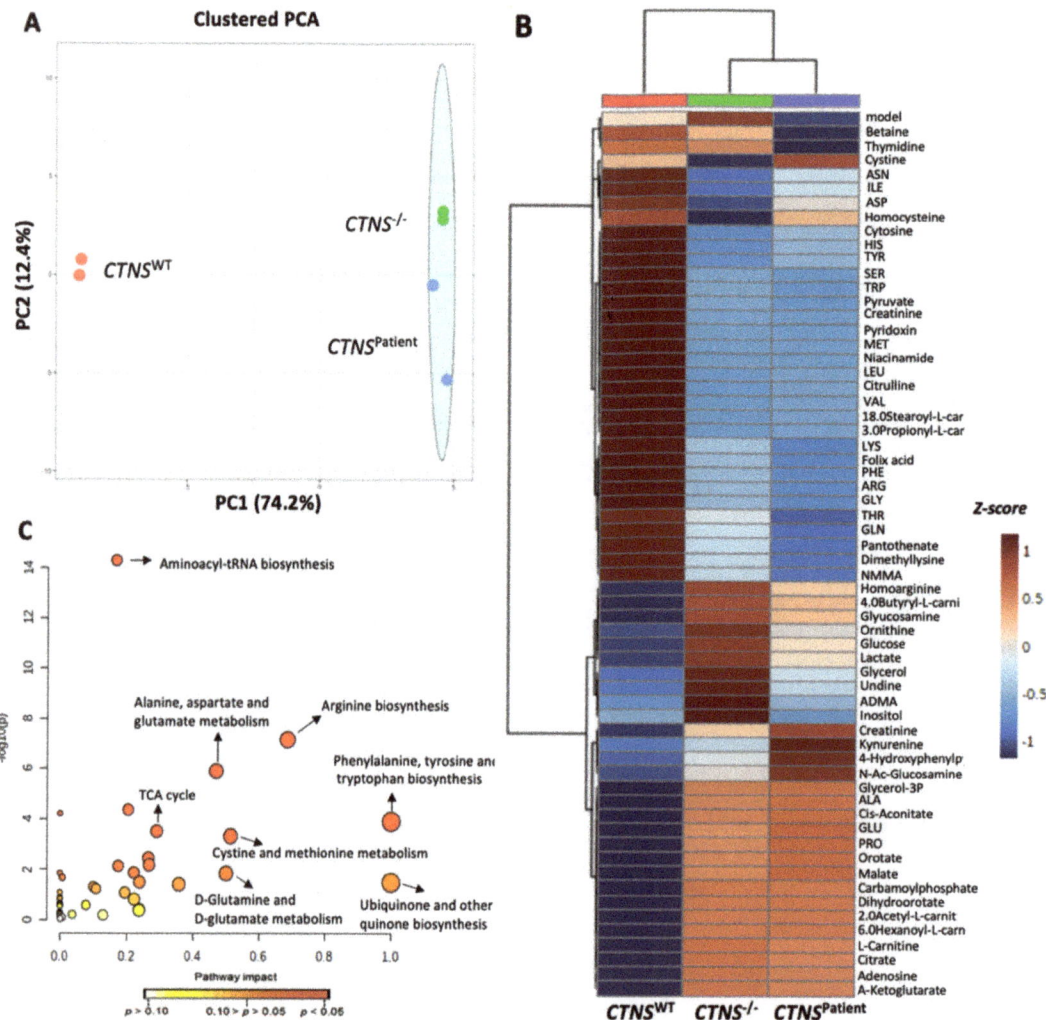

Figure 8. Metabolomic profiling of kidney tubules. Principal component analysis (PCA) of the ciPTEC $CTNS^{WT}$, $CTNS^{-/-}$, and $CTNS^{Patient}$ kidney tubule models based on the metabolites set measured. In the plot, the individual dots represent one biological repeat, and dots of the same color are the same experimental group (healthy ($CTNS^{WT}$, $CTNS^{-/-}$ and $CTNS^{Patient}$ kidney tubules) (**A**). Heatmap analysis of the top 60 metabolites differentially expressed in healthy and cystinotic kidney tubule models. Every row represents a different metabolite and its associated Z-score. Significantly increased metabolites ($p < 0.01$) are displayed in red, and significantly decreased metabolites ($p < 0.01$) are displayed in blue (**B**). Global pathway enrichment analysis of the metabolic pathways differentially expressed in the $CTNS^{-/-}$ compared to the healthy kidney tubules. The larger the circles and the further they appear from the y-axis, the higher the impact of that pathway in the $CTNS^{-/-}$ kidney tubules (**C**). Data was normalized to the median intensity. Data analysis was performed using univariate and multivariate analysis (N = 2; p-values < 0.05 were considered significant).

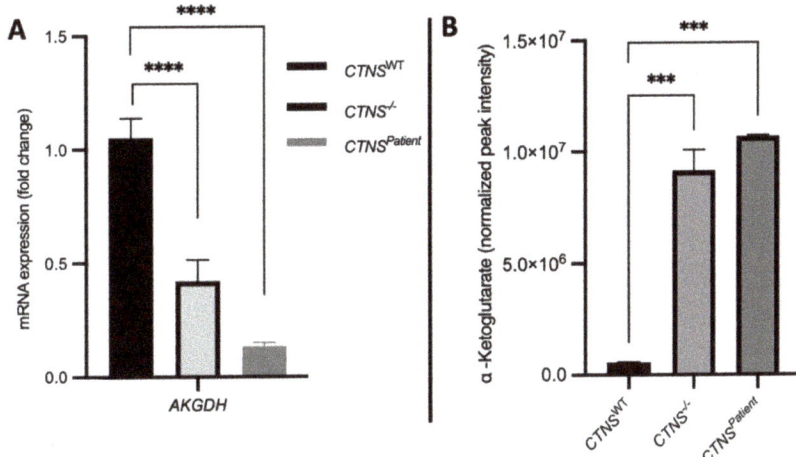

Figure 9. Cystinotic kidney tubules accumulate α-KG. Real-time PCR quantification show a significant 45% and 89% reduction ($CTNS^{-/-}$ and $CTNS^{Patient}$ kidney tubules, respectively) of the *AKGDH* gene (**A**). Cystinotic kidney tubules significantly accumulate α-KG in the cytoplasm (**B**). One-way ANOVA statistical analysis was performed (N = 3; *** p-value < 0.001; **** p-value < 0.0001).

4. Discussion

In this work, we developed and characterized 3-dimensional bioengineered proximal tubule models for studying nephropathic cystinosis. We compared two cystinotic kidney tubule models to a healthy proximal tubule. To avoid misleading results of the cystinotic phenotype due to the different genetic background between the cystinotic patient donor and the healthy donor, we included an isogenic cell line ($CTNS^{-/-}$), which was previously developed in-house using CRISPR/Cas9 from the healthy control cell line [9].

In comparison to the conventional 2-dimensional cultures, our HFM approach allows the cells to grow and develop in structures that mimic a tubule. All three cell lines cultured were able to proliferate and mature on the HFM and exhibit polarization markers, including the cilia and the Na^+/K^+-ATPase at the apical and basolateral side, respectively. This 3-dimensional tubular structure is crucial for studies that require molecular transport, since both the apical and the basolateral sides of the cells are accessible. Previous studies already demonstrated how the geometry of the culture surface affects the gene expression patterns and molecular pathways of the cells [38], including the kidney tubular cells [39]. Most studies reported a more mature cell differentiation when cultured in a 3-dimensional, microfluidics platform as compared to 2-dimensional cultures [9,40].

Cystinosis is mainly characterized by the loss or impairment of the *CTNS* gene, which leads to the intralysosomal accumulation of cystine [1]. Our results show a significant reduction (60%) and a total loss of *CTNS* gene expression in $CTNS^{-/-}$ and $CTNS^{Patient}$ kidney tubules, respectively. Consequently, the cystine accumulation found in both cystinotic models are more profound when compared to 2-dimensional cell cultures, especially in the $CTNS^{Patient}$ kidney tubules, which was 3-fold higher [9], and mimics the diagnostic testing results in the white blood cells of cystinotic patients [41]. We can hypothesize that growing these cells in the HFM 3-dimensional configuration enhances the cystinotic phenotype caused by the complete loss of cystinosin in these cells.

Both cystinotic models exhibit a loss of organization of the cell monolayer and a significantly higher leakage when compared to the healthy kidney tubules. Clinically, the renal presentation of cystinosis includes a dilated and atrophic proximal tubule [42], a direct consequence of a loss of monolayer tightness and epithelial organization [43].

This phenotype was clearly observed in our cystinotic kidney tubules and was more profound in the $CTNS^{Patient}$ model, which harbors the 57kb deletion in $CTNS$. Furthermore, *in vivo* cystinosis studies reported abnormal levels of autophagy [44,45], with changes in the expression of key autophagy genes such as *TFEB*, *LC3II*, and *SQSTM1*. Our results show a significant increase of p62 and LC3 protein in both cystinotic tubules, consistent with increased autophagy in both models of cystinosis. Furthermore, our data reveals that the mTOR/LAMP1protein complex is dissociated in both cystinotic kidney tubule models when compared to the heathy control. The inactivation of mTOR is expected to activate the translocation of the transcription factor TFEB to the nucleus, which in turn will downregulate its own mRNA levels, which is also what we observed in our system. The mRNA levels of p62 were more puzzling. In line with increased protein levels, the expression of p62 was increased in the $CTNS^{-/-}$ tubules when compared to the $CTNS^{WT}$. In the $CTNS^{Patient}$ tubules, on the other hand, p62 mRNA levels were consistently down. This may be due to a (slight) difference in autophagic flux. We previously found that, after blocking, the autophagic flux with bafilomycin the autophagy markers LC3 and p63 would rise, and to a higher extend in $CTNS^{-/-}$ cells compared to $CTNS^{Patient}$ cells [9]. In this case the $CTNS^{-/-}$ tubules also have to produce and degrade higher levels of autophagic cargo (including p62), whereas in the $CTNS^{Patient}$ cells the cargo degradation may be delayed. As p62 is accumulating and not efficiently degraded there may be no need for the $CTNS^{Patient}$ cells to keep producing more p63 mRNA (resulting in lower mRNA levels). In the literature there is also conflicting evidence to what extent the increase in autophagy seen in cystinosis is accompanied by a block in autophagy or that the autophagic flux is actually increased. This also suggests that the outcome of this assay may depend on the model system used and other factors, such as genetic background, may play a role. Overall, our data on vesicle trafficking impairment is consistent with the phenotype previously observed in cystinosis [4,43,46,47].

Despite the gap in understanding the link between cystine accumulation and its implication in the molecular pathways leading to nephropathy, cystinosis has been extensively described as a metabolic disease [48,49]. Our metabolomic analysis displays the impact of *CTNS* loss in the intra-cellular pathways in cystinotic kidney tubules, showcasing that cystinosis is not only a lysosomal storage disease, but a condition that significantly affects many metabolic processes such as glucose, glutamine, and alanine metabolism and the TCA cycle. Some of these pathways are directly related while others are not, but the accumulation of cystine seems to be the key element in such a metabolic impairment. As previously mentioned, renal Fanconi syndrome appears in early stages in cystinotic patients. The clinical presentation includes the loss of amino acids and proteins, which leads to proteinuria/aminoaciduria, glycosuria, and hypophosphatemia/hyperphosphaturia [50,51]. Therefore, kidney tubules are a powerful instrument to study in depth the metabolic pathways underlying cystinosis and, hence, offer a promising platform to further study the metabolic and proteomic disturbances in renal Fanconi syndrome.

Autophagy is a digestion process that fuels the cells with essential aminoacids that will eventually enter the TCA cycle. One metabolite involved in the TCA cycle and that has been described previously in increased autophagy is α-KG, which appears to play a role in key pathways in cystinosis, such as glucose, glutamine, and alanine metabolism. Numerous studies have described the close relationship between α-KG and cystine [52,53], including its downstream effect on oxidative stress and role in the glucose, glutamine and other aminoacids metabolism. Moreover, under healthy conditions, α-KG is degraded by the mitochondrial enzyme *AKGDH*, which we observed significantly reduced in both cystinotic kidney tubule models. Mitochondrial dysfunction has also been reported for cystinotic cell lines [54], which could lead to the downregulation of *AKGDH* and, subsequently, the induction of α-KG accumulation. Both cystinotic kidney tubules demonstrated a significant accumulation of α-KG and a downregulation of *AKGDH* when compared to the healthy kidney tubules. The metabolic analysis of the cystinotic kidney tubules showcased the similarities between the isogenic $CTNS^{-/-}$ and $CTNS^{Patient}$ 3D models. Similarly, the differences in the metabolic pathways between the cystinosis models and the healthy bioengineered kidney tubules were also better represented in 3D than what has been previously seen in 2-dimensional cell culture studies [9].

The enhancement of the hallmarks of the disease or the better representation of the clinical condition in 3D models is a recurrent observation in the literature for many disorders. For instance, reproducing the cell-to-extracellular matrix interaction, recapitulating the expression of apoptosis-related genes, the increase of drug sensitivity, and mimicking tumor invasion processes are some of the traits that have shown to be better represented in 3D cancer models [55–57]. 3D liver disease models have also been reported advantageous over 2D cultures since they allow for the study of biliary excretion of metabolites, the functional establishment of cell polarity, and crucial processes in liver disease such as inflammation and fibrosis [58–60]. Additionally, having 3D cultures made it possible to study the metabolic interaction between diseased lung cells and cancer-associated fibroblasts [61], but many more examples have been published.

In this study, we aimed to establish the added benefit of culturing cystinotic cells in 3-dimensions on an HFM. In addition to the phenotypical characteristics that these cells show in a 2-dimensional setting, we could now also observe differences in cell organization and the alignment of cells along the direction of the fiber. Furthermore, growing the cells on a porous membrane allowed us to perform a leakage assay, which showed that the monolayer of the cystinotic cells was less tight compared to control cells. That said, culturing the cells on an HFM also comes with some drawbacks. You need more cells because only part of the cells will adhere the membrane in contrast with 2-dimensional culturing where all the seeded cells will end up in the well. Additionally, care must be taken to not disrupt the kidney tubule monolayer during handling, and imaging must be conducted with one fiber at the time, making this approach more labor intensive and less suitable for high throughput applications. Furthermore, assays that require a larger number of cells (such as western blotting) remain challenging. Therefore, growing cells as a kidney tubule may not be the best option for all types of analysis, but rather adds to the toolbox of methods available for the study of proximal tubule diseases, especially when cell transport and cellular organization are involved.

In summary, our bioengineered kidney tubule models mimic the pathophysiology and the morphological abnormalities of nephropathic cystinosis better than the 2-dimensional cell culture models available to study this disease. In addition, the HFM platform offers a complex system that allows for perfusion, which facilitates the assessment of metabolites transport and encourages drug testing in a proximal tubule-imitating architecture. Hence, transitioning from 2-dimensional cell cultures to complex, microphysiological models that better mimic the disease is crucial to advance our understanding of the molecular mechanisms of the disease of interest and paves the way to personalized medicine.

Author Contributions: Conceptualization, E.S.G., R.M. and M.J.J.; methodology, E.S.G., R.M. and M.J.J.; software, E.S.G. and M.J.J.; validation, E.S.G., R.M. and M.J.J.; formal analysis E.S.G.; investigation, E.S.G.; resources, R.M.; data curation, E.S.G.; writing—original draft preparation, E.S.G.; writing—review and editing, E.S.G., R.M. and M.J.J.; visualization, E.S.G.; supervision, R.M. and M.J.J.; project administration, R.M.; funding acquisition, M.J.J. and R.M. All authors have read and agreed to the published version of the manuscript.

Funding: This research received funding from the IMAGEN project, which is co-funded by the PPP Allowance made available by Health~Holland, Top Sector Life Sciences & Health, to stimulate public–private partnerships (IMplementation of Advancements in GENetic Kidney Disease, LSHM20009; E.S.G., M.J.J. and R.M.).

Institutional Review Board Statement: The three cell lines used in this study were obtained from Cell4Pharma (Nijmegen, The Netherlands, MTA #A16-0147). The ciPTEC line was developed in 2008 at Radboudumc from a healthy human volunteer who donated a urine sample, strictly following the medical ethical guidelines and with approval as published in Wimer et al. 2010 [24]. The cell line is patented as 'A novel conditionally immortalized human proximal tubule cell line expressing functional influx and efflux transporters', Patent P6057046PCT; PCT/EP2016/080026, by Radboudumc.

Since 2019, Radboudumc gave the exclusive licence for the use of the cell line by Cell4Pharma, who now provides the cells; www.cell4pharma.com, Oss, The Netherlands.

Informed Consent Statement: Not applicable.

Data Availability Statement: The raw data for the metabolomics analysis is currently being uploaded to a public data depository.

Acknowledgments: The authors would like to gratefully thank João Faria and Marta Valverde for the training and the input provided for the hollow fiber membrane set-up and the chambers preparation. Additionally, we thank Sabbir Ahmed for the support provided for the LC-MS measurements. We would also like to thank Koen Westphal for the training provided for the confocal microscopy. We thank Esther Zaal and Celia Berkers from the Metabolism Expertise Center (Utrecht University, Utrecht, The Netherlands) for their guidance on and support for the metabolomics work. Lastly, we would like to thank Rosalie Haak for the support with the experiments during her internship in our group.

Conflicts of Interest: The authors declare no conflict of interest.

References

1. Gahl, W.A.; Thoene, J.G.; Schneider, J.A. Cystinosis. *N. Engl. J. Med.* **2002**, *347*, 111–121. [CrossRef] [PubMed]
2. Town, M.; Jean, G.; Cherqui, S.; Attard, M.; Forestier, L.; Whitmore, S.A.; Callen, D.F.; Gribouval, O.; Broyer, M.; Bates, G.P.; et al. A novel gene encoding an integral membrane protein is mutated in nephropathic cystinosis. *Nat. Genet.* **1998**, *18*, 319–324. [CrossRef] [PubMed]
3. Touchman, J.W.; Anikster, Y.; Dietrich, N.L.; Maduro, V.V.B.; McDowell, G.; Shotelersuk, V.; Bouffard, G.G.; Beckstrom-Sternberg, S.M.; Gahl, W.A.; Green, E.D. The genomic region encompassing the nephropathic cystinosis gene (CTNS): Complete sequencing of a 200-kb segment and discovery of a novel gene within the common cystinosis-causing deletion. *Genome Res.* **2000**, *10*, 165–173. [CrossRef] [PubMed]
4. Ivanova, E.A.; De Leo, M.G.; Van Den Heuvel, L.; Pastore, A.; Dijkman, H.; De Matteis, M.A.; Levtchenko, E.N. Endo-lysosomal dysfunction in human proximal tubular epithelial cells deficient for lysosomal cystine transporter cystinosin. *PLoS ONE* **2015**, *10*, e0120998. [CrossRef]
5. Steinherz, R.; Tietze, F.; Gahl, W.A.; Triche, T.J.; Chiang, H.; Modesti, A.; Schulman, J.D. Cystine accumulation and clearance by normal and cystinotic leukocytes exposed to cystine dimethyl ester. *Proc. Natl. Acad. Sci. USA* **1982**, *79*, 4446–4450. [CrossRef]
6. Gahl, W.A.; Tietze, F.; Bashan, N.; Steinherz, R.; Schulman, J.D. Defective cystine exodus from isolated lysosome-rich fractions of cystinotic leukocytes. *J. Biol. Chem.* **1982**, *257*, 9570–9575. [CrossRef]
7. Cherqui, S.; Courtoy, P.J. The renal Fanconi syndrome in cystinosis: Pathogenic insights and therapeutic perspectives. *Nat. Rev. Nephrol.* **2017**, *13*, 115–131. [CrossRef]
8. Jamalpoor, A.; Othman, A.; Levtchenko, E.N.; Masereeuw, R.; Janssen, M.J. Molecular Mechanisms and Treatment Options of Nephropathic Cystinosis. *Trends Mol. Med.* **2021**, *27*, 673–686. [CrossRef]
9. Jamalpoor, A.; van Gelder, C.A.; Yousef Yengej, F.A.; Zaal, E.A.; Berlingerio, S.P.; Veys, K.R.; Pou Casellas, C.; Voskuil, K.; Essa, K.; Ammerlaan, C.M.; et al. Cysteamine–bicalutamide combination therapy corrects proximal tubule phenotype in cystinosis. *EMBO Mol. Med.* **2021**, *13*, e13067. [CrossRef]
10. Hollywood, J.A.; Przepiorski, A.; D'Souza, R.; Yengej, F.A.; Zaal, E.A.; Berlingerio, S.P.; Wolvetang, E.J.; Harrison, P.T.; Davidson, A.J.; Holm, T.M. Use of human induced pluripotent stem cells and kidney organoids to develop a cysteamine/mTOR inhibition combination therapy for cystinosis. *J. Am. Soc. Nephrol.* **2020**, *31*, 962–982. [CrossRef]
11. Sansanwal, P.; Sarwal, M.M. p62/SQSTM1 prominently accumulates in renal proximal tubules in nephropathic cystinosis. *Pediatr. Nephrol.* **2012**, *27*, 2137–2144. [CrossRef]
12. Bellomo, F.; Signorile, A.; Tamma, G.; Ranieri, M.; Emma, F.; De Rasmo, D. Impact of atypical mitochondrial cyclic-AMP level in nephropathic cystinosis. *Cell. Mol. Life Sci.* **2018**, *75*, 3411–3422. [CrossRef]
13. Luciani, A.; Festa, B.P.; Chen, Z.; Devuyst, O. Defective autophagy degradation and abnormal tight junction-associated signaling drive epithelial dysfunction in cystinosis. *Autophagy* **2018**, *14*, 1157–1159. [CrossRef]
14. Cassiman, D.; Cornelissen, E.A.M.; Janssen, M.; Levtchenko, E.N.; Bos, M.; Boullart, K.; Sondag, F. *Clinical Relevance and Patients Relevance of Delayed-Release Cysteamine Bitartrate for Patients with Nephropathic Cystinosis: Clinical and Patient/Caregiver Perspective*; Europe-ExPro: Munich, Germany, 2016.
15. Schulman, J.D.; Bradley, K.H. Cystinosis: Therapeutic implications of in vitro studies of cultured fibroblasts. *J. Pediatr.* **1971**, *78*, 833–836. [CrossRef]
16. Pisoni, R.L.; Thoene, J.G.; Christensen, H.N. Detection and characterization of carrier-mediated cationic amino acid transport in lysosomes of normal and cystinotic human fibroblasts. Role in therapeutic cystine removal? *J. Biol. Chem.* **1985**, *260*, 4791–4798. [CrossRef]

17. Gorvin, C.M.; Wilmer, M.J.; Piret, S.E.; Harding, B.; van den Heuvel, L.P.; Wrong, O.; Jat, P.S.; Lippiat, J.D.; Levtchenko, E.N.; Thakker, R.V. Receptor-mediated endocytosis and endosomal acidification is impaired in proximal tubule epithelial cells of Dent disease patients. *Proc. Natl. Acad. Sci. USA* **2013**, *110*, 7014–7019. [CrossRef]
18. Festa, B.P.; Berquez, M.; Gassama, A.; Amrein, I.; Ismail, H.M.; Samardzija, M.; Staiano, L.; Luciani, A.; Grimm, C.; Nussbaum, R.L.; et al. OCRL deficiency impairs endolysosomal function in a humanized mouse model for Lowe syndrome and Dent disease. *Hum. Mol. Genet.* **2019**, *28*, 1931–1946. [CrossRef]
19. Peeters, K.; Wilmer, M.J.; Schoeber, J.P.; Reijnders, D.; van den Heuvel, L.P.; Masereeuw, R.; Levtchenko, E. Role of P-glycoprotein expression and function in cystinotic renal proximal tubular cells. *Pharmaceutics* **2011**, *3*, 782–792. [CrossRef]
20. Rossi, M.N.; Pascarella, A.; Licursi, V.; Caiello, I.; Taranta, A.; Rega, L.R.; Levtchenko, E.; Emma, F.; De Benedetti, F.; Prencipe, G. NLRP2 Regulates Proinflammatory and Antiapoptotic Responses in Proximal Tubular Epithelial Cells. *Front. Cell Dev. Biol.* **2019**, *7*, 252. [CrossRef]
21. Hall, G.; Gbadegesin, R.A.; Lavin, P.; Wu, G.; Liu, Y.; Oh, E.C.; Wang, L.; Spurney, R.F.; Eckel, J.; Lindsey, T.; et al. A novel missense mutation of Wilms' Tumor 1 causes autosomal dominant FSGS. *J. Am. Soc. Nephrol.* **2015**, *26*, 831–843. [CrossRef]
22. Reichold, M.; Klootwijk, E.D.; Reinders, J.; Otto, E.A.; Milani, M.; Broeker, C.; Laing, C.; Wiesner, J.; Devi, S.; Zhou, W.; et al. Glycine Amidinotransferase (GATM), Renal Fanconi Syndrome, and Kidney Failure. *J. Am. Soc. Nephrol.* **2018**, *29*, 1849–1858. [CrossRef] [PubMed]
23. Sasaki, S.; Hara, A.; Sakaguchi, M.; Nangaku, M.; Inoue, Y. Hepatocyte nuclear factor 4α regulates megalin expression in proximal tubular cells. *Biochem. Biophys. Rep.* **2019**, *17*, 87–92. [CrossRef] [PubMed]
24. Wilmer, M.J.; Saleem, M.A.; Masereeuw, R.; Ni, L.; van der Velden, T.J.; Russel, F.G.; Mathieson, P.W.; Monnens, L.A.; van den Heuvel, L.P.; Levtchenko, E.N. Novel conditionally immortalized human proximal tubule cell line expressing functional influx and efflux transporters. *Cell Tissue Res.* **2010**, *339*, 449–457. [CrossRef] [PubMed]
25. Yousef Yengej, F.A.; Jansen, J.; Rookmaaker, M.B.; Verhaar, M.C.; Clevers, H. Kidney organoids and tubuloids. *Cells* **2020**, *9*, 1326. [CrossRef]
26. Freedman, B.S. Modeling Kidney Disease with iPS Cells. Supplementary Issue: Stem Cell Biology. *Biomark. Insights* **2015**, *10*, 153–169. [CrossRef]
27. De Carvalho Ribeiro, P.; Oliveira, L.F.; Caldas, H.C. Differentiating Induced Pluripotent Stem Cells into Renal Cells: A New Approach to Treat Kidney Diseases. *Stem Cells Int.* **2020**, *2020*, 8894590. [CrossRef]
28. Lau, R.W.; Wang, B.; Ricardo, S.D. Gene editing of stem cells for kidney disease modelling and therapeutic intervention. *Nephrology* **2018**, *23*, 981–990. [CrossRef]
29. Schophuizen, C.M.; De Napoli, I.E.; Jansen, J.; Teixeira, S.; Wilmer, M.J.; Hoenderop, J.G.; Van den Heuvel, L.P.; Masereeuw, R.; Stamatialis, D. Development of a living membrane comprising a functional human renal proximal tubule cell monolayer on polyethersulfone polymeric membrane. *Acta Biomater.* **2015**, *14*, 22–32. [CrossRef]
30. Englezakis, A.; Gozalpour, E.; Kamran, M.; Fenner, K.; Mele, E.; Coopman, K. Development of a hollow fibre-based renal module for active transport studies. *J. Artif. Organs* **2021**, *24*, 473–484. [CrossRef]
31. Jochems, P.G.; van Bergenhenegouwen, J.; van Genderen, A.M.; Eis, S.T.; Versprille, L.J.W.; Wichers, H.J.; Jeurink, P.V.; Garssen, J.; Masereeuw, R. Development and validation of bioengineered intestinal tubules for translational research aimed at safety and efficacy testing of drugs and nutrients. *Toxicol. In Vitro* **2019**, *60*, 1–11. [CrossRef]
32. Jansen, J.; De Napoli, I.E.; Fedecostante, M.; Schophuizen, C.M.S.; Chevtchik, N.V.; Wilmer, M.J.; van Asbeck, A.H.; Croes, H.J.; Pertijs, J.C.; Wetzels, J.F.; et al. Human proximal tubule epithelial cells cultured on hollow fibers: Living membranes that actively transport organic cations. *Sci. Rep.* **2015**, *5*, 16702. [CrossRef]
33. Chevtchik, N.V.; Mihajlovic, M.; Fedecostante, M.; Bolhuis-Versteeg, L.; Sastre Toraño, J.; Masereeuw, R.; Stamatialis, D. A bioartificial kidney device with polarized secretion of immune modulators. *J. Tissue Eng. Regen. Med.* **2018**, *12*, 1670–1678. [CrossRef]
34. Wilmer, M.J.; Kluijtmans, L.A.; van der Velden, T.J.; Willems, P.H.; Scheffer, P.G.; Masereeuw, R.; Monnens, L.A.; van den Heuvel, L.P.; Levtchenko, E.N. Cysteamine restores glutathione redox status in cultured cystinotic proximal tubular epithelial cells. *Biochim. Biophys. Acta (BBA)-Mol. Basis Dis.* **2011**, *1812*, 643–651. [CrossRef]
35. Oo, Z.Y.; Deng, R.; Hu, M.; Ni, M.; Kandasamy, K.; Bin Ibrahim, M.S.; Ying, J.Y.; Zink, D. The performance of primary human renal cells in hollow fiber bioreactors for bioartificial kidneys. *Biomaterials* **2011**, *32*, 8806–8815. [CrossRef]
36. Jansen, J.; Fedecostante, M.; Wilmer, M.J.; Peters, J.G.; Kreuser, U.M.; Van Den Broek, P.H.; Mensink, R.A.; Boltje, T.J.; Stamatialis, D.; Wetzels, J.F.; et al. Bioengineered kidney tubules efficiently excrete uremic toxins. *Sci. Rep.* **2016**, *6*, 1–12. [CrossRef]
37. Jamalpoor, A.; Sparidans, R.W.; Pou Casellas, C.; Rood, J.J.; Joshi, M.; Masereeuw, R.; Janssen, M.J. Quantification of cystine in human renal proximal tubule cells using liquid chromatography–tandem mass spectrometry. *Biomed. Chromatogr.* **2018**, *32*, e4238. [CrossRef]
38. Yu, S.M.; Oh, J.M.; Lee, J.; Lee-Kwon, W.; Jung, W.; Amblard, F.; Granick, S.; Cho, Y.K. Substrate curvature affects the shape, orientation, and polarization of renal epithelial cells. *Acta Biomater.* **2018**, *77*, 311–321. [CrossRef]
39. Shen, C.; Meng, Q.; Zhang, G. Increased curvature of hollow fiber membranes could up-regulate differential functions of renal tubular cell layers. *Biotechnol. Bioeng.* **2013**, *110*, 2173–2183. [CrossRef]

40. Luca, A.C.; Mersch, S.; Deenen, R.; Schmidt, S.; Messner, I.; Schäfer, K.L.; Baldus, S.E.; Huckenbeck, W.; Piekorz, R.P.; Knoefel, W.T.; et al. Impact of the 3D microenvironment on phenotype, gene expression, and EGFR inhibition of colorectal cancer cell lines. *PLoS ONE* **2013**, *8*, e59689. [CrossRef]
41. Avani, S.L.; Samantha, C.; Kumar, S.J.; Prasobh, G.R. Cystinosis: A Review. *World J. Pharm. Res.* **2021**, *10*, 332–342.
42. Servais, A.; Moriniere, V.; Grünfeld, J.P.; Noël, L.H.; Goujon, J.M.; Chadefaux-Vekemans, B.; Antignac, C. Late-onset nephropathic cystinosis: Clinical presentation, outcome, and genotyping. *Clin. J. Am. Soc. Nephrol.* **2008**, *3*, 27–35. [CrossRef]
43. Raggi, C.; Luciani, A.; Nevo, N.; Antignac, C.; Terryn, S.; Devuyst, O. Dedifferentiation and aberrations of the endolysosomal compartment characterize the early stage of nephropathic cystinosis. *Hum. Mol. Genet.* **2014**, *23*, 2266–2278. [CrossRef]
44. Napolitano, G.; Johnson, J.L.; He, J.; Rocca, C.J.; Monfregola, J.; Pestonjamasp, K.; Cherqui, S.; Catz, S.D. Impairment of chaperone-mediated autophagy leads to selective lysosomal degradation defects in the lysosomal storage disease cystinosis. *EMBO Mol. Med.* **2015**, *2*, 158–174. [CrossRef]
45. Sansanwal, P.; Yen, B.; Gahl, W.A.; Ma, Y.; Ying, L.; Wong, L.J.; Sarwal, M.M. Mitochondrial autophagy promotes cellular injury in nephropathic cystinosis. *J. Am. Soc. Nephrol.* **2010**, *21*, 272–283. [CrossRef]
46. Johnson, J.L.; Napolitano, G.; Monfregola, J.; Rocca, C.J.; Cherqui, S.; Catz, S.D. Upregulation of the Rab27a-dependent trafficking and secretory mechanisms improves lysosomal transport, alleviates endoplasmic reticulum stress, and reduces lysosome overload in cystinosis. *Mol. Cell. Biol.* **2013**, *33*, 2950–2962. [CrossRef]
47. Puertollano, R. mTOR and lysosome regulation. *F1000Prime Rep.* **2014**, *6*, 52. [CrossRef]
48. Cinotti, E.; Perrot, J.L.; Labeille, B.; Espinasse, M.; Ouerdane, Y.; Boukenter, A.; Thuret, G.; Gain, P.; Campolmi, N.; Douchet, C.; et al. Optical diagnosis of a metabolic disease: Cystinosis. *J. Biomed. Opt.* **2013**, *18*, 046013. [CrossRef]
49. Okuno, R.; Ito, Y.; Eid, N.; Otsuki, Y.; Kondo, Y.; Ueda, K. Upregulation of autophagy and glycolysis markers in keloid hypoxic-zone fibroblasts: Morphological characteristics and implications. *Histol. Histopathol.* **2018**, *33*, 1075–1087.
50. Roth, K.S.; Foreman, J.W.; Segal, S. The Fanconi syndrome and mechanisms of tubular transport dysfunction. *Kidney Int.* **1981**, *20*, 705–716. [CrossRef]
51. Vilasi, A.; Cutillas, P.R.; Maher, A.D.; Zirah, S.F.; Capasso, G.; Norden, A.W.; Holmes, E.; Nicholson, J.K.; Unwin, R.J. Combined proteomic and metabonomic studies in three genetic forms of the renal Fanconi syndrome. *Am. J. Physiol. Ren. Physiol.* **2007**, *293*, F456–F467. [CrossRef]
52. Shibuya, N.; Koike, S.; Tanaka, M.; Ishigami-Yuasa, M.; Kimura, Y.; Ogasawara, Y.; Fukui, K.; Nagahara, N.; Kimura, H. A novel pathway for the production of hydrogen sulfide from D-cysteine in mammalian cells. *Nat. Commun.* **2013**, *4*, 1366. [CrossRef] [PubMed]
53. Ribas, V.; Garcia-Ruiz, C.; Fernandez-Checa, J.C. Glutathione and mitochondria. *Front. Pharmacol.* **2014**, *5*, 151. [CrossRef] [PubMed]
54. Starkov, A.A. An update on the role of mitochondrial alpha-ketoglutarate dehydrogenase in oxidative stress. *Mol. Cell. Neurosci.* **2013**, *55*, 13–16. [CrossRef] [PubMed]
55. Mazzoleni, G.; Di Lorenzo, D.; Steimberg, N. Modelling tissues in 3D: The next future of pharmaco-toxicology and food research? *Genes Nutr.* **2009**, *4*, 13. [CrossRef] [PubMed]
56. Ghosh, S.; Spagnoli, G.C.; Martin, I.; Ploegert, S.; Demougin, P.; Heberer, M.; Reschner, A. Three-dimensional culture of melanoma cells profoundly affects gene expression profile: A high density oligonucleotide array study. *J. Cell. Physiol.* **2005**, *204*, 522–531. [CrossRef] [PubMed]
57. Frieboes, H.B.; Zheng, X.; Sun, C.H.; Tromberg, B.; Gatenby, R.; Cristini, V. An integrated computational/experimental model of tumor invasion. *Cancer Res.* **2006**, *66*, 1597–1604. [CrossRef] [PubMed]
58. Duriez, M.; Jacquet, A.; Hoet, L.; Roche, S.; Bock, M.D.; Rocher, C.; Haussy, G.; Vigé, X.; Bocskei, Z.; Slavnic, T.; et al. A 3D human liver model of nonalcoholic steatohepatitis. *J. Clin. Transl. Hepatol.* **2020**, *8*, 359. [CrossRef]
59. Berthiaume, F.; Moghe, P.V.; Toner, M.; Yarmush, M.L. Effect of extracellular matrix topology on cell structure, function, and physiological responsiveness: Hepatocytes cultured in a sandwich configuration. *FASEB J.* **1996**, *10*, 1471–1484. [CrossRef]
60. Semino, C.E.; Merok, J.R.; Crane, G.G.; Panagiotakos, G.; Zhang, S. Functional differentiation of hepatocyte-like spheroid structures from putative liver progenitor cells in three-dimensional peptide scaffolds. *Differentiation* **2003**, *71*, 262–270. [CrossRef]
61. Koukourakis, M.I.; Kalamida, D.; Mitrakas, A.G.; Liousia, M.; Pouliliou, S.; Sivridis, E.; Giatromanolaki, A. Metabolic cooperation between co-cultured lung cancer cells and lung fibroblasts. *Lab. Investig.* **2017**, *97*, 1321–1331. [CrossRef]

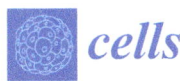

Review

Programmed Cell Death in Cystinosis

Elizabeth G. Ames and Jess G. Thoene *

Division of Pediatric Genetics, Metabolism, and Genomic Medicine, Department of Pediatrics, University of Michigan Health System, Ann Arbor, MI 48109, USA; amese@med.umich.edu
* Correspondence: jthoene@med.umich.edu

Abstract: Cystinosis is a lethal autosomal recessive disease that has been known clinically for over 100 years. There are now specific treatments including dialysis, renal transplantation and the orphan drug, cysteamine, which greatly improve the duration and quality of patient life, however, the cellular mechanisms responsible for the phenotype are unknown. One cause, programmed cell death, is clearly involved. Study of extant literature via Pubmed on "programmed cell death" and "apoptosis" forms the basis of this review. Most of such studies involved apoptosis. Numerous model systems and affected tissues in cystinosis have shown an increased rate of apoptosis that can be partially reversed with cysteamine. Proposed mechanisms have included changes in protein signaling pathways, autophagy, gene expression programs, and oxidative stress.

Keywords: cystinosis; apoptosis; programmed cell death

1. Introduction

Programmed cell death is such an essential cell function that it is uniquely challenging to dissect out the contributions to the development of the complex clinical phenotype of cystinosis. Here we present a summary and analysis of literature pertaining to the role of apoptosis in cystinosis obtained by searching PubMed for all articles identified with the searches "cystinosis and apoptosis" as well as "cystinosis and programmed cell death".

Cystinosis is a pan-systemic disease which causes severe failure to thrive, retinopathy, keratopathy, renal Fanconi syndrome, and progressive renal dysfunction that results in renal failure by age 10 years. It was first described in 1903 in two sibs as "Familiare Cystindiathese". In addition to severe failure to thrive, these children displayed increased urination and ultimately kidney failure. On microscopic examination at autopsy, the children were found to have prominent tissue crystals, identified as cystic oxide, now known to be cystine [1]. In 1967 it was demonstrated that the cystine was intracellular within leukocytes from patients with cystinosis, and that the cystine content reflected a Mendelian distribution [2], which enabled discovery of defective cystine lysosomal transport as the genesis of the disease in 1982 [3].

This was followed by development of cysteamine as the first effective specific therapy for cystinosis [4]. It is effective because cysteamine reacts with cystine within the lysosomes to form a product exported by the intact lysine carrier [5], reducing the cystine concentration to the level of the obligate heterozygous parents who do not develop any of the phenotypic features. That transporter has been characterized as closely related to the yeast PQ loop family of vacuolar membrane transporters, and designated PQLC2 [6].

Cysteamine, one of the first US FDA-approved orphan drugs (1994), has a beneficial effect on the course of the disease (see elsewhere in this paper). However, as noted by many authors, cysteamine does not prevent renal failure, but merely delays it, nor does it improve the renal Fanconi Syndrome [7].

2. The Role of Apoptosis in Cystinosis and Response to Cysteamine

Failure of cystinosin results in cystine accumulation that is confined to lysosomes and precludes cystine from interacting with intracellular metabolism. Therefore, the first

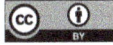

obvious challenge is to determine how cystine could interfere to such an extent as to cause the lethal phenotype. A first step toward explaining this enigma came in 2002 [8] with the observation that cystinotic fibroblasts display a 2 to 3-fold increase in the apoptotic rate compared to normal fibroblasts, and that normalization of the cystine content by pre-treatment with cysteamine also normalizes the apoptosis rate. Moreover, when normal cells are pre-loaded with cystine dimethylester to increase the lysosomal cystine content to the levels seen in cystinotic cells, the apoptosis rate increases to that seen in cystinotic cells. Similar results were found in renal proximal tubule epithelial cells as well [8]. The toxicity of CDME in normal cultured fibroblasts via a toxic effect on mitochondria has been raised [9]. However this study employed 1–5 mM CDME, whereas the study cited above showing increased apoptosis after loading normal cells with CDME used 0.25–0.5 mmM CDME. This lower concentration showed little effect on cells in the Wilmer study.

The next step occurred in 2006 when it was shown that due to lysosomal permeabilization, which occurs early in the apoptosis cascade, and before the cell is irreversibly committed to cell death, cystine can leave the lysosomes and thiolate a crucial disulfide in the proapoptotic kinase, PKC∂. It had previously been shown that such cysteinylation increases the activity of this kinase [10]. Further, inhibition of PKC∂ via siRNA silencing or with 12-O-tetradecanoylphorbol-13-acetate treatment markedly diminishes the apoptotic rate in parallel with the diminution in kinase activity [11]. A plot of lysosomal cystine concentration versus the rate of apoptosis including both normal and cystinotic cultured fibroblasts has the form of a rectangular hyperbola with a K_m of 0.2 nmol/mg protein, which approximates the normal lysosomal cystine content. Fibroblast lines from intermediate and ocular cystinosis do not lie on this curve, but display less apoptosis for a given cystine content [12].

Currently, increased apoptosis in cystinotic tissues has been described by several laboratories, which have confirmed that decreasing lysosomal cystine storage also decreases the elevated rate of apoptosis [7,8,13]. One group found a relatively minor increase in apoptosis (1.4-fold) in stem cells and organoids which was not reduced by cysteamine treatment [14]. This raises the issue of how well model systems mimic the clinical, biochemical, and cellular phenotypes, and which of these cell and animal systems are most faithful to the human disease. Apoptosis studies have been conducted in genetically-created cystinotic systems or via utilization of cystine dimethylester to create lysosomal cystine loading in human, mouse, and rat fibroblasts [12] (See Table). A study showing an increased rate of apoptosis in cystinotic proximal tubule cells found glutathione (GSH) depletion and failure to increase mitochondrial activity and maintain ATP levels under hypoxic conditions [13]. Increased apoptosis with correction by cysteamine was shown in the zebrafish model of cystinosis [7]. Using this model, this study showed elevated lysosomal cystine, increased apoptosis, and tubular dysfunction progressing to renal failure. Similar findings were reported in human induced pluripotent stem cells and kidney organoids [14] in which significantly elevated cystine and increased apoptosis was observed. Cystine was decreased by treatment with cysteamine, but the elevated rate of apoptosis was not. The cells displayed enlarged lysosomes, attributed to the osmotic effect of cystine, because treatment with cysteamine partially restored lysosomal size. However, since cystine is the least soluble amino acid (112 mg/L at 25 degrees centigrade and neutral pH, and has minimum solubility at the lysosomal pH of 5.0 [15], it precipitates at 0.46 mM. Induced vacuolation of lysosomes using membrane-impermeant sucrose requires 24 h exposure at 100 mM [16], hence the enlarged lysosomes may have occurred from other effects. No abnormalities in ATP or GSH concentration were found in these cells.

Increased apoptosis in cystinotic tissues can account for much of the clinical phenotype seen in cystinosis. Progressive loss of renal proximal tubular epithelial cells via abnormal apoptosis results in the "Swan Neck" deformity [17], and such progression can subsequently lead to non-functional atubular glomeruli [18] that can progress to overt renal failure over time. The renal tubule and retina are highly sensitive to apoptosis [8], and these two tissues are the first to be affected in nephropathic cystinosis [1], hence it is feasible that the order of tissues involved in the disease reflects the intrinsic sensitivity of each to apoptosis. It should be noted that abnormal apoptosis contributes to many birth defects [19], however dysmorphism is not part of the cystinosis phenotype. It therefore appears that increased apoptosis in cystinotic tissues is a regulated multi-step process, not just an "ON" switch for immediate cell death.

3. Autophagy in Cystinosis

Autophagy is a specialized cellular process that can both promote survival of a cell or promote programmed cell death. Autophagy has an entwined relationship with apoptosis due to shared regulatory genes and cellular machinery, which can confound experimental isolation of one cell death mechanism compared to another [20]. The role of autophagy in cystinosis has been specifically reviewed elsewhere, but there are several studies that examine the interplay between apoptosis and autophagy within model systems of cystinosis. One of the most basic observations initially showed that autophagy was increased in cystinotic tissues. Renal biopsies and cultured fibroblasts identified morphological and protein signaling markers of increased mitochondrial autophagy and autophagosomes while observing fewer total mitochondria in patients with nephropathic cystinosis compared to other forms of cystinosis and normal cells. The use of an autophagy inhibitor (3-methyl adenine) normalized the increased rate of apoptosis seen in the cystinotic cell lines. These results are consistent with autophagy both leading to and promoting apoptosis in cystinosis [21].

In a screen for compounds which reduce levels of specific markers of impaired autophagy (p62/SQSTM1), luteolin was shown to ameliorate several of the phenotypic abnormalities in constitutively-induced *CTNS*-null renal proximal tubular epithelial cells, including the aberrant autophagy-lysosomal degradative pathway, abnormalities in redox status, and increased sensitivity to apoptosis [22].

Analysis of renal biopsies and cultured fibroblasts identified morphological and protein signaling markers of mitochondrial autophagy in patients with nephropathic cystinosis compared to other forms of cystinosis and normal cells. These findings led to the hypothesis that autophagy leads to and synergistically promotes apoptosis in cystinosis [21].

4. Gene Expression Profiling and Signal Cascades

Gene expression studies of blood samples from cystinosis patients shows increased gene expression of apoptosis, mitochondrial dysfunction, and oxidative stress markers [23].

Rossi et al. reported that *NLRP2* is overexpressed in cystinotic proximal tubule epithelial cells compared to healthy subject cells. Using *NLRP2* overexpression, they noted a lower apoptotic rate. When *NLRP2* was silenced with siRNA, the apoptotic rate increased, which seems to contradict what is commonly observed in cystinosis [24].

5. Oxidative Stress

The issue of abnormal redox potential in cystinotic cells and tissues, and more recently, as a mediator of aberrant apoptosis, is challenging due to the multiple systems employed and interpretation of results. In 1978, Oshima et al. reported the GSH content of cystinotic fibroblasts was 91% of the content found in normal fibroblasts [25]. In three cystinotic fibroblast lines, Chol et al. found GSH content was 70% of that found in control cells [26]. Studies in matched, low passage number cystinotic fetal skin, cystinotic fetal lung, and normal fetal lung fibroblasts, found the concentration of GSH, and the GSH/GSSG ratio were comparable [27]. It is not expected that the abnormally increased cystine accumulations in cystinotic cells would alter cellular redox potential given that the lysosomal cystine pool is physically separated from the cystosolic compartment. Without functioning cystinosin, cystine remains intralysosomal until exocystosed. Lysosomes represent only about 10% of cell volume in cystinotic fibroblasts [28], and since cystine is very insoluble, with a solubility limit of about 0.5 mM in aqueous solution to 1.66 mM in plasma [1], instantaneous dilution into the total cytosol of a saturating solution of cystine would yield a final cytosolic cystine concentration of 0.05–0.166 mM. Given the GSH concentration in the cytosol of ~10 mM [29], it is unlikely that cystine would greatly alter the global redox status of the cytosol. Any GSSG formed by reaction with cystine would be rapidly reduced back to GSH by cytosolic reductases [1]. These observations were extended by Wilmer et al. who found, using a proximal tubular epithelial cell model, no difference in GSH between control and cystinotic cells, ATP production, or the oxidation state of proteins or lipids. They also found that cysteamine increased GSH in both normal and control cells, but did not improve sodium-dependent phoshate uptake. This last finding is consistent with the clinical observation that cysteamine therapy does not improve the renal Fanconi syndrome, a component of which is failure of sodium reabsorption [30]. Bellomo et al. showed that in HK-2 cells CTNS gene expression was correlated with intracellular cysteine level and with the cysteine/cystine equilibrium, implying a regulated role for CTNS in maintaining the intracellular redox state [31].

Studies by Sumayao et al. involving redox potential and apoptosis used a variety of cell and tissue models. With *CTNS* silencing of a proximal tubular epithelial cell line, they found an increase in apoptosis and ROS which was decreased by cysteamine [32]. GSH was reported in an earlier publication [33] as being two-fold decreased in the *CTNS* knockout cells. However, GSH was measured using a non-specific reagent, 5,5′-dithio-bis-2-nitrobenzoic acid, which reacts with all thiols. It is also not surprising that the concentration of ROS is diminished in the presence of cysteamine, since it is a known free-radical scavenger that is oxidized to the disulfide, cystamine, which can then be regenerated to cysteamine by GSH [34].

A recent paper shows that a disulfide, disulfiram, forms mixed disulfides with cystine, and has cystine-depleting and anti-apoptotic effects [35] Presumably, like the disulfide cystamine [4], reduction of disulfiram to the free thiol diethyldithiocarbamate occurs in the cytosol via GSH which then enters lysosomes where disulfide interchange occurs, permitting the mixed disulfides to exit, and causing cystine depletion [5].

Laube et.al studied GSH in native cystinotic proximal tubular epithelial cells obtained from patient urine. They found an increased apoptotic rate of approximately 200% after TNF alpha stimulation as measured by TUNEL. Cystinotic proximal tubular cells had 6.8 nmol GSH/mg protein, whereas the controls had 11.8 nmol ($p < 0.001$) and impaired recovery from hypoxic stress [11]. These cells had a two-fold increase in apoptosis rate without an exogenous trigger, not seen in other studies in fibroblasts or RPTE cells [8,11,36]. GSH was measured specifically in Laube's study via HPLC with electrochemical detection [37]. In extensive studies in cystinotic ciPTEC, tubuloids and zebrafish, a connection between ROS, apoptosis, and alpha ketogluterate was established. These characteristics of Ctns$^{-/-}$ tissues were ameliorated by co-treatment with cysteamine and bicalutamide. This suggests a possible clinical use in patients which might improve the renal tubule defect [38].

6. Thyroid Effects of Apoptosis

Along with the more prominent effects of cystinosin deficiency in the kidney, untreated cystinosis is associated with hypothyroidism during childhood [39,40]. Studies using thyrocytes from *CTNS* knockout mice, determined that the basis of the hypothyroidism seen in cystinosis is multifactorial and that apoptosis plays a large role in this aspect of the phenotype. In addition to defective thyroglobulin synthesis, which is driven by the endoplasmic reticulum stress response, and unfolded protein response, there is progressive colloid exhaustion and impaired thyroglobulin proteolytic processing within lysosomes. Further, *CTNS*-deficient thyrocytes demonstrated a 4.5 fold increase in cell proliferation and an even more markedly increased rate of apoptosis [41]. This increased apoptosis is also likely triggered by the unfolded protein response limiting synthesis and secretion of thyroglobulin. Together these effects within thyrocytes provide an explanation for the hypothyroidism seen in individuals with cystinosis.

7. Pancreatic Effects of Apoptosis

Abnormal insulin secretion represents one of the later manifestations of cystinosis. Adults with cystinosis have been noted to have higher rates of diabetes post-transplant compared to adults who have undergone renal transplantation for other causes even when factors like corticosteroid use have been considered [42]. The role of apoptosis in pancreatic dysfunction was studied using *CTNS* knockdown within a beta-cell line. When *CTNS* was knocked down, the cells were noted to have cystine accumulation and altered redox potential suggesting that this model system appropriately captured the phenotype within this organ. Reactive oxygen species were hypothesized to have multiple effects including increased NFκB expression and within the mitochondria, there was reduced mitochondrial membrane potential and decreased ATP generation. Both increased NFκB expression and decreased mitochondrial membrane potential led to increased rates of apoptosis. In turn, increased apoptosis, in addition to decreased ATP generation led to decreased rates of insulin release [43].

8. Summary and Future Directions

As described in this review, the role of apoptosis in the pathogenesis of cystinosis is established. Other abnormalities that have been noted in cystinosis cell physiology include altered gene expression, increased autophagy, increased oxidative stress, inappropriate mitochondrial stress response, and abnormal lysosomal function. As shown in Table 1, this review has outlined how these mechanisms affect programmed cell death within specific experimental systems and what the effects cysteamine had on apoptosis.

What remains to be determined is the role of these other non-apoptotic paths, and if they also contribute to cell death. Unanswered questions include: What is primary in causing increased gene expression in cystinotic cells? Is lysosomal cystine storage essential for causing increased apoptosis or does the increased intralysosomal cystine content simply represent an epiphenomenon of the disease? If the increased lysosomal cystine content is not required for pathogenesis, why does long-term cysteamine depletion of cystine in patients yield an average doubling of native kidney survival? If elevated lysosomal molarity isn't the cause of increased lysosomal size, what is? What is the primary trigger in the apoptotic cascade? If GSH concentration is normal in cystinotic tissue, how is a redox imbalance initiated and maintained? What accounts for the milder phenotypes in intermediate and ocular cystinosis, and why do they show a lower elevation in apoptosis for a given cystine content than the nephropathic lines? Does increased apoptosis cause increased autophagy or does increased autophagy cause increased apoptosis [44]? Which cells/tissues/organ systems/organisms, such as the $Ctns^{-/-}$ mouse [45], best model the pathological abnormalities in the patient? What moderates the increased apoptosis so that generalized dysmorphology does not occur? New molecular biology techniques and imaging technology are promising methods to address these questions and possibly shed new light on additional treatment strategies.

Table 1. Summary of Cell Death in Cystinosis.

Model System	Mediator	Target	Effect on Apoptosis or Necrosis	Effect of Cysteamine	References (Year)
Human cystinotic fibroblasts	Native lysosomal cystine	PKC δ	Increased apoptosis 3 fold	Lowered cystine and normalized apoptosis	[7,9] (2002, 2006)
Human normal fibroblasts	CDME-induced increased lysosomal cystine	PKC δ	-	N/A	[7,9] (2002, 2006)
Human normal RPTC	CDME	PKC δ	Increased apoptosis 8 fold	N/A	[7,9] (2002, 2006)
Normal rat fibroblasts	CDME	N/A	Increase apoptosis 16 fold	N/A	[10] (2005)
Normal mouse fibroblasts	CDME	N/A	Increase apoptosis 5 fold	N/A	[10] (2005)
Cystinosis patient-derived induced pluripotent stem cells	Native lysosomal cystine	N/A	Increased apoptosis 1.4 fold	No effect	[12] (2020)
Ctns$^{-/-}$ Zebrafish	Native lysosomal cystine	N/A	Increased apoptosis 7 fold	Decreased apoptosis	[6] (2017)
Cystinotic RPTC	Native lysosomal cystine	N/A	Increased apoptosis 2 fold	N/A	[11] (2006)
Cystinotic RPTC	Native lysosomal cystine	Caspase 4	Increased apoptosis 3 fold	N/A	[19] (2010)
Cystinotic RPTC	NLRP2	NF-κB	Increased apoptosis	N/A	[22] (2019)
Ctns(−/−) mice	N/A	Atubular glomeruli	Increased necrosis, apoptosis, and autophagy	N/A	[15] (2015)
siRNA knockdown of CTNS in normal RPTC	ROS	GSH, Redox capacity	Increased early and late apoptosis, and necrosis	Decreased apoptosis and necrosis	[33] (2016)
Cystinotic ciRPTC Ctns$^{-/-}$ Zebra-fish larva	ROS	p62/SQSTM1	Increased apoptosis 3.5 fold Increased apoptosis 5 fold	Cysteamine not done Reversed by luteolin	[20] (2020)
Cystinotic ciRPTC Ctns$^{-/-}$ mice Zebrafish	ROS	N/A	Increased apoptosis 7 fold	Reversed by cysteamine and disulfiram	[36] (2021)

CDME: Cystine dimethyl ester; RPTC: Renal proximal tubular cells; ciRPTC: Conditionally immortalized proximal tubule epithelial cells; ROS: Reactive oxygen species.

Funding: This research received no external funding.

Conflicts of Interest: The authors declare no conflict of interest.

Abbreviations

GSH	reduced glutathione
GSSG	oxidized glutathione
PKC∂	protein kinase C delta
ROS	reactive oxygen species
ciPTEC	conditionally immortalized proximal tubule epithelial cell

References

1. Gahl, W.A.; Thoene, J.G.; Schneider, J.A. A Disorder of Lysosomal Memebrane Transport. In *The Metabolic and Molecular Basis of Inherited Diseases*, 8th ed.; Scriver, C.R., Beaudet, A.L., Sly, W.S., Valle, D., Eds.; McGraw Hill: New York, NY, USA, 2001; pp. 5085–5108.
2. Schulman, J.D.; Bradley, K.H.; Seegmiller, J.E. Cystine: Compartmentalization within Lysosomes in Cystinotic Leukocytes. *Science* **1969**, *166*, 1152–1154. [CrossRef] [PubMed]
3. Gahl, W.A.; Bashan, N.; Tietze, F.; Bernardini, I.; Schulman, J.D. Cystine Transport is Defective in Isolated Leukocyte Lysosomes from Patients with Cystinosis. *Science* **1982**, *217*, 1263–1265. [CrossRef]
4. Thoene, J.G.; Oshima, R.G.; Crawhall, J.C. Intracellular Cystine Depletion by Aminothiols In Vitro and In Vivo. *J. Clin. Investig.* **1976**, *58*, 180–189. [CrossRef] [PubMed]
5. Pisoni, R.L.; Thoene, J.G.; Christensen, H.N. Detection and Characterization of Carrier-Mediated Cationic Amino Acid Transport in Lysosomes of Normal and Cystinotic Human Fibroblasts. Role in Therapeutic Cystine Removal? *J. Biol. Chem.* **1985**, *260*, 4791–4798. [CrossRef]
6. Jeźégou, A.; Llinares, E.; Anne, C.; Kieffer-Jaquinod, S.; O'Regan, S.; Aupetit, J.; Chabli, A.; Sagné, C.; Debacker, C.; Chadefaux-Vekemans, B.; et al. Heptahelical Protein PQLC2 Is a Lysosomal Cationic Amino Acid Exporter Underlying the Action of Cysteamine in Cystinosis Therapy. *Proc. Natl. Acad. Sci. USA* **2012**, *109*, E3434–E3443. [CrossRef]
7. Elmonem, M.; Khalil, R.; Khodaparast, L.; Khodaparast, L.; Arcolino, F.; Morgan, J.; Pastore, A.; Tylzanowski, P.; Ny, A.; Lowe, M.; et al. Cystinosis (ctns) Zebrafish Mutant Shows Pronephric Glomerular and Tubular Dysfunction. *Sci. Rep.* **2017**, *7*, 42583. [CrossRef]
8. Park, M.; Helip-Wooley, A.; Thoene, J. Lysosomal Cystine Storage Augments Apoptosis in Cultured Human Fibroblasts and Renal Tubular Epithelial Cells. *J. Am. Soc. Nephrol.* **2002**, *13*, 2878–2887. [CrossRef]
9. Wilmer, M.J.; Willems, P.H.; Verkaart, S.; Visch, H.J.; De Graaf-Hess, A.; Blom, H.J.; Monnens, L.A.; van den Heuvel, L.P.; Levtchenko, E.N. Cystine Dimethylester Model of Cystinosis: Still Reliable? *Pediatr. Res.* **2007**, *62*, 151–155. [CrossRef]
10. Chu, F.; Ward, N.E.; O'Brian, C.A. PKC Isozyme S-Cysteinylation by Cystine Stimulates the Pro-Apoptotic Isozyme PKCδ and Inactivates the Oncogenic Isozyme PKCε. *Carcinogenesis* **2003**, *24*, 317–325. [CrossRef]
11. Park, M.A.; Pejovic, V.; Kerisit, K.G.; Junius, S.; Thoene, J.G. Increased Apoptosis in Cystinotic Fibroblasts and Renal Proximal Tubule Epithelial Cells Results from Cysteinylation of Protein Kinase Cδ. *J. Am. Soc. Nephrol.* **2006**, *17*, 3167–3175. [CrossRef]
12. Park, M.A.; Thoene, J.G. Potential role of apoptosis in development of the cystinotic phenotype. *Pediatr. Nephrol.* **2005**, *20*, 441–446. [CrossRef] [PubMed]
13. Laube, G.; Shah, V.; Stewart, V.; Hargreaves, I.; Haq, M.; Heales, S.; van't Hoff, W.G. Glutathione Depletion and Increased Apoptosis Rate in Human Cystinotic Proximal Tubular Cells. *Pediatr. Nephrol.* **2006**, *21*, 503–509. [CrossRef] [PubMed]
14. Hollywood, J.A.; Przepiorski, A.; D'Souza, R.F.; Sreebhavan, S.; Wolvetang, E.J.; Harrison, P.T.; Davidson, A.J.; Holm, T.M. Use of Human Induced Pluripotent Stem Cells and Kidney Organoids to Develop a Cysteamine/Mtor Inhibition Combination Therapy for Cystinosis. *J. Am. Soc. Nephrol.* **2020**, *31*, 962–982. [CrossRef] [PubMed]
15. Sano, K. Uber die Loselichkeit der Aminosauren bei variierter Wasserstoffzahl. *Biochem. Zeit.* **1926**, *168*, 14.
16. Helip-Wooley, A.; Thoene, J.G. Sucrose-Induced Vacuolation Results in Increased Expression of Cholesterol Biosynthesis and Lysosomal Genes. *Exp. Cell. Res.* **2004**, *292*, 89–100. [CrossRef]
17. Galarreta, C.; Forbes, M.; Thornhill, B.; Antignac, C.; Gubler, M.; Nevo, N.; Murphy, M.P.; Chevalier, R.L. The Swan-Neck Lesion: Proximal Tubular Adaptation to Oxidative Stress in Nephropathic Cystinosis. *Am. J. Physiol. Ren. Physiol.* **2015**, *308*, F1155–F1166. [CrossRef]
18. Larsen, C.P.; Walker, P.D.; Thoene, J.G. The Incidence of Atubular Glomeruli in Nephropathic Cystinosis Renal Biopsies. *Mol. Genet. Metab.* **2010**, *101*, 417–420. [CrossRef]
19. Edwards, M.J. Apoptosis, the heat shock response, hyperthermia, with defects, disease and cancer. Where are the common links? *Cell Stress Chaperones* **1998**, *3*, 213–220. [CrossRef]
20. Eisenberg-Lerner, A.; Bialik, S.; Simon, H.U.; Kimchi, A. Life and Death Partners: Apoptosis, Autophagy and the Cross-Talk between Them. *Cell Death Differ.* **2009**, *16*, 966–975. [CrossRef]
21. Sansanwal, P.; Yen, B.; Gahl, W.; Ma, Y.; Ying, L.; Wong, L.; Sarwal, M.M. Mitochondrial Autophagy Promotes Cellular Injury in Nephropathic Cystinosis. *J. Am. Soc. Nephrol.* **2010**, *21*, 272–283. [CrossRef]
22. De Leo, E.; Elmonem, M.; Berlingerio, S.; Berquez, M.; Festa, B.; Raso, R.; Bellomo, F.; Starborg, T.; Janssen, M.J.; Abbaszadeh, Z.; et al. Cell-Based Phenotypic Drug Screening Identifies Luteolin as Candidate Therapeutic for Nephropathic Cystinosis. *J. Am. Soc. Nephrol.* **2020**, *31*, 1522–1537. [CrossRef] [PubMed]
23. Sansanwal, P.; Li, L.; Hsieh, S.; Sarwal, M. Insights into Novel Cellular Injury Mechanisms by Gene Expression Profiling in Nephropathic Cystinosis. *J. Inherit. Metab. Dis.* **2010**, *33*, 775–786. [CrossRef] [PubMed]
24. Rossi, M.; Pascarella, A.; Licursi, V.; Caiello, I.; Taranta, A.; Rega, L.; Levtchenko, E.; Emma, F.; De Benedetti, F.; Prencipe, G. NLRP2 Regulates Proinflammatory and Antiapoptotic Responses in Proximal Tubular Epithelial Cells. *Front. Cell Dev. Biol.* **2019**, *7*, 252. [CrossRef] [PubMed]
25. Oshima, R.G.; Rhead, W.J.; Thoene, J.G.; Schneider, J.A. Cystine Metabolism in Human Fibroblasts. Comparison of Normal, Cystinotic, and γ Glutamylcysteine Synthetase Deficient cells. *J. Biol. Chem.* **1976**, *251*, 4287–4293. [CrossRef]

26. Chol, M.; Nevo, N.; Cherqui, S.; Antignac, C.; Rustin, P. Glutathione precursors replenish decreased glutathione pool in cystinotic cell lines. *Biochem. Biophys. Res. Commun.* **2004**, *324*, 231–235. [CrossRef]
27. Vitvitsky, V.; Witcher, M.; Banerjee, R.; Thoene, J. The Redox Status of Cystinotic Fibroblasts. *Mol. Genet. Metab.* **2010**, *99*, 384–388. [CrossRef]
28. Oude Elferink, R.P.J.; Harms, E.; Strijland, A.; Tager, J.M. The Intralysosomal pH in Cultured Human Skin Fibroblasts in Relation to Cystine Accumulation in Patients with Cystinosis. *Biochem. Biophys. Res. Commun.* **1983**, *116*, 154–161. [CrossRef]
29. Oestreicher, J.; Morgan, B. Glutathione: Subcellular Distribution and Membrane Transport. *Biochem. Cell Biol.* **2019**, *97*, 270–289. [CrossRef]
30. Wilmer, M.J.; Kluijtmans, L.A.J.; van der Velden, T.J.; Willems, P.H.; Scheffer, P.G.; Masereeuw, R.; Monnens, L.A.; van den Heuvel, L.P.; Levtchenko, E.N. Cysteamine restores glutathione redox status in cultured cystinotic proximal tubular epithelial cells. *Biochim. Biophys. Acta* **2011**, *1812*, 643–651. [CrossRef]
31. Bellomo, F.; Corallini, S.; Pastore, A.; Palma, A.; Laurenzi, C.; Emma, F.; Monnens, L.A.; Heuvel, L.P.V.D.; Levtchenko, E.N. Modulation of CTNS Gene Expression by Intracellular Thiols. *Free Radic. Biol. Med.* **2010**, *48*, 865–872. [CrossRef] [PubMed]
32. Sumayao, R.; McEvoy, B.; Newsholme, P.; McMorrow, T. Lysosomal Cystine Accumulation Promotes Mitochondrial Depolarization and Induction of Redox-Sensitive Genes in Human Kidney Proximal Tubular Cells. *J. Physiol.* **2016**, *594*, 3353–3370. [CrossRef] [PubMed]
33. Sumayao, R.; Mcevoy, B.; Martin-Martin, N.; Mcmorrow, T.; Newsholme, P. Cystine Dimethylester Loading Promotes Oxidative Stress and a Reduction in ATP Independent of Lysosomal Cystine Accumulation in a Human Proximal Tubular Epithelial Cell Line. *Exp. Physiol.* **2013**, *98*, 1505–1517. [CrossRef] [PubMed]
34. Sueishi, Y.; Nii, R. Monoterpene's Multiple Free Radical Scavenging Capacity as Compared with the Radioprotective Agent Cysteamine and Amifostine. *Bioorg. Med. Chem. Lett.* **2018**, *28*, 3031–3033. [CrossRef] [PubMed]
35. Taranta, A.; Elmonem, M.A.; Bellomo, F.; De Leo, E.; Boenzi, S.; Janssen, M.J.; Jamalpoor, A.; Cairoli, S.; Pastore, A.; De Stefanis, C.; et al. Benefits and Toxicity of Disulfiram in Preclinical Models of Nephropathic Cystinosis. *Cells* **2021**, *10*, 3294. [CrossRef] [PubMed]
36. Sansanwal, P.; Li, L.; Sarwal, M.M. Inhibition of Intracellular Clusterin Attenuates Cell Death in Nephropathic Cystinosis. *J. Am. Soc. Nephrol.* **2015**, *26*, 612–625. [CrossRef]
37. Riederer, P.; Sofic, E.; Rausch, W.-D.; Schmidt, B.; Reynolds, G.P.; Jellinger, K.; Youdim, M.B. Transition Metals, Ferritin, Glutathione, and Ascorbic Acid in Parkinsonian Brains. *J. Neurochem.* **1989**, *52*, 515–520. [CrossRef]
38. Jamalpoor, A.; Gelder, C.A.; Yousef Yengej, F.A.; Zaal, E.A.; Berlingerio, S.P.; Veys, K.R.; Casellas, C.P.; Voskuil, K.; Essa, K.; Ammerlaan, C.M.; et al. Cysteamine-Bicalutamide Combination Therapy Corrects Proximal Tubule Phenotype in Cystinosis. *EMBO Mol. Med.* **2021**, *13*, e13067. [CrossRef]
39. Lucky, A.W.; Howley, P.M.; Megyesi, K.; Spielberg, S.P.; Schulman, J.D. Endocrine Studies in Cystinosis: Compensated Primary Hypothyroidism. *J. Pediatr.* **1977**, *91*, 204–210. [CrossRef]
40. Chan, A.M.; Lynch, M.J.G.; Bailey, J.D.; Ezrin, C.; Fraser, D. Hypothyroidism in Cystinosis. A Clinical, Endocrinologic and Histologic Study Involving Sixteen Patients with Cystinosis. *Am. J. Med.* **1970**, *48*, 678–692. [CrossRef]
41. Gaide Chevronnay, H.; Janssens, V.; Van Der Smissen, P.; Liao, X.; Abid, Y.; Nevo, N.; Antignac, C.; Refetoff, S.; Cherqui, S.; Pierreux, C.E.; et al. A Mouse Model Suggests Two Mechanisms for Thyroid Alterations in Infantile Cystinosis: Decreased Thyroglobulin Synthesis Due to Endoplasmic Reticulum Stress/Unfolded Protein Response and Impaired Lysosomal Processing. *Endocrinology* **2015**, *156*, 2349–2364. [CrossRef]
42. Fivush, B.; Green, O.C.; Porter, C.C.; Balfe, J.W.; O'regan, S.; Gahl, W.A. Pancreatic Endocrine Insufficiency in Posttransplant Cystinosis. *Am. J. Dis. Child* **1987**, *141*, 1087–1089. [CrossRef] [PubMed]
43. McEvoy, B.; Sumayao, R.; Slattery, C.; McMorrow, T.; Newsholme, P. Cystine Accumulation Attenuates Insulin Release from the Pancreatic β-Cell Due to Elevated Oxidative Stress and Decreased ATP Levels. *J. Physiol.* **2015**, *593*, 5167–5182. [CrossRef] [PubMed]
44. De Rechter, S.; Decuypere, J.P.; Ivanova, E.; van den Heuvel, L.P.; De Smedt, H.; Levtchenko, E.; Mekahli, D. Autophagy in Renal Diseases. *Pediatr. Nephrol.* **2016**, *31*, 737–752. [CrossRef] [PubMed]
45. Gaide Chevronnay, H.; Janssens, V.; Van Der Smissen, P.; N'Kuli, F.; Nevo, N.; Guiot, Y.; Levtchenko, E.; Marbaix, E.; Pierreux, C.E.; Cherqui, S.; et al. Time Course of Pathogenic and Adaptation Mechanisms in Cystinotic Mouse Kidneys. *J. Am. Soc. Nephrol.* **2014**, *25*, 1256–1269. [CrossRef] [PubMed]

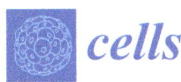

Review

Defective Cystinosin, Aberrant Autophagy—Endolysosome Pathways, and Storage Disease: Towards Assembling the Puzzle

Laura Rita Rega [1,*], Ester De Leo [1], Daniela Nieri [2] and Alessandro Luciani [2,*]

1. Renal Diseases Research Unit, Genetic and Rare Diseases Research Area, Bambino Gesù Children's Hospital, IRCCS, 00146 Rome, Italy; ester.deleo@opbg.net
2. Mechanisms of Inherited Kidney Diseases Group, Institute of Physiology, University of Zurich, 8057 Zurich, Switzerland; daniela.nieri@uzh.ch
* Correspondence: laurarita.rega@opbg.net (L.R.R.); alessandro.luciani@uzh.ch (A.L.); Tel.: +39-0668592997 (L.R.R.); +41-0446355070 (A.L.)

Abstract: Epithelial cells that form the kidney proximal tubule (PT) rely on an intertwined ecosystem of vesicular membrane trafficking pathways to ensure the reabsorption of essential nutrients—a key requisite for homeostasis. The endolysosome stands at the crossroads of this sophisticated network, internalizing molecules through endocytosis, sorting receptors and nutrient transporters, maintaining cellular quality control via autophagy, and toggling the balance between PT differentiation and cell proliferation. Dysregulation of such endolysosome-guided trafficking pathways might thus lead to a generalized dysfunction of PT cells, often causing chronic kidney disease and life-threatening complications. In this review, we highlight the biological functions of endolysosome-residing proteins from the perspectives of understanding—and potentially reversing—the pathophysiology of rare inherited diseases affecting the kidney PT. Using cystinosis as a paradigm of endolysosome disease causing PT dysfunction, we discuss how the endolysosome governs the homeostasis of specialized epithelial cells. This review also provides a critical analysis of the molecular mechanisms through which defects in autophagy pathways can contribute to PT dysfunction, and proposes potential interventions for affected tissues. These insights might ultimately accelerate the discovery and development of new therapeutics, not only for cystinosis, but also for other currently intractable endolysosome-related diseases, eventually transforming our ability to regulate homeostasis and health.

Keywords: autophagy; endolysosome; epithelial cell differentiation; homeostasis; lysosomal storage diseases; mitochondrial distress; kidney proximal tubule

Citation: Rega, L.R.; De Leo, E.; Nieri, D.; Luciani, A. Defective Cystinosin, Aberrant Autophagy—Endolysosome Pathways, and Storage Disease: Towards Assembling the Puzzle. Cells 2022, 11, 326. https://doi.org/10.3390/cells11030326

Academic Editor: Pei-Hui Lin

Received: 30 November 2021
Accepted: 11 January 2022
Published: 19 January 2022

Publisher's Note: MDPI stays neutral with regard to jurisdictional claims in published maps and institutional affiliations.

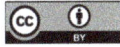

Copyright: © 2022 by the authors. Licensee MDPI, Basel, Switzerland. This article is an open access article distributed under the terms and conditions of the Creative Commons Attribution (CC BY) license (https://creativecommons.org/licenses/by/4.0/).

1. Introduction

Epithelial cells that line the proximal tubule (PT) of the kidney reabsorb a large variety of filtered macromolecules and low-molecular mass-nutrients through a particularly well-developed endolysosome system and through membrane trafficking pathways. Ever since its discovery by Christian De Duve in the 1960s, the endolysosome has come to be known as a single-membrane-enclosed organelle devoted to the degradation of damaged cellular constituents, including aged and/or misfolded proteins, and pathogens [1]. Extracellular and intracellular materials can reach the endolysosome through endocytosis and autophagy, respectively [2]. Fusion events subsequently enable the endolysosomes to recycle cargoes and/or substrates engulfed by endocytic and/or autophagic vesicles.

Beyond degradation and the disposal of cellular waste [3], the endolysosomes can also steer the metabolic trajectory of cells in response to nutrient availability, growth factors, and stress signals, hence guiding nearly every aspect of metabolic function, ultimately coordinating cell- and organism-wide growth [4]. As a consequence, dysregulation of endolysosomes and autophagy pathways might thus pose a devastating threat to many different cell types, eventually culminating in neurodegeneration, metabolic disease, cancer, and pathologies associated with ageing [2].

Over the last two decades, studies of rare inherited diseases, in combination with advances in technology and high-throughput omics, have provided novel insights into fundamental principles governing the contribution of the endolysosome to the maintenance of homeostasis [5,6]. Through converging approaches, these paradigms have helped to understand the pathogenesis of common kidney disease entities in which imbalances in the endolysosome system have been implicated in PT dysfunction [7]. Furthermore, the integration of genome-wide association studies (GWAS) with quantitative trait analyses (eQTLs) have identified that the expression of an endolysosome-residing enzyme, that is the beta-mannosidase (MANBA), is lower in the kidneys of subjects with chronic kidney disease (CKD), and that the MANBA risk allele shows evidence of structural and functional defects in endolysosome and autophagy pathways in kidney tubule cells [8]. In addition, common variants within genes closely linked to endolysosome function (e.g., CUBN, DAB2, RAB4, and LRP2) have recently been associated with proteinuria and CKD risk [9,10], highlighting the fundamental role of the endolysosome system in kidney health and its contribution to kidney disease risk within the population.

In this review, we discuss the biological functions of the endolysosome, not only as a "disposal-garbage system" of the cell, but also as a hub for homeostasis and signaling pathways, and delve into the breakdown and removal of damaged and/or dysfunctional mitochondria through autophagic pathways. Taking cystinosis as a paradigm of endolysosome disease causing PT dysfunction, we discuss how the endolysosome and autophagy govern the physiology of kidney tubule cells. We describe the cellular pathways and molecular underpinnings through which the absence of the endolysosome-residing transporter cystinosin might wreak havoc on autophagy, ultimately leading to dysfunction of the kidney PT. In the concluding section, we highlight potential new, attractive targets for therapeutically tackling cellular adversities linked to cystinosin dysfunction, offering new targetable pathways for this life-threatening disease.

2. Role of the Endolysosome System and Autophagy in Kidney Proximal Tubule

2.1. Receptor-Mediated Endocytosis and the Endolysosome

The kidney PT constitutes a paradigm of effective communication between the environment and endomembrane compartments, guiding the reabsorption of vital nutrients [5,6]. PT cells use receptor-mediated endocytosis and endolysosome-guided transport systems to efficiently reabsorb albumin and low molecular weight proteins (LMWPs) from the ultrafiltrate, preventing the urinary waste of essential proteins under physiological conditions [5,6]. The retrieval of albumin and LMWPs occurs through the multiligand receptors LRP2/megalin and cubilin [11–13], and the cooperating protein amnionless (AMN; Figure 1). The binding of filtered ligands to, and the interactions between both endocytic receptors, induces their internalization into clathrin-coated vesicles, and subsequent transport towards the endolysosomal compartments [14–16]. An essential component in this trafficking pathway is the apical endosomal compartment, where the ligands opportunely dissociate from their endocytic receptors through a process that requires sustained vesicular acidification (Figure 1) by the electrogenic vacuolar H^+-ATPase (v-ATPase) proton pump [17,18]. In the kidney PT, additional proteins appear to be involved in the maintenance of the endolysosomal acidification, such as the anion transporter chloride channel 5 and 7 (ClC5 and ClC7; [19]); the cystic fibrosis transmembrane conductance regulator (CFTR; [19]); and the cation transporters mucolipin 1 and two pore calcium channel 1 (TPC1) and TCP2, which mediate Ca^{2+} and Na^+ release from the endolysosome [20]. Once dissociated from their ligands, the endocytic receptors efficiently traffic to subapical Rab11$^+$ apical recycling endosomes and successively reach the apical membrane in a microtubule-dependent manner [16], sustaining new cycles of ligand binding and internalization (Figure 1). The generation and maintenance of the endolysosomal pH gradient sustains not only the progression of cargo-filled vesicles towards the endocytic route, but also the activation acid hydrolases within the degradative compartments [21]. Iterative rounds of cargo sorting, coupled with maturation of the early endosomes, result in the formation of late endosomes that fuse with the lysosomes to form endolysosomes (Figure 1), where their accompanying cargoes are eventually degraded [22].

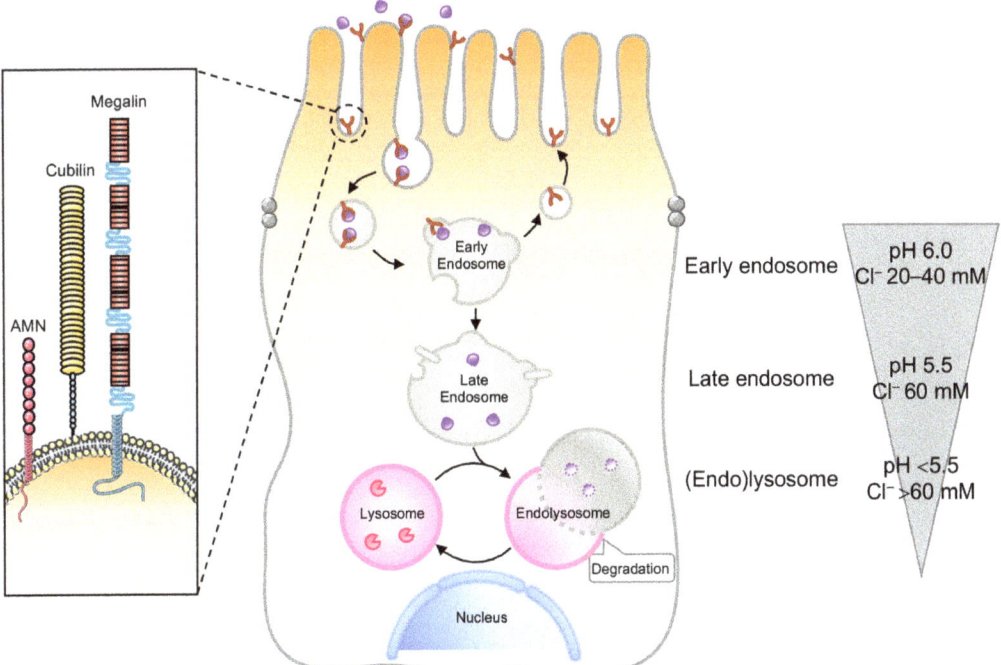

Figure 1. The endolysosome system in the kidney PT. Epithelial cells lining the kidney PT have multifunctional endocytic receptors and a highly developed endolysosome system to take up plasma proteins that are filtered by the glomerulus. The endocytic pathway in PT cells requires coated pits and vesicles, followed by early endosomes that form recycling endosomes or mature to late endosomes that fuse with the lysosome to form the endolysosomes. The luminal pH drops from 7.4 in the tubule lumen to 6.0 in early endosomes, 5.5 in late endosomes, and below 5.0 in endolysosomes. Such vesicular acidification enables the dissociation between receptors and their ligands, the recycling of receptors back to the apical membrane, and the progression of ligands towards the endolysosomal compartments. In parallel, the Cl^- concentrations drop from 110 mM in the extracellular space to 20–40 mM in early endosomes, 60 mM in late endosomes, and >80 mM in lysosomes, i.e., much higher than the 10–40 mM in the cytosol.

Accumulating evidence suggests that the endolysosome terminates autophagy—an evolutionary conserved pathway that degrades cellular components, such as defective organelles and misfolded proteins, to preserve homeostasis [1,23]. Furthermore, recent studies indicate that autophagy-mediated clearance pathways coordinate the renovation of cells and tissues during kidney development and differentiation, and are also involved in the prevention of genomic damage [24,25]. Therefore, its dysregulation might hasten not only PT dysfunction and kidney disease, but also other pathologies associated with kidney ageing [25,26].

Beyond its role in cellular destruction and quality control, the endolysosome system can steer the metabolic trajectories of cells in response to diverse microenvironmental cues in order to preserve homeostasis [2,4]. Crucial in this process is the (nutrient–dependent) recruitment of the evolutionarily conserved protein kinase called mTOR and its associated regulatory complex 1 (mTORC1) to the surface of the endolysosome through a multiprotein complex [27] comprising Rag guanosine triphosphatases (GTPases) [28,29], Ragulator [30,31], and vacuolar H^+-adenosine triphosphatase ATPase (v-ATPase) [32]. In the presence of nutrients, the complex localizes on the surface of the endolysosome, where the growth-factor-directed activation of the endolysosome-bound GTPase Rheb [33] allosterically stimulates mTORC1 activity. Signaling from endolysosomes, mTORC1 initiates anabolic programs enhancing growth and proliferation, while suppressing catabolic autophagy and cellular quality control [2,34,35]. In addition, recent studies in rat kidney cells suggest that the reactivation of mTORC1, in combination with the precise regulation of phosphoinositide production, also coordinates autophagic lysosomal reformation (ALR)—an essential process that helps recycle a full complement of functional lysosomes from auto/endolysosomes during prolonged starvation [36]. Furthermore, the cytosolic face of the endolysosome drives the dynamic association of MiT/TFE family basic helix−loop−helix (bHLH) transcription factors, including TFEB, TFE3, TFEC, and MiTF, which that regulate endolysosome biogenesis [34], autophagy [35], and energy metabolism [37], as well as tethering factors that promote endolysosome fusion [2] or contact with other organelles to carry out specific metabolic programs [38]. Intriguingly, the association between mTOR, endolysosome, and the reabsorptive dysfunction in PT cells lacking *Raptor* [39]—the scaffold protein that docks mTOR kinase on the surface of the endolysosome—suggests potential interactions between nutrient sensing, endolysosome-directed mTORC1 signaling, and the maintenance of the kidney PT integrity.

2.2. Types of Autophagy

Three major routes for the delivery of autophagic cargos to endolysosomes have been reported: macroautophagy, chaperone-mediated autophagy, and microautophagy (Figure 2). Macroautophagy—the best-characterized form of autophagy—involves the sequestration of cellular material within a double-membrane vesicle, termed an autophagosome [40]. Induction factors and stress signals determine the choice of the autophagosome content that can proceed in a relatively nonselective manner, that is the bulk autophagy [41], or entail the tightly regulated disposal of individual cellular components [42]. For instance, mitophagy removes dysfunctional and/or damaged mitochondria; "ribophagy" for ribosomes; "pexophagy" for peroxisomes; "reticulophagy" specifically dismantles portions of the endoplasmic reticulum; "nucleophagy" parts of the nucleus; "aggrephagy" selectively removes misfolded protein aggregates, "lipophagy" lipid droplets, and "xenophagy" specifically degrades intracellular bacteria that escape endosomes [42]. Irrespective of substrate specificity, selective autophagy relies on a set of cellular sensors that detect potentially dangerous cues and convert them into signals that are ultimately conveyed to the autophagic machinery [42].

Several distinct complexes containing autophagy-related proteins (ATGs) work with membrane trafficking components to regulate a well-oiled, multistep process that involves initiation, membrane nucleation and phagophore formation, phagophore elongation, cargo sequestration, expansion, autophagosome-lysosome fusion, and degradation. For example, a complex composed of serine/threonine protein kinases ULK1, ULK2, and other proteins stimulates the initiation of autophagy [43,44], while the class III phosphoinositide 3-kinase (PI3K) complex regulates the phagophore formation [45,46]. In addition, two ubiquitin-related systems, i.e., ATG12-ATG5-ATG16L and the microtubule-associated protein 1 light chain 3 (MAP1LC3, also known as LC3), govern the phagophore elongation and sealing of the autophagosome [47]. The autophagy-mediated turnover of damaged and/or dysfunctional mitochondria is required for protecting PT from a wide range of stimuli and insults, such as ischemia, acute kidney injury, sepsis, nutrient deprivation, exposure to toxins and/or pathogens, heat, radiation, hypoxia, and ureteral obstruction [20,48]. Conversely, the deletion of essential autophagy genes (e.g., *Atg5* or *Atg7*; [20,49]) damages PT cells through defective mitochondrial clearance and increased reactive oxygen species (ROS), further substantiating the fundamental role of autophagy in the maintenance of kidney PT integrity and normal physiology. A fascinating interplay between ATG proteins and the membrane dynamics and the nutrient and/or energy-dependent signaling networks that induce autophagy has extensively been described in detail elsewhere [50].

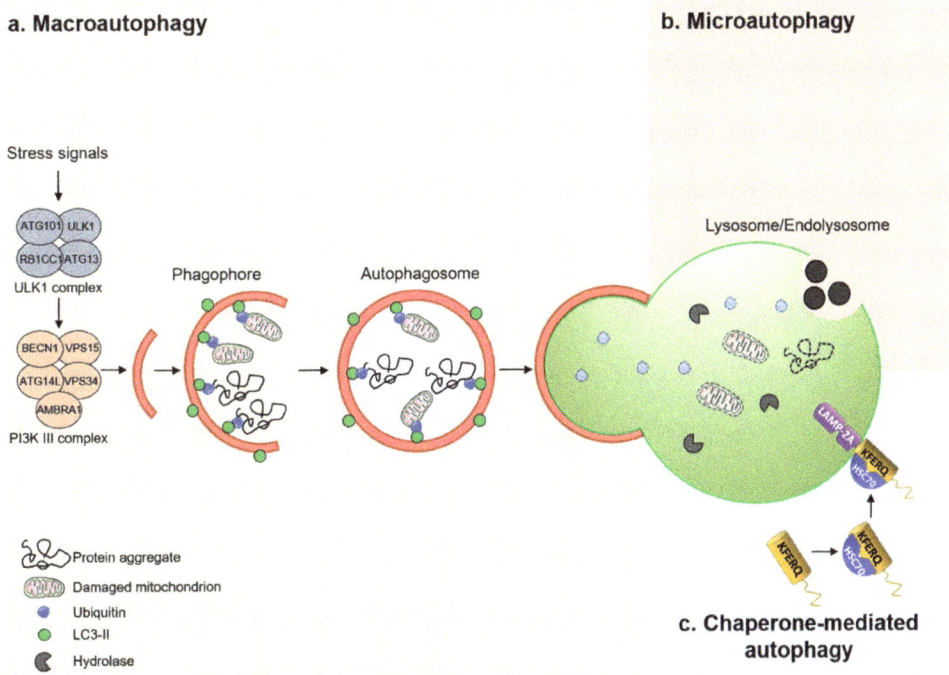

Figure 2. Different mechanisms of autophagy. (a) Macroautophagy is a nonselective bulk process that removes protein aggregates and/or damaged mitochondria. (b) Microautophagy captures cytoplasmic constituents through direct invagination of endolysosome membranes. Resulting vesicles are subsequently released into the lumen of the endolysosome for degradation. (c) CMA identifies proteins containing a KFERQ pentapeptide-related motif by a chaperone complex HSC70 that transports them into the lumen of the endolysosome through a receptor/translocon containing LAMP2A.

Conversely, chaperone-mediated autophagy (CMA) operates as a protein-exclusive type of autophagy, whereby KFERQ-like motif-bearing proteins are recognized by the heat-shock cognate protein HSPA8/HSC70 and cross the surface of the endolysosome through the binding to lysosomal-associated membrane protein 2A (LAMP2A). This triggers the assembly of receptor/translocon containing LAMP2A that targets the degradation of CMA-flagged substrates by endolysosomes [51]. In contrast to CMA and macroautophagy, microautophagy enwraps, sequesters, and transports cytosolic components into the lumen of endolysosomes without the formation of autophagosomes [52]. The resulting breakdown products generated by the endolysosome-based degradation are eventually exported to the cytoplasm through dedicated nutrient transporters that span the membrane of the endolysosome, and are further utilized for energy or in other metabolic reactions [53]. These recent discoveries are now putting autophagy–endolysosome degradative systems under the spotlight, as they play a key role in safeguarding the homeostasis, integrity, and physiology of the kidney PT.

3. Cystinosis as a Paradigm of Endolysosome Disease Causing PT Dysfunction

The dysregulation of the endolysosome system causes a generalized dysfunction of PT cells, ultimately triggering losses of essential nutrients into the urine, thereby causing CKD [54] and life-threatening complications. Such PT dysfunction can stem from rare inherited disorders, owing to the malfunctioning of endolysosome-residing proteins, particularly in cystinosis [5,6].

Cystinosis—one of a family of approximately 70 rare inborn diseases of the metabolism known as lysosomal storage diseases [55]—is caused by inactivating mutations in the *CTNS* gene encoding the proton-driven transporter cystinosin [56], which exports cystine from the endolysosome (Figure 3a). Given that the low abundance of cystinosin in the lysosomal membrane is the rate-limiting step for cystine transport, its functional loss leads cystine to accumulate within the endolysosomes of tissues across the body, culminating in severe multiorgan dysfunctions that affect primarily the brain, eyes, liver, muscles, pancreas, and kidneys.

The renal Fanconi syndrome is often the first manifestation of cystinosis, usually presenting within the first year of life and characterized by the early and severe dysfunction of PT cells, highlighting the unique vulnerability of kidney cell types [57]. Infantile (MIM #219800) and juvenile (MIM #219900) forms of cystinosis represent a frequent cause of inherited PT dysfunction and renal Fanconi syndrome. In addition, children with cystinosis display early deposition of cystine crystals in the cornea, thereby causing photophobia and painful corneal erosions [58]. In their second to third decade of life, patients with cystinosis can also develop hypothyroidism, hypogonadism, diabetes, myopathy, and deterioration of fine vision and decline of the central nervous system [59–61].

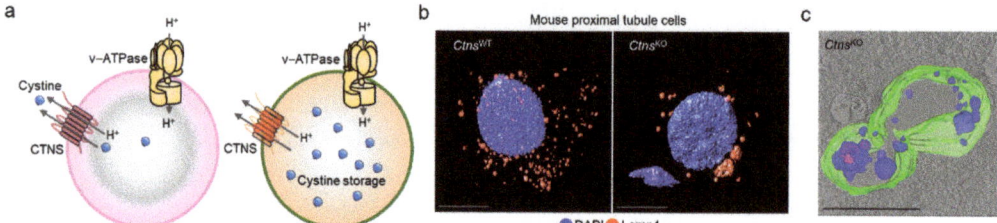

Figure 3. Cystinosin: from endolysosome to disease. (**a**) Cystinosin works in tandem with v-ATPase to transport cystine from the endolysosome, and its absence triggers (**b**,**c**) the storage of cystine within enlarged endolysosomes in primary proximal tubule cells derived from mouse kidneys. Adapted from Festa et al. [62].

The only available strategy to counteract cystine storage is the oral administration of cysteamine, which allows cystine to exit from the endolysosomes [63]. However, cysteamine treatment is hampered by side effects and poor tolerance, and it does not prevent or treat PT dysfunction [63]. Stem cells and gene therapy treatments, which rescued the eyes, kidneys, and thyroid in *Ctns* knockout (KO) mice, and are currently being tested in cystinosis patients, are limited by complexity and high costs [57,64]. Thus, there is an urgent need to identify safe and cost-effective therapeutics for patients with cystinosis. The advent of a growing number of animal and cell-based models that reproduce the human disease pathology has improved our understanding of disease mechanisms and the cellular pathways underlying PT dysfunction and renal Fanconi syndrome, ultimately accelerating the discovery and development of promising new therapeutic approaches. This progress and the recent discoveries are discussed in detail in the next sections.

4. Insights into Disease Pathways—The Role of Impaired Autophagy

Recent studies using a $Ctns^{KO}$ mouse model that recapitulates multiple features of cystinosis have suggested that the absence of cystinosin in PT cells leads cystine to accumulate within enlarged endolysosomes that move to the perinuclear region and exhibit structural, trafficking, and functional defects (Figure 3b,c). This presumably activates a signaling cascade that drives abnormal cell growth and apical dedifferentiation, ultimately leading to defective receptor-mediated endocytosis and urinary loss of LMW proteins in vivo [65,66]. The tight integration between endolysosome system, regulation of growth signaling pathways, and maintenance of PT differentiation suggests that endolysosome dysfunction driven by cystinosin loss might disrupt the homeostasis in cystinosis-affected PT cells. How, mechanistically, the absence of cystinosin wreaks havoc on cellular homeostasis has remained incompletely understood.

Accumulating evidence suggests that the endolysosome can capture and degrade aged and/or malfunctioning cellular constituents through macroautophagy/autophagy—an evolutionarily conserved, "self–eating" process through which potentially dangerous cytosolic entities are sequestered within autophagosomes and subsequently delivered to endolysosomes for degradation [1,67,68]. This homeostatic process is particularly active in PT cells, whose intense reabsorptive properties require the maintenance of the mitochondrial network [25,69]. Given the structural and functional defects of cystinosis-affected endolysosomes and considering that autophagy relies on catabolic properties of endolysosomes, the cystinosin loss-induced storage of cystine might compromise the degradation of autophagosomes in kidney PT cells. Using differentiated PT cell culture systems, which closely reproduce the key features of the in vivo disease phenotype [62,70] in combination with bona fide autophagy biosensors and assay technologies, Festa and colleagues revealed that primary cells derived from microdissected PT segments of $Ctns^{KO}$ (henceforward referred to as mPTCs) mice fail to dismantle Lc3b-flagged autophagosomes [62,71]. Evidence supporting incomplete autophagy flux in cystinosin-deficient PT cells include the following: (i) abnormally high numbers of autophagosomes under-normal growth conditions; (ii) failure to clear autophagic vesicles (AVs) formed after starvation-induced autophagy, mimicking bafilomycin (Bfn) A1 action; (iii) inability of BfnA1 to further elevate the Lc3-II and Sqstm1/p62 protein levels and the numbers of punctate Lc3b-flagged autophagosomes; (iv) and impaired degradation of the resting autophagosomes in $Ctns^{KO}$ mPTCs with a selective PI3K3/Vps34 inhibitor [62,71]. Similar autophagy defects (e.g., accumulation of AVs and their defective degradation, and increased p62 levels) have also been observed in several other LSDs (Table 1 [72–90]). Defects in autophagy–endolysosome degradative pathways, which are also encountered in ctns-deficient zebrafish, are reverted by exogenously expressing wild-type cystinosin in mutant cells [62,71]. Of note, treatment with the oral drug cysteamine, which efficiently depletes the storage of cystine within endolysosomes, does not restore the functioning of endolysosomes nor the catabolic autophagy in patient cells [91,92]. Thus, cystinosin—beyond its function in cystine transport—might act as an evolutionarily conserved, metabolic rheostat that regulates the response of endolysosomes to the arrival of endocytosed and autophagy cargoes, hence safeguarding the integrity and the physiological homeostasis of kidney tubule cells [62,71].

Conversely, Napolitano and colleagues indicate that the macroautophagy/autophagy flux seems to be fully normal, despite the increased number of autophagosomes in mutant cells [93]. Thus, it is plausible that elevated numbers of autophagosome could stem from compensatory mechanisms due to defects in CMA. Indeed, studies in cultured cells (e.g., hepatocytes and T cells) have indicated a functional crosstalk between macroautophagy and CMA, whereby cells respond to the failure of one of these pathways by activating the other [94,95]. In line with this concept, studies on lysosomes purified from livers of starved $Ctns^{KO}$ mice unveil defects in the degradation of glyceraldehyde-3-posphate dehydrogenase (GADPH)—a well-established substrate for the CMA pathway [51]. These abnormalities are reflected by dislodgement of the lysosomal receptor Lamp2a required for CMA from its natural binding partner Lamp1 and co-localization with Rab11a-positive recycling endosomes. These trafficking defects appear to be specific for Lamp2a, as other Lamp proteins can normally reach the endolysosomes in cystinosis-affected fibroblasts [93]. The small GTPase Ras-related protein Rab-11A (RAB11), and the RAB7 effector Rab-interacting lysosomal protein (RILP), seem to be part of this trafficking machinery, as the correction of the lower levels observed for both proteins in patient cells is sufficient to repair LAMP2A mistargeting, and hence the CMA pathway in diseased cells [96]. Such an apparent discrepancy might be attributed to: (i) differential biochemistry of distinct cell types in the body; (ii) turnover rates of autophagy cargos and substrates; (iii) cell type and tissue/organ-dependent adaptive responses to counteract the primary storage defect, and (iv) whether the cells are renewing or terminally differentiated; and (v) differential threshold triggered by cystine storage to induce dysfunction in distinct cell types, and affected tissues and organs. However, in some studies, exogenous expression of the dynein subunit, e.g., DYNC1LI2 (dynein, cytoplasmic 1 light intermediate chain 2)—a key cytoskeletal motor protein involved intracellular transport of cargo, organelle trafficking, mitotic spindle assembly, and positioning—rescues the localization of the chaperone-mediated autophagy (CMA) receptor LAMP2A, CMA activity, and the cellular homeostasis in cystinosis-affected PT cells [97]. Regardless of the mechanisms involved, the concept that defects in endolysosomes and autophagy pathways might contribute to cystinosis pathogenesis is in line with recent studies that indicate an accumulation of autophagosomes engulfing damaged and/or dysfunction mitochondria, and increased formation of aggregate-prone SQSTM1/p62 inclusions in both kidney biopsies [98,99] and patient cells [100].

Table 1. Autophagy pathways in lysosomal storage diseases.

Mechanisms of Lysosomal Storage	Disease Examples	Lysosomal Protein Defect	Substrate	AV Accumulation	Defective AV Degradation	CMA Activity	Increased SQSTM1/p62	Refs.
Lysosomal enzyme deficiencies	Fabry	α-Galactosidase	(Lyso-) Globotriaosylceramide	Yes	Yes	??	Yes	[81]
	Gaucher	β-Glucocerebrosidase	Glucosylceramide, glucosylsphingosine	Yes	Yes	??	Yes	[80,85,86]
	Mucopolysaccharidoses	Enzymes involved in Mucopolysaccharide catabolism	Mucopolysaccharides	Yes	Yes	??	Yes	[75–77]
	Multiple sulfatase deficiency	SUMF1 (Activator of sulfatases)	Multiple, including sulfated glycosaminoglycans	Yes	Yes	??	Yes	[75,76]
	Pompe	α-Glucosidase	Glycogen	Yes	Yes	??	Yes	[72,73,87,88]
Defects in soluble non-enzymatic lysosomal proteins	Niemann-Pick disease type C2	NPC2	Cholesterol and sphingolipids	Yes	Yes	??	Yes	[78,79]
	Cystinosis	Cystinosin	Cystine	Yes	Yes	Reduced	Yes	[62,71,93,97,100,101]
Defects in lysosomal membrane proteins	Danon	Lysosomal-associated membrane protein 2, splicing variant A (LAMP2)	Glycogen and other autophagic components	Yes	Yes	??	Yes	[74]
	Mucolipidosis IV	Mucolipin-1	Mucopolysaccharides and lipids	Yes	Yes	Reduced	Yes	[82–84]
	Niemann-Pick disease type C1	NPC1	Cholesterol and sphingolipids	Yes	Yes	??	Yes	[78,79,88]

5. Autophagy, Mitochondria, and Epithelial Dysfunction in Cystinosis

The conjugation of defective endolysosome dynamics and impaired catabolic properties is strikingly similar to cellular alterations stemming from the accumulation of monoclonal light chains (κLCs) within the endolysosomes of PT cells, causing a similar epithelial dysfunction [7]. Furthermore, the uncontrolled increase in the endolysosomal PtdIns(4,5)P$_2$ pool that arises from loss-of-function of the PtdIns(4,5)P$_2$ 5-phosphatase OCRL triggers endolysosome dysfunction and autophagosome accumulation of patients with Lowe syndrome [102,103]—another rare inherited disorders causing PT dysfunction and renal Fanconi syndrome. The storage of either cystine or κLCs or PtdIns(4,5)P$_2$ might thus tamp down the homeostasis and transport functions of PT cells, emphasizing the crucial role of autophagy–endolysosome degradative systems in preserving the homeostasis and physiology of the kidney PT.

As a direct consequence of defective autophagy–endolysosome degradation systems, $Ctns^{KO}$ PT cells remarkably accumulate SQSTM1- and ubiquitin-forming aggregates with damaged and/or dysfunctional mitochondria within enlarged, non-degradative endolysosomes, ultimately overproducing mitochondrial-derived reactive oxygen species (ROS) [62,71]. Genetic (e.g., short hairpin RNA interference targeting $Atg7$) and pharmacological (e.g., inhibition of Beclin1/Vps-34 complex by using SAR-405 or Spautin-1) suppression of autophagy dampens the functioning of the mitochondrial network, inducing oxidative stress, while repressing the receptor-mediated endocytosis and transport properties of PT cells [62,71]. This evidence further reinforces the mechanistic connection between defective mitochondrial quality control, oxidative stress, and cellular dysfunction. Thus, the maintenance of degradative autophagy might serve as a bona fide (homeostasis-modifying) process that regulates the identity of the kidney tubule cells. How, mechanistically, defects in degradative autophagy disrupting the differentiation of PT cells have remained to be fully elucidated.

Recent insights have illuminated the biological functions of tight junction proteins in safeguarding the epithelial cell behavior and phenotype. In particular, tight junction adaptor protein 1 (Tjp1) represses the nuclear translocation of an Y box binding protein 3 (Ybx3) —a transcriptional factor that promotes cell proliferation while repressing PT differentiation during kidney development [104]. As oxidative stress damages tight junction integrity [105], the excessive mitochondrial ROS induced by cystinosin loss might trigger an abnormal activation of the tight junction associated Ybx3 (Y box binding protein) signaling, which would, in turn, lead to epithelial dysfunction in cystinosis PT cells. In line with this model, increased levels of mitochondrial ROS stimulate Gna12/Ga12-SRC-mediated phosphorylation of Tjp1 and its subsequent misrouting to enlarged, non-degradative endolysosomes. The disruption of tight junction integrity triggers the hyperactivation of tight junction-associated Ybx3 signaling, with increased proliferation (e.g., $Ccnd1$ and $Pcna$) and reduced apical differentiation (e.g., $Lrp2$), ultimately disabling receptor-mediated endocytosis and epithelial functions in $Ctns^{KO}$ cells [62,71] (Figure 4). Gain- and loss-of-function approaches targeting $Gna12$ or $Tjp1$ or $Ybx3$, or pharmacological interventions impeding activation of the Gna12-Src-directed signaling (e.g., with the mitochondrial-targeted antioxidant Mito-TEMPO or with the SRC inhibitor SU6656) restore epithelial functions in $Ctns^{KO}$ cells [62,71]. By regulating autophagy and the Tjp1-Yxb3 signaling, the crosstalk between cystinosin and the endolysosome system might thus dictate the balance between proliferation and differentiation of PT cells, and hence their role in homeostasis.

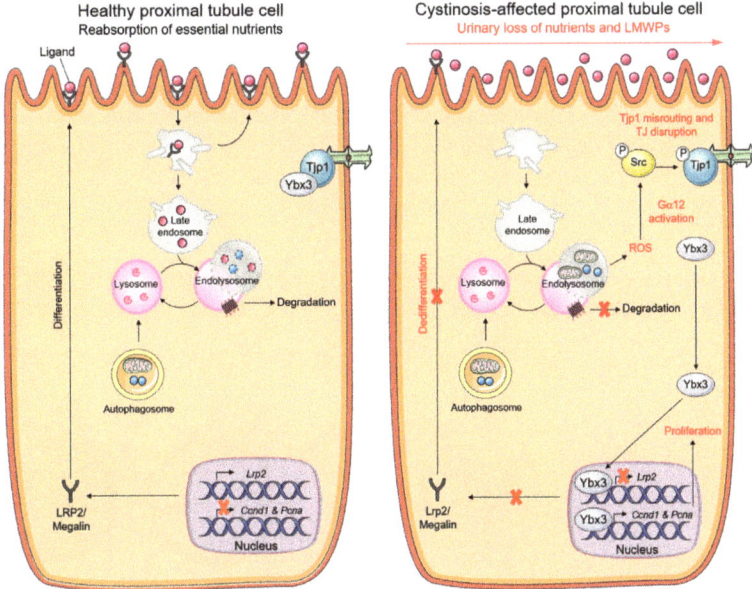

Figure 4. Pathogenic cascade driving PT dysfunction in cystinosis cells. Graphical schematic illustrating that cystinosin-deficient PT cells accumulate dysfunctional mitochondria and reactive-oxygen species (ROS), triggering an abnormal activation of the tight junction—associated signalling that stimulates proliferation while suppressing apical dedifferentiation. Reprinted with permission from Ref. [6]. Copyright 2021 Springer Nature.

6. Pharmacological Modulation of Autophagy as a Targetable Pathway in Cystinosis

There are no curative treatments for cystinosis, and the current supportive care approaches have substantially decreased mortality and overall morbidity. For example, supplementation with water, bicarbonate, citrate, phosphate, salts, and vitamin D can rapidly attenuate the metabolic complications associated with renal Fanconi syndrome, and hence maintain an adequate body fluid and electrolyte homeostasis [6,57]. Beyond management care, patients with cystinosis can benefit from treatment with cysteamine [58]—an FDA-approved drug that depletes the endolysosomal cystine storage by cleaving cystine into free cysteine and cysteamine–cysteine mixed sulphide. These metabolites are subsequently exported from the endolysosome to cytoplasm through cationic amino acid transporter 2 (PQLC2), which spans the endolysosomal membrane [106]. Despite an improvement in patients' quality of life, treatment is hampered by adverse effects, poor tolerance, and a strict dosing schedule, and it does not prevent or treat the renal Fanconi syndrome and kidney failure [58,63]. Therefore, there is an urgent need to yield promising new targetable interventions in the early course of cystinosis.

The molecular understanding of regulatory circuitries coupling endolysosome disease, autophagy, and epithelial dysfunction might thus guide the discovery and development of targeted therapeutics for cystinosis patients [57,64]. In this case, interventions that are aimed to target each step of the pathogenic cascade might mediate beneficial effects and potentially counteract the homeostatic perturbations imposed by cystinosin loss and the resulting cystine storage. For example, small molecule compounds that either activate CMA [107] or boost the excretion [108] of cystine-loaded endolysosomes might ameliorate clinical outcomes if they are used concomitantly with the cystine-depleting drug cysteamine [93,109] (Figure 5). Boosting CMA with small-molecule activators (e.g., QX77) increases the lifetime of the endocytic receptor megalin at the plasma membrane, ultimately improving the epithelial functions in human PT cells lacking cystinosin (e.g., CRISPR-Cas9-induced gene deletion) [101]. Consistent with these observations, combinatorial strategies using an mTORC1 inhibitor (e.g., everolimus) and cysteamine rescues the homeostasis and functioning of autophagy–endolysosome degradation systems in cystinosis patient-derived pluripotent stem cells (iPSCs) and kidney organoid models of the disease [110] (Figure 5).

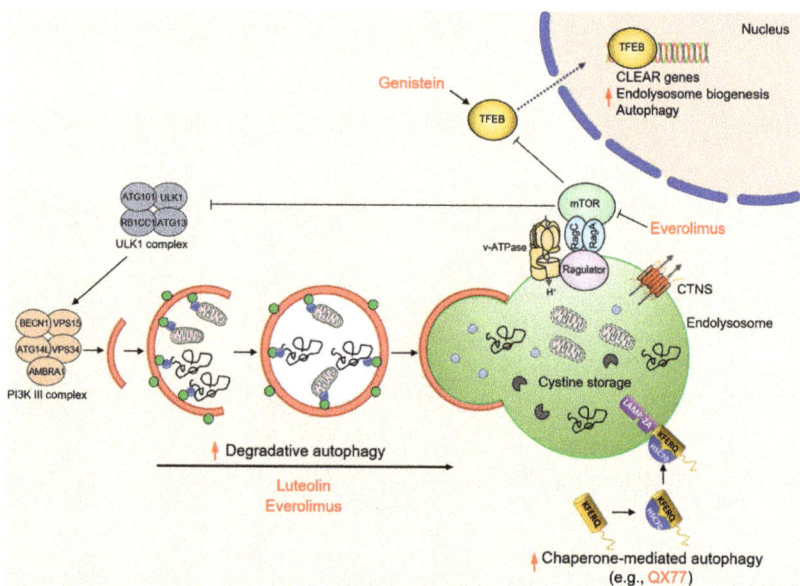

Figure 5. Summary of emerging therapeutic strategies targeting autophagy pathways in cystinosis.

Despite normal mTORC1 activity in cystinotic iPSCs and their derived kidney organoids, the molecular mechanisms behind the beneficial effects of the combo treatment remain largely elusive. In this setting, a potential mediator could be the activation of TFEB—a master regulator that controls the expression of the genes involved in autophagy and endolysosome biogenesis [2,34,35] (Figure 5). Recent work showing that cystinosin might physically interact with many components of the v-ATPase–Ragulator–Rag complex [110,111], which regulates the mTORC1 lifetime and its activation at the surface of the endolysosome, and that the reconstitution of TFEB signaling stimulates the catabolic properties of endolysosomes and the completion of autophagy in conditionally immortalized PT epithelial cells (ciPTEC) derived from the urine of a cystinotic patient [92], further substantiate the concept. Indeed, the pharmacological induction (e.g., genistein) of nuclear translocation and the activation of TFEB-dependent transcriptional programs has recently been shown to empty cystine storage, to restore the functioning of endolysosomes and degradative autophagy, and to improve the processing of endocytosed cargos in cystinotic ciPTEC [92] (Figure 5).

Recently, drug discovery and repurposing strategies are gaining momentum as a default tool for providing affordable therapies in rare inherited diseases [112,113]. With the possibility to screen approved and investigational products, the process is well adapted to the curiosity-driven research culture in academia, hence mitigating the risk inherent in preclinical drug discovery. With this lag in mind, De Leo and colleagues recently identified small molecule drug candidates [100] that decrease the accumulation of the autophagy substrate p62/SQSTM1 and restore the autophagy–endolysosome degradative pathways, which are compromised in different models and cell systems of cystinosis [100]. Among several positive hits, luteolin—a natural flavonoid that is present in various fruits and vegetables—has emerged as the most interesting candidate. This compound has a good safety profile, owing to its similarity to genistein, and improves the endolysosome-mediated degradation of autophagy cargoes and substrates, including damaged and dysfunctional (ROS-overproducing) mitochondria [100] (Figure 5). In addition, treating cystinotic ciPTEC, mPTCs derived from mouse $Ctns^{KO}$ kidneys, and zebrafish models of cystinosis with luteolin not only repaired endolysosomes, autophagy degradation, and mitochondrial redox homeostasis and cellular distress, but also restored megalin expression at the plasma membrane, ultimately stimulating protein absorption and hence transport functions [100]. These findings extend previous observations demonstrating that structural and functional deformities of the kidney PT could be delayed in $Ctns^{KO}$ mice by administrating mitochondria-targeted ROS scavengers such as mitoquinone [114] or mito-TEMPO [62]. Thus, the modulation of autophagy–endolysosome degradative systems might offer a promising new therapeutic avenue not only for cystinosis, but also for other currently intractable diseases related to endolysosome storage.

7. Concluding Remarks

The maintenance of a healthy endolysosomal system is particularly crucial for preserving the homeostasis and physiology of kidney tubule cells, and loss-of-function mutations that impair the functioning of the endolysosome system can invariably lead to PT dysfunction and kidney disease. Rare inherited defects in an endolysosome-residing protein and the storage materials, as exemplified here by cystinosis, might disable autophagy and organelle quality control, triggering a level of mitochondrial distress that drives the dysfunction of the kidney PT. Further studies will be required for understanding whether other LSDs might have various degrees of PT dysfunction and kidney disease. In most cases, kidney disease manifestations might be overshadowed by more severe symptoms affecting the brain, underestimating the prevalence of kidney involvement in these disorders.

The mechanisms by which cystinosin deficiency wreaks havoc on homeostasis and function of the endolysosome system remain largely elusive. These defects could stem from defects in mannose-6-phosphate (M6P)-dependent trafficking [115] or megalin-directed reuptake of filtered lysosomal cathepsins [116] or endolysosome acidification [117]. Alternatively, the storage of cystine wrought by cystinosin loss might affect the folding of disulphide-bonded substrates for endoproteolytic attack or thiol-active catalytic sites of endolysosomal cathepsins, ultimately affecting processing and their lasting maturation [57,118].

As the endolysosome is the site for nutrient sensing and the activation of mTORC1 signaling—the master regulator that represses autophagy and endolysosome biogenesis—it will be important to evaluate whether cystinosin deficiency and cystine storage might contribute to hyperactive mTORC1. This might in turn inhibit endolysosome and autophagosome biogenesis, thus generating a vicious cycle that boosts metabolic dyshomeostasis and dysfunction in cystinosis cells. Although cystinosin could physically interact with many components of the v-ATPase–Ragulator–Rag complex [111] that regulates mTORC1 activity, the contribution of dysregulated nutrient sensing and mTOR signaling to disease pathogenesis remains an open question. The recent development of model organisms [62] and primary PT cell culture systems [65,70], which closely reproduce the key features of the disease phenotype, and mass spectrometry-based profiling of intact endolysosomes [119], presents an opportunity to address this critical point.

Decline in endolysosome function and mitochondrial autophagy are clear hallmarks of ageing, and correlate with metabolic dysfunction [3]. Indeed, the behavior of "aged" endolysosomes mimics the cellular phenotypes encountered in cystinosis and other LSD cells. We suspect that the dysregulation of adaptive response to mitochondrial distress might also contribute to maladaptation and disease in patients with cystinosis, and this will require further studies to understand the effects of *CTNS* mutations on organelle repair pathways, such as mitochondrial unfolded protein response (UPRmt) and mitochondrial biogenesis. The increasing power of organelle-specific purification and profiling via proteomic, lipidomic, and metabolomic-based approaches will be useful in filling these missing knowledge gaps. These questions are just examples of all the exciting work that lies ahead to comprehensively dissect the biological functions of cystinosin in the context of tissue homeostasis and disease.

A current challenge is to translate the knowledge gained from fundamental studies of endolysosome biology to the treatment of cystinosis and other endolysosome-related diseases. In this regard, the use of informative preclinical models, coupled with improved knowledge of disease signatures and the recent advances in multi-omics technologies, might accelerate the discovery and development of "first-in-class" therapeutics that can halt the progression of cystinosis, as well as other rare and more common diseases related to endolysosome dysfunction.

Author Contributions: L.R.R. and A.L. conceptualized the article. L.R.R., E.D.L. and A.L. wrote the article. D.N. and E.D.L. researched the data for the article and drew the figures under the supervision of L.R.R. and A.L. All of the authors contributed substantially to the discussion of the content and reviewed the article before submission. L.R.R. and A.L. edited the article. All authors have read and agreed to the published version of the manuscript.

Funding: A.L. is supported by Cystinosis Research Foundation (Irvine, CA, USA) and the Swiss National Centre of Competence in Research (NCCR) Kidney Control of Homeostasis (Kidney.CH). A.L. received financial support from the University Research Priority Program of the University of Zurich (URPP) ITINERARE—Innovative Therapies in Rare Diseases. The funders had no role in study design, data collection, and interpretation, or the decision to submit the work for publication. L.R. and E.D.L. are supported by Cystinosis Research Foundation (Irvine, CA, USA) and Italian Ministry of Health.

Conflicts of Interest: The authors declare no conflict of interest.

References

1. Levine, B.; Kroemer, G. Biological Functions of Autophagy Genes: A Disease Perspective. *Cell* **2019**, *176*, 11–42. [CrossRef] [PubMed]
2. Ballabio, A.; Bonifacino, J.S. Lysosomes as dynamic regulators of cell and organismal homeostasis. *Nat. Rev. Mol. Cell Biol.* **2020**, *21*, 101–118. [CrossRef] [PubMed]
3. Aman, Y.; Schmauck-Medina, T.; Hansen, M.; Morimoto, R.I.; Simon, A.K.; Bjedov, I.; Palikaras, K.; Simonsen, A.; Johansen, T.; Tavernarakis, N.; et al. Autophagy in healthy aging and disease. *Nat. Aging* **2021**, *1*, 634–650. [CrossRef]
4. Shin, H.R.; Zoncu, R. The Lysosome at the Intersection of Cellular Growth and Destruction. *Dev. Cell* **2020**, *54*, 226–238. [CrossRef]
5. van der Wijst, J.; Belge, H.; Bindels, R.J.M.; Devuyst, O. Learning physiology from inherited kidney disorders. *Physiol. Rev.* **2019**, *99*, 1575–1653. [CrossRef] [PubMed]
6. Festa, B.P.; Berquez, M.; Nieri, D.; Luciani, A. Endolysosomal Disorders Affecting the Proximal Tubule of the Kidney: New Mechanistic Insights and Therapeutics. *Rev. Physiol. Biochem. Pharmacol.* **2021**. [CrossRef]
7. Luciani, A.; Sirac, C.; Terryn, S.; Javaugue, V.; Prange, J.A.; Bender, S.; Bonaud, A.; Cogné, M.; Aucouturier, P.; Ronco, P.; et al. Impaired lysosomal function underlies monoclonal light chain–associated renal Fanconi syndrome. *J. Am. Soc. Nephrol.* **2016**, *27*, 2049–2061. [CrossRef]
8. Gu, X.; Yang, H.; Sheng, X.; Ko, Y.A.; Qiu, C.; Park, J.; Huang, S.; Kember, R.; Judy, R.L.; Park, J.; et al. Kidney disease genetic risk variants alter lysosomal beta-mannosidase (MANBA) expression and disease severity. *Sci. Transl. Med.* **2021**, *13*, eaaz1458. [CrossRef] [PubMed]
9. Pattaro, C.; Teumer, A.; Gorski, M.; Chu, A.Y.; Li, M.; Mijatovic, V.; Garnaas, M.; Tin, A.; Sorice, R.; Li, Y.; et al. Genetic associations at 53 loci highlight cell types and biological pathways relevant for kidney function. *Nat. Commun.* **2016**, *7*, 10023. [CrossRef] [PubMed]
10. Wuttke, M.; Li, Y.; Li, M.; Sieber, K.B.; Feitosa, M.F.; Gorski, M.; Tin, A.; Wang, L.; Chu, A.Y.; Hoppmann, A.; et al. A catalog of genetic loci associated with kidney function from analyses of a million individuals. *Nat. Genet.* **2019**, *51*, 957–972. [CrossRef]
11. Christensen, E.I.; Birn, H. Megalin and cubilin: Multifunctional endocytic receptors. *Nat. Rev. Mol. Cell Biol.* **2002**, *3*, 256–266. [CrossRef]
12. Eshbach, M.L.; Weisz, O.A. Receptor-Mediated Endocytosis in the Proximal Tubule. *Annu. Rev. Physiol.* **2017**, *79*, 425–448. [CrossRef]
13. Nielsen, R.; Christensen, E.I.; Birn, H. Megalin and cubilin in proximal tubule protein reabsorption: From experimental models to human disease. *Kidney Int.* **2016**, *89*, 58–67. [CrossRef] [PubMed]
14. Mishra, S.K.; Keyel, P.A.; Hawryluk, M.J.; Agostinelli, N.R.; Watkins, S.C.; Traub, L.M. Disabled-2 exhibits the properties of a cargo-selective endocytic clathrin adaptor. *EMBO J.* **2002**, *21*, 4915–4926. [CrossRef] [PubMed]
15. Gekle, M. Renal tubule albumin transport. *Annu. Rev. Physiol.* **2005**, *67*, 573–594. [CrossRef] [PubMed]

16. Kaksonen, M.; Roux, A. Mechanisms of clathrin-mediated endocytosis. *Nat. Rev. Mol. Cell Biol.* **2018**, *19*, 313–326. [CrossRef] [PubMed]
17. Faundez, V.; Hartzell, H.C. Intracellular chloride channels: Determinants of function in the endosomal pathway. *Sci. STKE* **2004**, *2004*, re8. [CrossRef]
18. Abbas, Y.M.; Wu, D.; Bueler, S.A.; Robinson, C.V.; Rubinstein, J.L. Structure of V-ATPase from the mammalian brain. *Science* **2020**, *367*, 1240–1246. [CrossRef]
19. Devuyst, O.; Luciani, A. Chloride transporters and receptor-mediated endocytosis in the renal proximal tubule. *J. Physiol.* **2015**, *593*, 4151–4164. [CrossRef] [PubMed]
20. Xu, H.; Ren, D. Lysosomal physiology. *Annu. Rev. Physiol.* **2015**, *77*, 57–80. [CrossRef] [PubMed]
21. Hurtado-Lorenzo, A.; Skinner, M.; El Annan, J.; Futai, M.; Sun-Wada, G.H.; Bourgoin, S.; Casanova, J.; Wildeman, A.; Bechoua, S.; Ausiello, D.A.; et al. V-ATPase interacts with ARNO and Arf6 in early endosomes and regulates the protein degradative pathway. *Nat. Cell Biol.* **2006**, *8*, 124–126. [CrossRef]
22. Cullen, P.J.; Steinberg, F. To degrade or not to degrade: Mechanisms and significance of endocytic recycling. *Nat. Rev. Mol. Cell Biol.* **2018**, *19*, 679–696. [CrossRef]
23. Pohl, C.; Dikic, I. Cellular quality control by the ubiquitin-proteasome system and autophagy. *Science* **2019**, *366*, 818–822. [CrossRef] [PubMed]
24. Jiang, P.; Mizushima, N. Autophagy and human diseases. *Cell Res.* **2014**, *24*, 69–79. [CrossRef] [PubMed]
25. Tang, C.; Livingston, M.J.; Liu, Z.; Dong, Z. Autophagy in kidney homeostasis and disease. *Nat. Rev. Nephrol.* **2020**, *16*, 489–508. [CrossRef] [PubMed]
26. Klionsky, D.J.; Petroni, G.; Amaravadi, R.K.; Baehrecke, E.H.; Ballabio, A.; Boya, P.; Bravo-San Pedro, J.M.; Cadwell, K.; Cecconi, F.; Choi, A.M.K.; et al. Autophagy in major human diseases. *EMBO J.* **2021**, *40*, e108863. [CrossRef] [PubMed]
27. Liu, G.Y.; Sabatini, D.M. mTOR at the nexus of nutrition, growth, ageing and disease. *Nat. Rev. Mol. Cell Biol.* **2020**, *21*, 183–203. [CrossRef] [PubMed]
28. Rogala, K.B.; Gu, X.; Kedir, J.F.; Abu-Remaileh, M.; Bianchi1, L.F.; Bottino1, A.M.S.; Dueholm1, R.; Niehaus1, A.; Overwijn1, D.; Priso Fils1, A.C.; et al. Structural basis for the docking of mTORC1 on the lysosomal surface. *Science* **2019**, *366*, 468–475. [CrossRef] [PubMed]
29. Sancak, Y.; Peterson, T.R.; Shaul, Y.D.; Lindquist, R.A.; Thoreen, C.C.; Bar-Peled, L.; Sabatini, D.M. The rag GTPases bind raptor and mediate amino acid signaling to mTORC1. *Science* **2008**, *320*, 1496–1501. [CrossRef]
30. Sancak, Y.; Bar-Peled, L.; Zoncu, R.; Markhard, A.L.; Nada, S.; Sabatini, D.M. Ragulator-rag complex targets mTORC1 to the lysosomal surface and is necessary for its activation by amino acids. *Cell* **2010**, *141*, 290–303. [CrossRef] [PubMed]
31. Lawrence, R.E.; Cho, K.F.; Rappold, R.; Thrun, A.; Tofaute, M.; Kim, D.J.; Moldavski, O.; Hurley, J.H.; Zoncu, R. A nutrient-induced affinity switch controls mTORC1 activation by its Rag GTPase–Ragulator lysosomal scaffold. *Nat. Cell Biol.* **2018**, *20*, 1052–1063. [CrossRef] [PubMed]
32. Zoncu, R.; Bar-Peled, L.; Efeyan, A.; Wang, S.; Sancak, Y.; Sabatini, D.M. mTORC1 senses lysosomal amino acids through an inside-out mechanism that requires the vacuolar H+-ATPase. *Science* **2011**, *334*, 678–683. [CrossRef] [PubMed]
33. Yang, H.; Jiang, X.; Li, B.; Yang, H.J.; Miller, M.; Yang, A.; Dhar, A.; Pavletich, N.P. Mechanisms of mTORC1 activation by RHEB and inhibition by PRAS40. *Nature* **2017**, *552*, 368–373. [CrossRef]
34. Sardiello, M.; Palmieri, M.; Di Ronza, A.; Medina, D.L.; Valenza, M.; Gennarino, V.A.; Di Malta, C.; Donaudy, F.; Embrione, V.; Polishchuk, R.S.; et al. A gene network regulating lysosomal biogenesis and function. *Science* **2009**, *325*, 473–477. [CrossRef]
35. Settembre, C.; Di Malta, C.; Polito, V.A.; Arencibia, M.G.; Vetrini, F.; Erdin, S.; Erdin, S.U.; Huynh, T.; Medina, D.; Colella, P.; et al. TFEB links autophagy to lysosomal biogenesis. *Science* **2011**, *332*, 1429–1433. [CrossRef] [PubMed]
36. Yu, L.; McPhee, C.K.; Zheng, L.; Mardones, G.A.; Rong, Y.; Peng, J.; Mi, N.; Zhao, Y.; Liu, Z.; Wan, F.; et al. Termination of autophagy and reformation of lysosomes regulated by mTOR. *Nature* **2010**, *465*, 942–946. [CrossRef] [PubMed]
37. Settembre, C.; De Cegli, R.; Mansueto, G.; Saha, P.K.; Vetrini, F.; Visvikis, O.; Huynh, T.; Carissimo, A.; Palmer, D.; Klisch, T.J.; et al. TFEB controls cellular lipid metabolism through a starvation-induced autoregulatory loop. *Nat. Cell Biol.* **2013**, *15*, 647–658. [CrossRef] [PubMed]
38. Wong, Y.C.; Ysselstein, D.; Krainc, D. Mitochondria-lysosome contacts regulate mitochondrial fission via RAB7 GTP hydrolysis. *Nature* **2018**, *554*, 382–386. [CrossRef]
39. Grahammer, F.; Ramakrishnan, S.K.; Rinschen, M.M.; Larionov, A.A.; Syed, M.; Khatib, H.; Roerden, M.; Sass, J.O.; Helmstaedter, M.; Osenberg, D.; et al. MTOR regulates endocytosis and nutrient transport in proximal tubular cells. *J. Am. Soc. Nephrol.* **2017**, *28*, 230–241. [CrossRef]
40. Mizushima, N. A brief history of autophagy from cell biology to physiology and disease. *Nat. Cell Biol.* **2018**, *20*, 521–527. [CrossRef]
41. Mizushima, N.; Levine, B. Autophagy in Human Diseases. *N. Engl. J. Med.* **2020**, *383*, 1564–1576. [CrossRef] [PubMed]
42. Sica, V.; Galluzzi, L.; Bravo-San Pedro, J.M.; Izzo, V.; Maiuri, M.C.; Kroemer, G. Organelle-Specific Initiation of Autophagy. *Mol. Cell* **2015**, *59*, 522–539. [CrossRef]
43. Park, J.M.; Jung, C.H.; Seo, M.; Otto, N.M.; Grunwald, D.; Kim, K.H.; Moriarity, B.; Kim, Y.M.; Starker, C.; Nho, R.S.; et al. The ULK1 complex mediates MTORC1 signaling to the autophagy initiation machinery via binding and phosphorylating ATG14. *Autophagy* **2016**, *12*, 547–564. [CrossRef]

44. Park, J.M.; Seo, M.; Jung, C.H.; Grunwald, D.; Stone, M.; Otto, N.M.; Toso, E.; Ahn, Y.; Kyba, M.; Griffin, T.J.; et al. ULK1 phosphorylates Ser30 of BECN1 in association with ATG14 to stimulate autophagy induction. *Autophagy* **2018**, *14*, 584–597. [CrossRef]
45. Kihara, A.; Noda, T.; Ishihara, N.; Ohsumi, Y. Two distinct Vps34 phosphatidylinositol 3-kinase complexes function in autophagy and carboxypeptidase y sorting in Saccharomyces cerevisiae. *J. Cell Biol.* **2001**, *153*, 519–530. [CrossRef]
46. Zhong, Y.; Wang, Q.J.; Li, X.; Yan, Y.; Backer, J.M.; Chait, B.T.; Heintz, N.; Yue, Z. Distinct regulation of autophagic activity by Atg14L and Rubicon associated with Beclin 1-phosphatidylinositol-3-kinase complex. *Nat. Cell Biol.* **2009**, *11*, 468–476. [CrossRef]
47. Walczak, M.; Martens, S. Dissecting the role of the Atg12-Atg5-Atg16 complex during autophagosome formation. *Autophagy* **2013**, *9*, 424–425. [CrossRef] [PubMed]
48. Havasi, A.; Dong, Z. Autophagy and Tubular Cell Death in the Kidney. *Semin. Nephrol.* **2016**, *36*, 174–188. [CrossRef] [PubMed]
49. Yamamoto, T.; Takabatake, Y.; Kimura, T.; Takahashi, A.; Namba, T.; Matsuda, J.; Minami, S.; Kaimori, J.Y.; Matsui, I.; Kitamura, H.; et al. Time-dependent dysregulation of autophagy: Implications in aging and mitochondrial homeostasis in the kidney proximal tubule. *Autophagy* **2016**, *12*, 801–813. [CrossRef]
50. Dikic, I.; Elazar, Z. Mechanism and medical implications of mammalian autophagy. *Nat. Rev. Mol. Cell Biol.* **2018**, *19*, 349–364. [CrossRef]
51. Kaushik, S.; Cuervo, A.M. The coming of age of chaperone-mediated autophagy. *Nat. Rev. Mol. Cell Biol.* **2018**, *19*, 365–381. [CrossRef]
52. Mijaljica, D.; Prescott, M.; Devenish, R.J. Microautophagy in mammalian cells: Revisiting a 40-year-old conundrum. *Autophagy* **2011**, *7*, 673–682. [CrossRef] [PubMed]
53. Lawrence, R.E.; Zoncu, R. The lysosome as a cellular centre for signalling, metabolism and quality control. *Nat. Cell Biol.* **2019**, *21*, 133–142. [CrossRef] [PubMed]
54. Eckardt, K.U.; Coresh, J.; Devuyst, O.; Johnson, R.J.; Köttgen, A.; Levey, A.S.; Levin, A. Evolving importance of kidney disease: From subspecialty to global health burden. *Lancet* **2013**, *382*, 158–169. [CrossRef]
55. Platt, F.M. Emptying the stores: Lysosomal diseases and therapeutic strategies. *Nat. Rev. Drug Discov.* **2018**, *17*, 133–150. [CrossRef]
56. Town, M.; Jean, G.; Cherqui, S.; Attard, M.; Forestier, L.; Whitmore, S.A.; Gallen, D.F.; Gribouval, O.; Broyer, M.; Bates, G.P.; et al. A novel gene encoding an integral membrane protein is mutated in nephropathic cystinosis. *Nat. Genet.* **1998**, *18*, 319–324. [CrossRef] [PubMed]
57. Cherqui, S.; Courtoy, P.J. The renal Fanconi syndrome in cystinosis: Pathogenic insights and therapeutic perspectives. *Nat. Rev. Nephrol.* **2017**, *13*, 115–131. [CrossRef] [PubMed]
58. Gahl, W.A.; Thoene, J.G.; Schneider, J.A. Cystinosis. *N. Engl. J. Med.* **2002**, *347*, 111–121. [CrossRef]
59. Nesterova, G.; Gahl, W. Nephropathic cystinosis: Late complications of a multisystemic disease. *Pediatr. Nephrol.* **2008**, *23*, 863–878. [CrossRef] [PubMed]
60. Trauner, D.A.; Williams, J.; Ballantyne, A.O.; Spilkin, A.M.; Crowhurst, J.; Hesselink, J. Neurological impairment in nephropathic cystinosis: Motor coordination deficits. *Pediatr. Nephrol.* **2010**, *25*, 2061–2066. [CrossRef] [PubMed]
61. Viltz, L.; Trauner, D.A. Effect of age at treatment on cognitive performance in patients with cystinosis. *J. Pediatr.* **2013**, *163*, 489–492. [CrossRef] [PubMed]
62. Festa, B.P.; Chen, Z.; Berquez, M.; Debaix, H.; Tokonami, N.; Prange, J.A.; van de Hoek, G.; Alessio, C.; Raimondi, A.; Nevo, N.; et al. Impaired autophagy bridges lysosomal storage disease and epithelial dysfunction in the kidney. *Nat. Commun.* **2018**, *9*, 161. [CrossRef] [PubMed]
63. Brodin-Sartorius, A.; Tête, M.J.; Niaudet, P.; Antignac, C.; Guest, G.; Ottolenghi, C.; Charbit, M.; Moyse, D.; Legendre, C.; Lesavre, P.; et al. Cysteamine therapy delays the progression of nephropathic cystinosis in late adolescents and adults. *Kidney Int.* **2012**, *81*, 179–189. [CrossRef]
64. Jamalpoor, A.; Othman, A.; Levtchenko, E.N.; Masereeuw, R.; Janssen, M.J. Molecular Mechanisms and Treatment Options of Nephropathic Cystinosis. *Trends Mol. Med.* **2021**, *27*, 673–686. [CrossRef] [PubMed]
65. Raggi, C.; Luciani, A.; Nevo, N.; Antignac, C.; Terryn, S.; Devuyst, O. Dedifferentiation and aberrations of the endolysosomal compartment characterize the early stage of nephropathic cystinosis. *Hum. Mol. Genet.* **2014**, *23*, 2266–2278. [CrossRef] [PubMed]
66. Gaide Chevronnay, H.P.; Janssens, V.; Van Der Smissen, P.; N'Kuli, F.; Nevo, N.; Guiot, Y.; Levtchenko, E.; Marbaix, E.; Pierreux, C.E.; Cherqui, S.; et al. Time course of pathogenic and adaptation mechanisms in cystinotic mouse kidneys. *J. Am. Soc. Nephrol.* **2014**, *25*, 1256–1269. [CrossRef] [PubMed]
67. Mizushima, N.; Komatsu, M. Autophagy: Renovation of cells and tissues. *Cell* **2011**, *147*, 728–741. [CrossRef] [PubMed]
68. Galluzzi, L.; Baehrecke, E.H.; Ballabio, A.; Boya, P.; Bravo-San Pedro, J.M.; Cecconi, F.; Choi, A.M.; Chu, C.T.; Codogno, P.; Colombo, M.I.; et al. Molecular definitions of autophagy and related processes. *EMBO J.* **2017**, *36*, 1811–1836. [CrossRef]
69. Fougeray, S.; Pallet, N. Mechanisms and biological functions of autophagy in diseased and ageing kidneys. *Nat. Rev. Nephrol.* **2015**, *11*, 34–45. [CrossRef] [PubMed]
70. Berquez, M.; Krohn, P.; Luciani, A.; Devuyst, O. Receptor-mediated endocytosis and differentiation in proximal tubule cell systems. *J. Am. Soc. Nephrol.* **2021**, *32*, 1265–1267. [CrossRef] [PubMed]
71. Luciani, A.; Festa, B.P.; Chen, Z.; Devuyst, O. Defective autophagy degradation and abnormal tight junction-associated signaling drive epithelial dysfunction in cystinosis. *Autophagy* **2018**, *14*, 1157–1159. [CrossRef]

72. Raben, N.; Hill, V.; Shea, L.; Takikita, S.; Baum, R.; Mizushima, N.; Ralston, E.; Plotz, P. Suppression of autophagy in skeletal muscle uncovers the accumulation of ubiquitinated proteins and their potential role in muscle damage in Pompe disease. *Hum. Mol. Genet.* **2008**, *17*, 3897–3908. [CrossRef]
73. Raben, N.; Schreiner, C.; Baum, R.; Takikita, S.; Xu, S.; Xie, T.; Myerowitz, R.; Komatsu, M.; Van Der Meulen, J.H.; Nagaraju, K.; et al. Suppression of autophagy permits successful enzyme replacement therapy in a lysosomal storage disorder—Murine Pompe disease. *Autophagy* **2010**, *6*, 1078–1089. [CrossRef]
74. Tanaka, Y.; Guhde, G.; Suter, A.; Eskelinen, E.L.; Hartmann, D.; Lüllmann-Rauch, R.; Janssen, P.M.L.; Blanz, J.; Von Figura, K.; Saftig, P. Accumulation of autophagic vacuoles and cardiomyopathy LAMP-2-deficient mice. *Nature* **2000**, *406*, 902–906. [CrossRef]
75. Settembre, C.; Fraldi, A.; Jahreiss, L.; Spampanato, C.; Venturi, C.; Medina, D.; de Pablo, R.; Tacchetti, C.; Rubinsztein, D.C.; Ballabio, A. A block of autophagy in lysosomal storage disorders. *Hum. Mol. Genet.* **2008**, *17*, 119–129. [CrossRef] [PubMed]
76. Fraldi, A.; Annunziata, F.; Lombardi, A.; Kaiser, H.J.; Medina, D.L.; Spampanato, C.; Fedele, A.O.; Polishchuk, R.; Sorrentino, N.C.; Simons, K.; et al. Lysosomal fusion and SNARE function are impaired by cholesterol accumulation in lysosomal storage disorders. *EMBO J.* **2010**, *29*, 3607–3620. [CrossRef]
77. Tessitore, A.; Pirozzi, M.; Auricchio, A. Abnormal autophagy, ubiquitination, inflammation and apoptosis are dependent upon lysosomal storage and are useful biomarkers of mucopolysaccharidosis VI. *Pathogenetics* **2009**, *2*, 4. [CrossRef] [PubMed]
78. Ko, D.C.; Milenkovic, L.; Beier, S.M.; Manuel, H.; Buchanan, J.A.; Scott, M.P. Cell-autonomous death of cerebellar purkinje neurons with autophagy in niemann-pick type C disease. *PLoS Genet.* **2005**, *1*, 81–95. [CrossRef] [PubMed]
79. Pacheco, C.D.; Elrick, M.J.; Lieberman, A.P. Tau deletion exacerbates the phenotype of Niemann-Pick type C mice and implicates autophagy in pathogenesis. *Hum. Mol. Genet.* **2009**, *18*, 956–965. [CrossRef] [PubMed]
80. Sun, Y.; Liou, B.; Ran, H.; Skelton, M.R.; Williams, M.T.; Vorhees, C.V.; Kitatani, K.; Hannun, Y.A.; Witte, D.P.; Xu, Y.H.; et al. Neuronopathic Gaucher disease in the mouse: Viable combined selective saposin C deficiency and mutant glucocerebrosidase (V394L) mice with glucosylsphingosine and glucosylceramide accumulation and progressive neurological deficits. *Hum. Mol. Genet.* **2010**, *19*, 1088–1097. [CrossRef] [PubMed]
81. Chévrier, M.; Brakch, N.; Lesueur, C.; Genty, D.; Ramdani, Y.; Moll, S.; Djavaheri-Mergny, M.; Brasse-Lagnel, C.; Laquerrière, A.; Barbey, F.; et al. Autophagosome maturation is impaired in Fabry disease. *Autophagy* **2010**, *6*, 589–599. [CrossRef] [PubMed]
82. Vergarajauregui, S.; Connelly, P.S.; Daniels, M.P.; Puertollano, R. Autophagic dysfunction in mucolipidosis type IV patients. *Hum. Mol. Genet.* **2008**, *17*, 2723–2737. [CrossRef] [PubMed]
83. Venugopal, B.; Mesires, N.T.; Kennedy, J.C.; Curcio-Morelli, C.; Laplante, J.M.; Dice, J.F.; Slaugenhaupt, S.A. Chaperone-mediated autophagy is defective in mucolipidosis type IV. *J. Cell. Physiol.* **2009**, *219*, 344–353. [CrossRef]
84. Curcio-Morelli, C.; Charles, F.A.; Micsenyi, M.C.; Cao, Y.; Venugopal, B.; Browning, M.F.; Dobrenis, K.; Cotman, S.L.; Walkley, S.U.; Slaugenhaupt, S.A. Macroautophagy is defective in mucolipin-1-deficient mouse neurons. *Neurobiol. Dis.* **2010**, *40*, 370–377. [CrossRef]
85. Kinghorn, K.J.; Grönke, S.; Castillo-Quan, J.I.; Woodling, N.S.; Li, L.; Sirka, E.; Gegg, M.; Mills, K.; Hardy, J.; Bjedov, I.; et al. A Drosophila model of neuronopathic gaucher disease demonstrates lysosomal-autophagic defects and altered mTOR signalling and is functionally rescued by rapamycin. *J. Neurosci.* **2016**, *36*, 11654–11670. [CrossRef] [PubMed]
86. Brown, R.A.; Voit, A.; Srikanth, M.P.; Thayer, J.A.; Kingsbury, T.J.; Jacobson, M.A.; Lipinski, M.M.; Feldman, R.A.; Awad, O. MTOR hyperactivity mediates lysosomal dysfunction in Gaucher's disease iPSC-neuronal cells. *DMM Dis. Model. Mech.* **2019**, *12*. [CrossRef] [PubMed]
87. Fukuda, T.; Ahearn, M.; Roberts, A.; Mattaliano, R.J.; Zaal, K.; Ralston, E.; Plotz, P.H.; Raben, N. Autophagy and Mistargeting of Therapeutic Enzyme in Skeletal Muscle in Pompe Disease. *Mol. Ther.* **2006**, *14*, 831–839. [CrossRef] [PubMed]
88. Nascimbeni, A.C.; Fanin, M.; Masiero, E.; Angelini, C.; Sandri, M. Impaired autophagy contributes to muscle atrophy in glycogen storage disease type II patients. *Autophagy* **2012**, *8*, 1697–1700. [CrossRef] [PubMed]
89. Chi, C.; Leonard, A.; Knight, W.E.; Beussman, K.M.; Zhao, Y.; Cao, Y.; Londono, P.; Aune, E.; Trembley, M.A.; Small, E.M.; et al. LAMP-2B regulates human cardiomyocyte function by mediating autophagosome–lysosome fusion. *Proc. Natl. Acad. Sci. USA* **2019**, *116*, 556–565. [CrossRef]
90. Davis, O.B.; Shin, H.R.; Lim, C.Y.; Wu, E.Y.; Kukurugya, M.; Maher, C.F.; Perera, R.M.; Ordonez, M.P.; Zoncu, R. NPC1-mTORC1 Signaling Couples Cholesterol Sensing to Organelle Homeostasis and Is a Targetable Pathway in Niemann-Pick Type C. *Dev. Cell* **2021**, *56*, 260–276. [CrossRef]
91. Ivanova, E.A.; De Leo, M.G.; Van Den Heuvel, L.; Pastore, A.; Dijkman, H.; De Matteis, M.A.; Levtchenko, E.N. Endo-Lysosomal Dysfunction in Human Proximal Tubular Epithelial Cells Deficient for Lysosomal Cystine Transporter Cystinosin. *PLoS ONE* **2015**, *10*, e0120998. [CrossRef]
92. Rega, L.R.; Polishchuk, E.; Montefusco, S.; Napolitano, G.; Tozzi, G.; Zhang, J.; Bellomo, F.; Taranta, A.; Pastore, A.; Polishchuk, R.; et al. Activation of the transcription factor EB rescues lysosomal abnormalities in cystinotic kidney cells. *Kidney Int.* **2016**, *89*, 862–873. [CrossRef] [PubMed]
93. Napolitano, G.; Johnson, J.L.; He, J.; Rocca, C.J.; Monfregola, J.; Pestonjamasp, K.; Cherqui, S.; Catz, S.D. Impairment of chaperone-mediated autophagy leads to selective lysosomal degradation defects in the lysosomal storage disease cystinosis. *EMBO Mol. Med.* **2015**, *7*, 158–174. [CrossRef] [PubMed]

94. Massey, A.C.; Kaushik, S.; Sovak, G.; Kiffin, R.; Cuervo, A.M. Consequences of the selective blockage of chaperone-mediated autophagy. *Proc. Natl. Acad. Sci. USA* **2006**, *103*, 5805–5810. [CrossRef] [PubMed]
95. Kaushik, S.; Massey, A.C.; Mizushima, N.; Cuervo, A.M. Constitutive activation of chaperone-mediated autophagy in cells with impaired macroautophagy. *Mol. Biol. Cell* **2008**, *19*, 2179–2192. [CrossRef] [PubMed]
96. Zhang, J.; Johnson, J.L.; He, J.; Napolitano, G.; Ramadass, M.; Rocca, C.; Kiosses, W.B.; Bucci, C.; Xin, Q.; Gavathiotis, E.; et al. Cystinosin, the small GTPase Rab11, and the Rab7 effector RILP regulate intracellular trafficking of the chaperone-mediated autophagy receptor LAMP2A. *J. Biol. Chem.* **2017**, *292*, 10328–10346. [CrossRef] [PubMed]
97. Rahman, F.; Johnson, J.L.; Zhang, J.; He, J.; Pestonjamasp, K.; Cherqui, S.; Catz, S.D. DYNC1LI2 regulates localization of the chaperone-mediated autophagy receptor LAMP2A and improves cellular homeostasis in cystinosis. *Autophagy* **2021**, 1–19. [CrossRef]
98. Sansanwal, P.; Sarwal, M.M. Abnormal mitochondrial autophagy in nephropathic cystinosis. *Autophagy* **2010**, *6*, 971–973. [CrossRef] [PubMed]
99. Sansanwal, P.; Sarwal, M.M. P62/SQSTM1 prominently accumulates in renal proximal tubules in nephropathic cystinosis. *Pediatr. Nephrol.* **2012**, *27*, 2137–2144. [CrossRef] [PubMed]
100. De Leo, E.; Elmonem, M.A.; Berlingerio, S.P.; Berquez, M.; Festa, B.P.; Raso, R.; Bellomo, F.; Starborg, T.; Janssen, M.J.; Abbaszadeh, Z.; et al. Cell-based phenotypic drug screening identifies luteolin as candidate therapeutic for nephropathic cystinosis. *J. Am. Soc. Nephrol.* **2020**, *31*, 1522–1537. [CrossRef]
101. Zhang, J.; He, J.; Johnson, J.L.; Rahman, F.; Gavathiotis, E.; Cuervo, A.M.; Catz, S.D. Chaperone-mediated autophagy upregulation rescues megalin expression and localization in cystinotic proximal tubule cells. *Front. Endocrinol.* **2019**, *10*, 21. [CrossRef]
102. De Leo, M.G.; Staiano, L.; Vicinanza, M.; Luciani, A.; Carissimo, A.; Mutarelli, M.; Di Campli, A.; Polishchuk, E.; Di Tullio, G.; Morra, V.; et al. Autophagosome-lysosome fusion triggers a lysosomal response mediated by TLR9 and controlled by OCRL. *Nat. Cell Biol.* **2016**, *18*, 839–850. [CrossRef] [PubMed]
103. Festa, B.P.; Berquez, M.; Gassama, A.; Amrein, I.; Ismail, H.M.; Samardzija, M.; Staiano, L.; Luciani, A.; Grimm, C.; Nussbaum, R.L.; et al. OCRL deficiency impairs endolysosomal function in a humanized mouse model for Lowe syndrome and Dent disease. *Hum. Mol. Genet.* **2019**, *28*, 1931–1946. [CrossRef] [PubMed]
104. Lima, W.R.; Parreira, K.S.; Devuyst, O.; Caplanusi, A.; N'Kuli, F.; Marien, B.; Van Der Smissen, P.; Alves, P.M.S.; Verroust, P.; Christensen, E.I.; et al. ZONAB promotes proliferation and represses differentiation of proximal tubule epithelial cells. *J. Am. Soc. Nephrol.* **2010**, *21*, 478–488. [CrossRef] [PubMed]
105. Yu, W.; Beaudry, S.; Negoro, H.; Boucher, I.; Tran, M.; Kong, T.; Denker, B.M. H 2O 2 activates G protein, α 12 to disrupt the junctional complex and enhance ischemia reperfusion injury. *Proc. Natl. Acad. Sci. USA* **2012**, *109*, 6680–6685. [CrossRef] [PubMed]
106. Jézégou, A.; Llinares, E.; Anne, C.; Kieffer-Jaquinod, S.; O'Regan, S.; Aupetit, J.; Chabli, A.; Sagné, C.; Debacker, C.; Chadefaux-Vekemans, B.; et al. Heptahelical protein PQLC2 is a lysosomal cationic amino acid exporter underlying the action of cysteamine in cystinosis therapy. *Proc. Natl. Acad. Sci. USA* **2012**, *109*, E3434–E3443. [CrossRef] [PubMed]
107. Anguiano, J.; Garner, T.P.; Mahalingam, M.; Das, B.C.; Gavathiotis, E.; Cuervo, A.M. Chemical modulation of chaperone-mediated autophagy by retinoic acid derivatives. *Nat. Chem. Biol.* **2013**, *9*, 374–382. [CrossRef] [PubMed]
108. McNeill, A.; Magalhaes, J.; Shen, C.; Chau, K.Y.; Hughes, D.; Mehta, A.; Foltynie, T.; Cooper, J.M.; Abramov, A.Y.; Gegg, M.; et al. Ambroxol improves lysosomal biochemistry in glucocerebrosidase mutation-linked Parkinson disease cells. *Brain* **2014**, *137*, 1481–1495. [CrossRef]
109. Johnson, J.L.; Napolitano, G.; Monfregola, J.; Rocca, C.J.; Cherqui, S.; Catz, S.D. Upregulation of the Rab27a-Dependent Trafficking and Secretory Mechanisms Improves Lysosomal Transport, Alleviates Endoplasmic Reticulum Stress, and Reduces Lysosome Overload in Cystinosis. *Mol. Cell. Biol.* **2013**, *33*, 2950–2962. [CrossRef]
110. Hollywood, J.A.; Przepiorski, A.; D'Souza, R.F.; Sreebhavan, S.; Wolvetang, E.J.; Harrison, P.T.; Davidson, A.J.; Holm, T.M. Use of human induced pluripotent stem cells and kidney organoids to develop a cysteamine/mtor inhibition combination therapy for cystinosis. *J. Am. Soc. Nephrol.* **2020**, *31*, 962–982. [CrossRef]
111. Andrzejewska, Z.; Nevo, N.; Thomas, L.; Chhuon, C.; Bailleux, A.; Chauvet, V.; Courtoy, P.J.; Chol, M.; Chiara Guerrera, I.; Antignac, C. Cystinosin is a component of the vacuolar H+-ATPase-ragulator-rag complex controlling mammalian target of rapamycin complex 1 signaling. *J. Am. Soc. Nephrol.* **2016**, *27*, 1678–1688. [CrossRef]
112. Bellomo, F.; De Leo, E.; Taranta, A.; Giaquinto, L.; Di Giovamberardino, G.; Montefusco, S.; Rega, L.R.; Pastore, A.; Medina, D.L.; Di Bernardo, D.; et al. Drug repurposing in rare diseases: An integrative study of drug screening and transcriptomic analysis in nephropathic cystinosis. *Int. J. Mol. Sci.* **2021**, *22*, 12829. [CrossRef]
113. Bellomo, F.; Medina, D.L.; De Leo, E.; Panarella, A.; Emma, F. High-content drug screening for rare diseases. *J. Inherit. Metab. Dis.* **2017**, *40*, 601–607. [CrossRef]
114. Galarreta, C.I.; Forbes, M.S.; Thornhill, B.A.; Antignac, C.; Gubler, M.C.; Nevo, N.; Murphy, M.P.; Chevalier, R.L. The swan-neck lesion: Proximal tubular adaptation to oxidative stress in nephropathic cystinosis. *Am. J. Physiol. Ren. Physiol.* **2015**, *308*, F1155–F1166. [CrossRef] [PubMed]
115. Bonam, S.R.; Wang, F.; Muller, S. Lysosomes as a therapeutic target. *Nat. Rev. Drug Discov.* **2019**, *18*, 923–948. [CrossRef] [PubMed]

116. Nielsen, R.; Courtoy, P.J.; Jacobsen, C.; Dom, G.; Lima, W.R.; Jadot, M.; Willnow, T.E.; Devuyst, O.; Christensen, E.I. Endocytosis provides a major alternative pathway for lysosomal biogenesis in kidney proximal tubular cells. *Proc. Natl. Acad. Sci. USA* **2007**, *104*, 5407–5412. [CrossRef]
117. Mindell, J.A. Lysosomal acidification mechanisms. *Annu. Rev. Physiol.* **2012**, *74*, 69–86. [CrossRef]
118. Arunachalam, B.; Phan, U.T.; Geuze, H.J.; Cresswell, P. Enzymatic reduction of disulfide bonds in lysosomes: Characterization of a gamma-interferon-inducible lysosomal thiol reductase (GILT). *Proc. Natl. Acad. Sci. USA* **2000**, *97*, 745–750. [CrossRef] [PubMed]
119. Abu-Remaileh, M.; Wyant, G.A.; Kim, C.; Laqtom, N.N.; Abbasi, M.; Chan, S.H.; Freinkman, E.; Sabatini, D.M. Lysosomal metabolomics reveals V-ATPase- and mTOR-dependent regulation of amino acid efflux from lysosomes. *Science* **2017**, *358*, 807–813. [CrossRef] [PubMed]

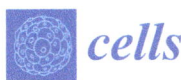 *cells*

Review

Nephropathic Cystinosis: Pathogenic Roles of Inflammation and Potential for New Therapies

Mohamed A. Elmonem [1,2,*], Koenraad R. P. Veys [3,4] and Giusi Prencipe [5]

1. Department of Clinical and Chemical Pathology, Faculty of Medicine, Cairo University, Cairo 11628, Egypt
2. Egypt Center for Research and Regenerative Medicine (ECRRM), Cairo 11517, Egypt
3. Laboratory of Pediatric Nephrology, Department of Development & Regeneration, KU Leuven, 3000 Leuven, Belgium; koenraad.veys@uzleuven.be
4. Department of Pediatrics, AZ Delta Campus, 8820 Torhout, Belgium
5. Laboratory of Immuno-Rheumatology, Bambino Gesù Children's Hospital, IRCCS, 00165 Rome, Italy; giusi.prencipe@opbg.net
* Correspondence: mohamed.abdelmonem@kasralainy.edu.eg

Abstract: The activation of several inflammatory pathways has recently been documented in patients and different cellular and animal models of nephropathic cystinosis. Upregulated inflammatory signals interact with many pathogenic aspects of the disease, such as enhanced oxidative stress, abnormal autophagy, inflammatory cell recruitment, enhanced cell death, and tissue fibrosis. Cysteamine, the only approved specific therapy for cystinosis, ameliorates many but not all pathogenic aspects of the disease. In the current review, we summarize the inflammatory mechanisms involved in cystinosis and their potential impact on the disease pathogenesis and progression. We further elaborate on the crosstalk between inflammation, autophagy, and apoptosis, and discuss the potential of experimental drugs for suppressing the inflammatory signals in cystinosis.

Keywords: macrophages; inflammasome; proximal tubular cells; endocytosis; autophagy; apoptosis; chitotriosidase; interleukins; galectin-3; cysteamine; novel therapies

Citation: Elmonem, M.A.; Veys, K.R.P.; Prencipe, G. Nephropathic Cystinosis: Pathogenic Roles of Inflammation and Potential for New Therapies. *Cells* 2022, *11*, 190. https://doi.org/10.3390/cells11020190

Academic Editor: Alfonso Eirin

Received: 28 December 2021
Accepted: 5 January 2022
Published: 6 January 2022

Publisher's Note: MDPI stays neutral with regard to jurisdictional claims in published maps and institutional affiliations.

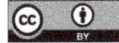

Copyright: © 2022 by the authors. Licensee MDPI, Basel, Switzerland. This article is an open access article distributed under the terms and conditions of the Creative Commons Attribution (CC BY) license (https:// creativecommons.org/licenses/by/ 4.0/).

1. Introduction

Crystallopathies, defined as diseases that involve the accumulation of intrinsic or environmental crystals or microparticles in the pathogenesis of tissue injury, are pathologically multifactorial syndromes that have been linked to the production of reactive oxygen species, immune cell recruitment and activation, and increased expression of various inflammatory cascade molecules [1,2]. The process of crystallization within cells is usually a very slow process, but when crystals form, they elicit direct cytotoxic effects, starting an auto-amplifying inflammatory loop commonly ending in cell death [2]. Crystals are commonly heavily deposited in the kidney, being the main excretory organ for most minerals and organic compounds that can form crystals. These include calcium oxalate, calcium phosphate, anhydrous uric acid, magnesium ammonium phosphate, sodium urate, and cystine. In many cases, crystal deposition is caused by lifestyle factors, such as poor dietary choices and improper hydration [3]. However, some of these disorders are hereditary in nature, including nephropathic cystinosis and primary hyperoxaluria, which are systemic diseases primarily affecting the kidney.

Nephropathic cystinosis is a monogenic autosomal recessive lysosomal storage disorder caused by variants in the *CTNS* gene, which codes for cystinosin—the cystine lysosomal symporter [4]. Defective cystinosin function leads to a multisystemic intra-lysosomal cystine accumulation. The disease commonly affects the kidneys during the first year of life through proximal tubular damage, leading to renal Fanconi syndrome, followed by progressive glomerular damage, and almost invariably ends in kidney failure. This usually requires kidney replacement therapy or kidney transplantation by the end of the first decade of life, if the child is not treated. Other affected organs include the eyes, thyroid, pancreas, gonads, muscles, and central nervous system (CNS), amongst others [5,6]. There are three major phenotypes: the infantile nephropathic phenotype (MIM #219800), which constitutes the majority of cases and appears during infancy and progresses to kidney failure rapidly if left untreated; the juvenile nephropathic phenotype (MIM #219900), which also affects the kidney but at a later age and is more slowly progressive; and the ocular or non-nephropathic phenotype (MIM #219750), which spares the kidney and usually manifests during adulthood [7].

Apart from the direct harmful effects of cystine crystal accumulation, several pathogenic processes affect cystinotic cells. Enhanced apoptosis is evident in vivo and in vitro in many cystinotic cell types, such as proximal tubular epithelial cells (PTECs), fibroblasts, and podocytes [8,9]. Both deficient ATP and cAMP levels were detected in cystinotic cells and were associated with mitochondrial dysfunction [10–12]. The enhanced motility and defective adhesion of cells leading to the loss of podocytes and PTECs in urine is a pathogenic process that contributes to the rapid progression towards kidney failure [9]. Defective endocytic trafficking and impaired proteolysis are commonly attributable to the evident lysosomal dysfunction in cystinosis [13]. Cystinosin further plays an important role in lysosomal homeostasis involving the mammalian target of the rapamycin complex 1 (mTORC1) and transcription factor EB (TFEB) [14,15]. When cystinosin is defective or missing, lysosomal signaling is disturbed resulting in altered regulation of lysosomal biogenesis and clearance and affecting both autophagy and anabolism [11,15,16].

Inflammation has recently been revealed as a major contributing mechanism to the pathogenesis and progression of both the renal and systemic involvement in cystinosis [17,18]. Cystine crystal accumulation, macrophage activation, enhanced oxidative stress, and inflammasome pathway activation are all driving factors behind the vicious cycle of cellular inflammation in cystinosis, which, no matter what the affected organ is, commonly ends in tissue fibrosis and loss of function. In the current review, we will discuss the different aspects of the inflammation process in cystinosis. We will detail the mechanisms behind inflammation, the effects of cysteamine, the current standard therapy for cystinosis on the inflammatory process, and, finally, the concept of targeting the inflammation in cystinosis as a novel potential therapeutic approach for the disease.

2. Role of Macrophages in Cystinosis

The kidneys of cystinotic patients and $Ctns^{-/-}$ mice are characterized by tubular atrophy and interstitial fibrosis, which are focally associated with inflammatory mononuclear infiltrates and largely consist of CD68 positive monocytes/macrophages [19–21]. Macrophages, together with dendritic cells, are the most abundant types of leukocytes present in the normal kidney [22]. In addition to playing a pivotal role in the innate immune responses, macrophages are critical mediators for regulating the maintenance of tissue homeostasis [23]. Indeed, they are versatile players in various processes, including balancing the development of fibrosis versus tissue repair and remodeling, clearance of cellular debris, angiogenesis, and various metabolic functions, such as glycolysis and oxidative phosphorylation [24]. In diseased kidneys, macrophages are increased in number and are key players in renal injury, inflammation, and the development of fibrosis [25].

Several bits of direct and indirect evidence strongly suggest a role for macrophages in the pathogenesis of cystinosis. Indeed, in cystinotic patients and in $Ctns^{-/-}$ mice, cystine crystals have been observed in the macrophages of most organs, including bone marrow, kidneys, liver, skin, and gastrointestinal mucosa [25–28] (Figure 1A). In in vitro studies, monocytes/macrophages displayed a great ability to phagocytize cystine crystal deposits [17,18] (Figure 1B), suggesting that, in these cells, cystine crystal accumulation is in part due to the dysfunction or absence of cystinosin, and in part due to the phagocytosis of the dying cells releasing their intracellular contents including cystine crystals. Cystinotic macrophages are unable to dissolve or get rid of the phagocytized cystine crystals because they have the same genetic and biochemical defect as other cytinotic cells, thus they tend to enter a non-ending cycle of cystine crystal deposition, wherein they send signals for the recruitment of other inflammatory cells and finally die [17].

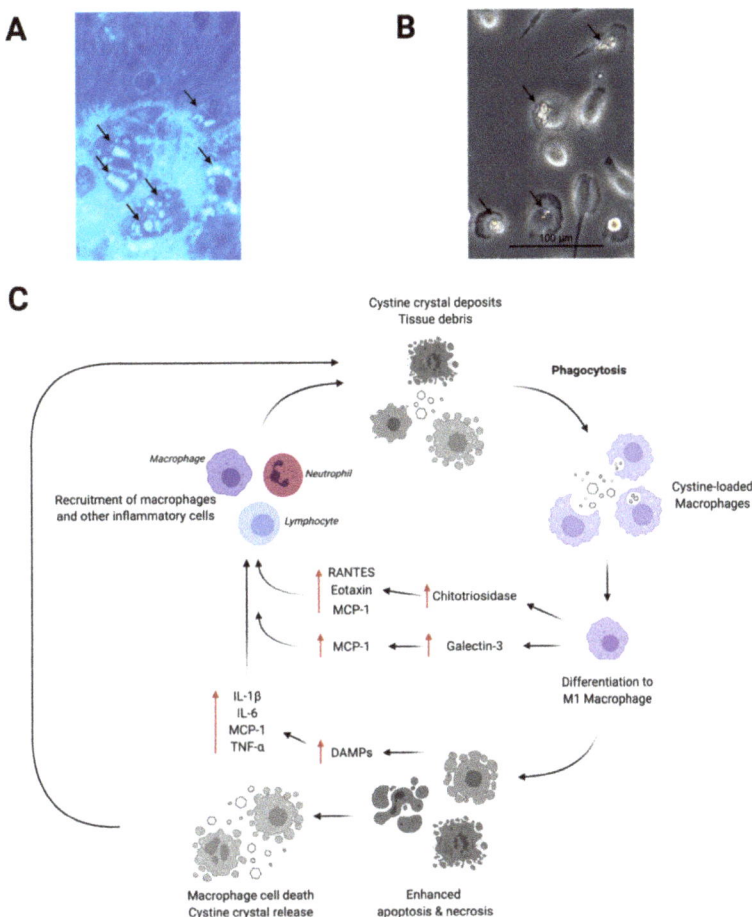

Figure 1. Macrophage activation and tissue injury in cystinosis. (**A**) Tissue cystine crystal accumulation in gastric mucosa (Toludine blue). Hexagonal and rhomboid cystine crystals are visible inside interstitial macrophages (arrows). (**B**) In vitro, incubation of macrophages with cystine crystals is followed by phagocytosis of the crystals (arrows). (**C**) A schematic diagram summarizing the mechanisms of macrophage recruitment and injury in tissues of nephropathic cystinosis patients. DAMPs, damage-associated molecular patterns; IL-1β, interleukin 1β; IL-6, interleukin 6; MCP-1, monocyte chemoattractant protein-1; RANTES, Regulated on Activation, Normal T Expressed and Secreted; TNF-α, tumor necrosis factor-α.

Based on their activation status and functions, macrophages are classified as classically activated macrophages (M1 macrophages), wound-healing macrophages (M2a macrophages), and regulatory macrophages (M2c macrophages) [29]. In $Ctns^{-/-}$ mouse kidneys, macrophages mainly display an M1-like pro-inflammatory profile [21]. Accordingly, phagocytosis of cystine crystals has been demonstrated to lead to the activation of monocytes/macrophages. Indeed, the uptake of cystine crystals by cultured human monocytes and mature macrophages induced the production of the pro-inflammatory cytokines, interleukin-1β (IL-1β) [18], and tumor necrosis factor-alpha (TNF-α) [17]. Consistent with the results obtained in vitro, cystinotic patients had significantly elevated plasma levels of IL-1β and an increase in *IL1B* mRNA expression levels in the peripheral blood mononuclear cells (PBMCs) was observed [18]. Moreover, a positive correlation between the intracellular cystine levels in polymorphonuclear leukocytes, at the time of blood sampling, and *IL1B* mRNA expression levels in PBMCs was also found [18].

Further supporting a role for cystine crystals as the activators of inflammatory responses in macrophages, the elevated levels of chitotriosidase enzyme activity were also reported in the supernatants of control macrophages incubated with an increasing concentration of cystine crystals recently [17,30]. Accordingly, an elevation in the chitotriosidase enzyme activity was also reported in patients with cystinosis, as well as in $Ctns^{-/-}$ mice [17] and in mutant zebrafish larvae (unpublished data). Chitotriosidase is an enzyme involved in the degradation of chitin (chitinase) that is expressed by activated macrophages, of which the activity has been found to be elevated in various lysosomal storage diseases, including Gaucher's disease, galactosialidosis, Niemann–Pick A/B and C diseases, cholesteryl ester storage disease, and several others [31,32]. Interestingly, chitotriosidase has been proposed as a novel biomarker for therapeutic monitoring and as a predictor of disease severity in nephropathic cystinosis [17]. Indeed, in a longitudinal study involving 61 cystinotic patients treated with cysteamine, the plasma chitotriosidase enzyme activity was significantly correlated with the white blood cells' cystine levels and with a number of extrarenal complications, suggesting that chitotriosidase enzyme activity, by reflecting the systemic cystine crystal-induced inflammation, gave better guidance on the whole-body cystine burden and, hence, compliance with cystine-depleting therapy [30].

Further supporting the role of macrophage-mediated inflammation in the progression of kidney disease in cystinosis, a recent study demonstrated a novel role for cystinosin, independent of the accumulation of cystine crystals, in regulating the localization and degradation of the β-galactosidase-binding protein family member Galectin-3 [21]. Galectin-3 is an inflammatory mediator that plays a role in acute and chronic inflammation by attracting monocytes/macrophages in diseased tissues. In $Ctns^{-/-}$ mice, the genetic deletion of *Gal3* led to decreased monocytes/macrophages infiltration in the kidney, amelioration of the renal functions, and to a significant reduction in the circulating levels of the monocyte chemoattractant protein-1 (MCP-1) cytokine. Accordingly, increased serum levels of MCP-1 also have been found in $Ctns^{-/-}$ mice and in patients with cystinosis, despite cysteamine treatment [21].

Although the exact nature of the immunostimulatory signals activating macrophages in cystinosis is still unknown, it is well documented that deposits of crystals, including cystine crystals, are able to induce cellular necroptosis, thereby leading to a release of damage-associated molecular patterns (DAMPs) [33]. DAMPs are endogenous danger molecules that initiate inflammatory responses by activating the pattern recognition receptors (PRRs), such as Toll-like and Nod-like receptors (TLRs and NLRs) [34]. Both TLRs and NLRs are expressed in the innate immune cells, such as macrophages and dendritic cells, as well as in non-immune cells, such as epithelial cells and fibroblasts. Therefore, it is reasonable to hypothesize that in cystinosis the cells damaged by the crystals release DAMPs that, in turn, initiate inflammatory responses by triggering various cells, including tissue-resident macrophages, and result in the release of pro-inflammatory cytokines and chemokines—such as IL-1β, IL-6, TNF-α, and MCP-1. The released cytokines and chemokines promote the recruitment of inflammatory cells that contribute to the exacerbation of the tissue injury (Figure 1C).

Altogether, this evidence strongly supports a role for the involvement of activated macrophages in the progression of tissue damage in cystinosis, particularly in the kidney.

3. Inflammasome Activation in Cystinosis

One of the most recently identified mechanisms of action, by which crystals induce kidney injury in both acute kidney injury (AKI) and chronic kidney disease (CKD), is the activation of the intracellular sensor inflammasome [35]. Inflammasomes are multiprotein complexes that play a major role in innate immune responses by controlling the caspase-1–dependent proteolytic maturation and release of the pro-inflammatory cytokines IL-1β and IL-18 [36].

Inflammasomes sense a wide variety of pathogen-associated molecular patterns as well as of DAMPs, including host-derived crystalline moieties [37,38]. Indeed, endogenous crystals or particles, such as monosodium urate, calcium phosphate, hydroxyapatite, silica, asbestos, cholesterol crystals, and calcium oxalate, have been found to act as agonists of the best characterized inflammasome, NLRP3 [39]. Although the exact mechanism by which NLRP3 is activated by several stimuli has not been fully clarified, NLRP3 activation by crystalline structures has been demonstrated to require lysosomal membrane destabilization, cathepsin B release into the cytosol, the generation of reactive oxygen species (ROS), an increase in cytosolic Ca^{2+}, and potassium efflux [40]. Similar to other crystalline inflammasome activators in in vitro experiments, cystine crystals are able to activate the inflammasome system in control of the monocytes and to induce caspase-1-dependent IL-1β secretion through a mechanism involving cathepsin B leakage, ROS production, and potassium efflux [18]. Consistent with this in vitro data in cystinotic patients, the circulating levels of the inflammasome-induced cytokines IL-1β and IL-18 were found to be significantly elevated when compared with those observed in healthy subjects. Further supporting a role for inflammasome activation in the pathogenesis of cystinosis in $Ctns^{-/-}$ mice, there was a significant increase in the renal expression of inflammasome-related genes, and an increase in the circulating levels of IL-18 was also observed [35]. Recently, the increased mRNA and protein levels of IL-1β were also found in the affected skeletal muscles of $Ctns^{-/-}$ mice [41]. However, to date, it remains to be studied in which cells, in vivo, in the cystinotic kidney and other affected organs, the inflammasome is activated. Several studies demonstrated that, in addition to the renal resident immune cells, PTECs, endothelial, and mesangial cells also express TLRs and NLRs and display the ability for releasing inflammatory molecules, including the IL-1β cytokine [42]. In this context, inflammasome-independent roles for NLRPs in the progression of chronic kidney diseases have also been reported [43]. Indeed, in addition to activating inflammasomes, NLRPs are also involved in the modulation of the inflammatory pathways in immune and non-immune cells, wherein they regulate the activity of the transcription factor NF-κB [44]. Recently, markedly elevated levels of the NOD-like receptor family member NLRP2 have been found in PTECs, both in primary cell cultures and in kidney biopsies, from cystinotic patients [45]. In particular, in vitro studies on cystinotic PTEC revealed a role for NLRP2 in amplifying the pro-inflammatory and profibrotic responses through the modulation of NF-kB activity, thereby unveiling an additional potential mechanism involving inflammation in the pathogenesis of cystinosis.

Altogether, these studies strongly support a role for inflammasome/NLRs-mediated inflammation in contributing to the pathogenesis and/or progression of cystinosis (Figure 2), and, therefore, provide the rationale for potential novel targets in the treatment of cystinosis.

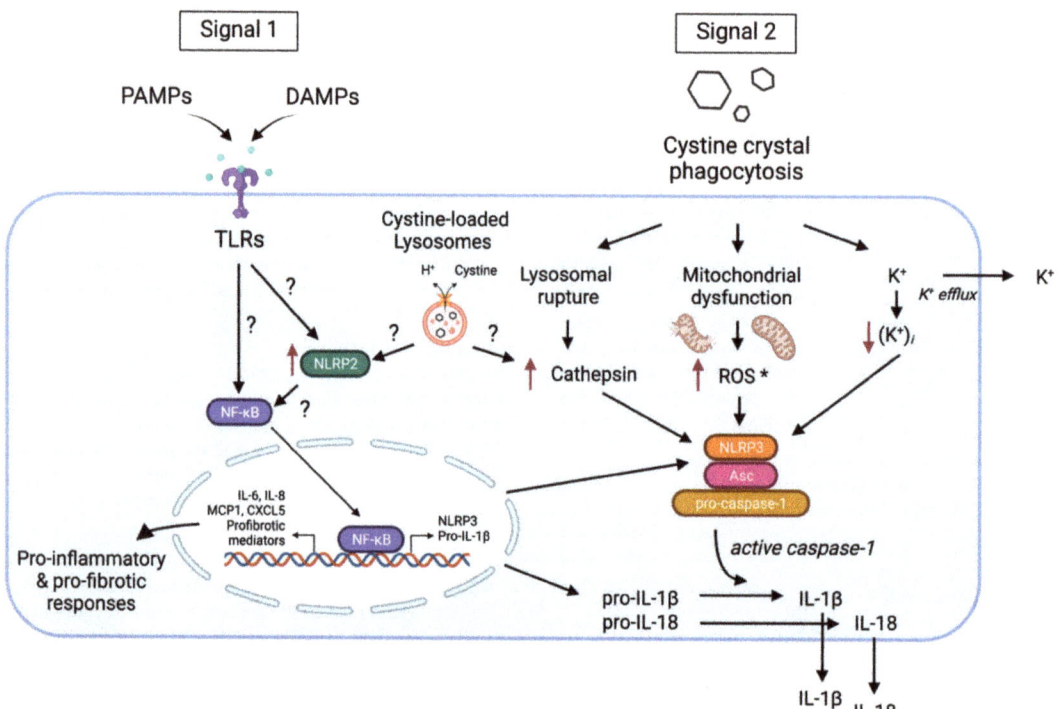

Figure 2. Activation of inflammasome-dependent and independent mechanisms in cystinosis. In vitro, in cultured monocytes, cystine crystals act as an NLRP3 agonist. Inflammasome activation requires two signals. Signal 1 is triggered by PAMPs or DAMPs through TLR/NLR activation and leads to NF-κB-dependent transcriptional activation of inflammasome components, including NLRP3, and IL-1β. Signal 2 is triggered by cystine crystals phagocytosis, causing K$^+$ efflux leading to hypokalemia, oxidative stress activation by ROS, or lysosomal rupture, and leads to the activation of the NLRP3 inflammasome, which ultimately results in the cleavage and secretion of the pro-inflammatory cytokines IL-1β and IL-18. A role for the cystine-loaded lysosome in activating inflammasomes has not been demonstrated. Inflammasome-independent mechanisms have also been described in human cystinotic PTECs, in which markedly high levels of NLRP2 have been observed. NLRP2 amplifies pro-inflammatory and profibrotic responses through activation of the NF-κB signaling pathway. CXCL5, C-X-C motif chemokine 5; DAMPs, damage-associated molecular patterns; IL, interleukin; MCP-1, monocyte chemoattractant protein-1; NF-κB, nuclear factor kappa light chain enhancer of activated B cells; NLRP3, NLR family pyrin domain containing 3; PAMPs, pathogen-associated molecular patterns; ROS, reactive oxygen species; TLRs, Toll-like receptors.

4. Interplay between Inflammation, Autophagy and Apoptosis in Cystinosis

Inflammatory cytokines, such as TNF-α and IL-1β, have long been associated with the stimulation of programmed cell death, or apoptosis, in various diseases [46–48], although the mechanisms for cell death in response to inflammatory cytokines are thought to be somehow distinct from those of genuine apoptosis [49]. Altered autophagy signals have recently been implicated in the crosstalk between inflammatory signals and apoptotic signals [50]. Autophagy is an important physiological cellular process involved in the restoration of energy homeostasis through the catabolism and recycling of dysfunctional or unneeded proteins and cellular organelles to improve cell survival upon exposure to various stress conditions. Furthermore, it may eliminate the specific stress triggered by damaged organelles, such as the endoplasmic reticulum (ER) or mitochondria [51,52]. Essentially, whether the cells survive or die during inflammation is largely dependent on the intricate balance between the pro-survival mechanisms of autophagy, when functioning properly, and the pro-death mechanisms of apoptosis or necroptosis [50].

In cystinosis, structurally and functionally abnormal mitochondria are an especially important aspect of the disease. As a major source of ROS, mitochondria are particularly susceptible to oxidative stress resulting from the inflammatory processes triggered by cystine accumulation and crystallization. This usually leads to the abnormal induction of mitochondrial autophagy (mitophagy), particularly in cystinotic PTECs and fibroblasts, with the enhanced expression of the microtubule-associated protein 1 light chain 3 (LC3-II/LC3-I) and beclin-1 [53]. This process was further associated with reduced mitochondrial ATP generation, cell starvation, increased generation of ROS, autophagic flux blockade, and enhanced apoptosis [53,54]. Moreover, mitochondrial dysfunction is usually associated with ER stress, which is a common pathogenic process that is linked to altered autophagy in various lysosomal storage disorders, including cystinosis [55,56]. Furthermore, caspase-4, the apoptotic cascade molecule, was stimulated by ER stress and was significantly enhanced in cystinotic PTECs [57].

Several inflammatory cytokines, such as IL-1β, TNF-α, and INF-γ, can enhance the process of autophagy through the activation of the mammalian target for rapamycin (mTOR) and AMP-activated protein kinase (AMPK) pathways [58]. Moreover, the important autophagy substrate, p62/SQSTM1, has been linked to the stimulation of chronic inflammation in the skin and myometrium through the activation of the NF-κB signaling pathway [59,60]. This molecule has been demonstrated as significantly elevated in the cellular models of cystinosis, particularly in PTECs [61–63].

Apoptotic signals can be initiated by both inflammatory cytokines and the autophagy substrate p62/SQSTM1. While p62/SQSTM1 can directly activate the extrinsic caspase pathway through the activation of caspase-8 and followed by caspase-3 [64,65], the inflammatory cytokines, such as IL-1β, IL-18, and TNF-α, stimulate apoptosis mainly by involving downstream signals, such as NF-κB, JAK/STAT, and p38/MAPK pathways, which may directly activate the caspase cascades or apoptosis induced by nitric oxide (NO) [46,66]. Figure 3 summarizes the important points of the crosstalk of inflammation, autophagy, and apoptosis in cystinotic cells.

In conclusion, inflammation in cystinosis disturbs the balance of the autophagy machinery, as both the inhibition of autophagy leading to the incomplete processing of autophagolysosomes and the abnormal induction of autophagy of certain organelles, such as mitochondria and the ER, can eventually lead to enhanced apoptosis.

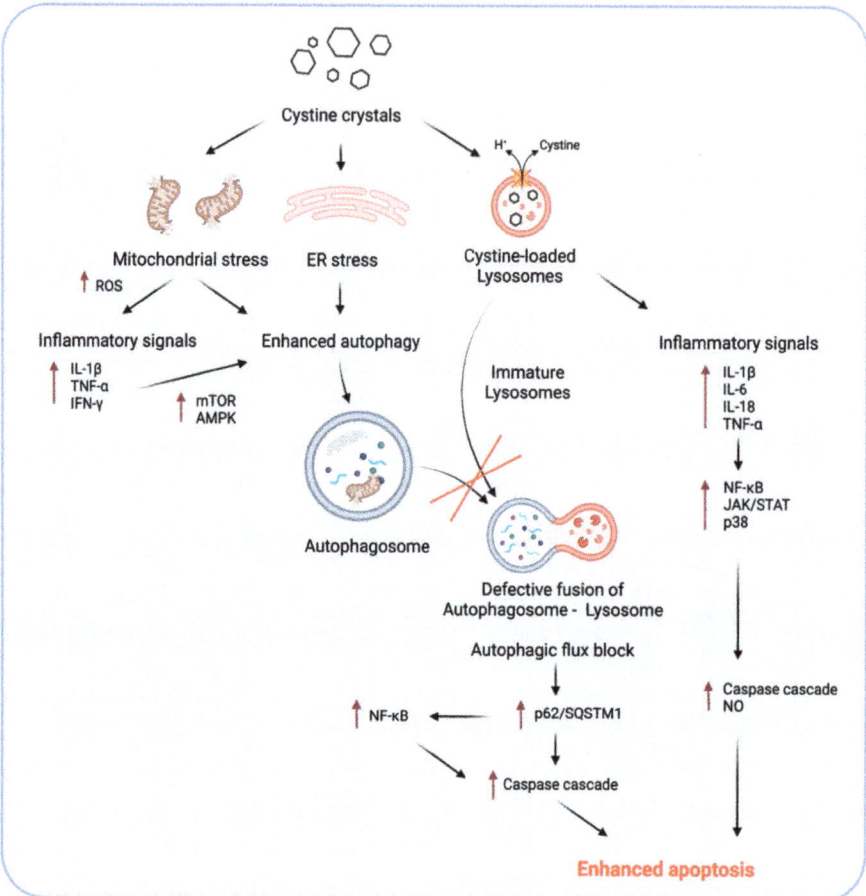

Figure 3. The interplay of inflammation, autophagy, and apoptosis in nephropathic cystinosis cells. A schematic representation of the effects of cystine crystals leading to the disturbance of inflammatory, autophagy, and apoptotic signals, and the disturbance of the crosstalk between these pathways. AMPK, AMP-activated protein kinase; INF-γ, interferon-γ; IL, interleukin; JAK/STAT, Januskinase/signal transducer and activator of transcription; mTOR, mammalian target of rapamycin; NF-κB, nuclear factor kappa light chain enhancer of activated B cells; NO, nitric oxide; p38, p38 mitogen activated protein kinase; p62/SQSTM1, Sequestosome-1; ROS, reactive oxygen species; TNF-α, tumor necrosis factor-α.

5. Response to Cysteamine Therapy in Cystinosis

The aminothiol cysteamine (beta-mercaptoethylamine) is currently the only approved specific therapy for nephropathic cystinosis. It was first applied for the treatment of cystinosis in 1976 and was approved by the FDA in 1994. It enters the lysosome and biochemically depletes the accumulated cystine very efficiently through its conversion into cysteine and cysteamine-cysteine–mixed disulfide, which can both exit the lysosome via different transporter mechanisms other than cystinosin, thus overcoming the main genetic and biochemical defects of the disease [4,67,68]. When initiated early in life at a proper dosage, cysteamine can improve the overall prognosis through delaying the development of end stage kidney disease and reducing the incidence of the major extra-renal complications, including hypothyroidism, myopathy, diabetes mellitus, neurological manifestations, and growth retardation. However, while it merely delays progressive kidney dysfunction, it cannot cure renal Fanconi syndrome, nor can it cure any other extra-renal complications when the drug is initiated late, during the course of the disease [69,70].

Apart from its cystine-lowering effects, which definitely have an enormous impact on decreasing the cellular inflammation, being one of its most powerful driving factors, cysteamine is also a potent antioxidant molecule that can suppress many of the inflammatory cascades following oxidative stress. It can reduce ROS generation, attenuates macrophage recruitment and activity, blocks myofibroblast proliferation and activation, and significantly decreases tissue fibrosis [71] (Figure 4). Cysteamine in low concentrations aids in the transport of the amino acid, cysteine, inside cells, which serves as replenishment machinery for the reduced glutathione—one of the most important intracellular antioxidants [72,73]. In PTECs, cysteamine was able to normalize both cystine levels and the glutathione redox status; however, it could not improve the mitochondrial ATP production or the decreased sodium-dependent phosphate uptake [74].

Interestingly, Okamura et al. demonstrated that, in two mouse models of CKD unrelated to cystinosis, cysteamine exerted its reno-protective effects by modulating oxidative stress [71]. Indeed, when macrophages were co-cultured in vitro with apoptotic renal tubular cells, intracellular ROS generation was reduced by 43–52% in the cysteamine-treated macrophages. In addition, cysteamine treatment attenuated the macrophage accumulation in the kidneys, inhibited myofibroblast differentiation and proliferation, and led to significant amelioration of renal fibrosis [71]. Therefore, although data regarding the effects of cysteamine on the inflammatory status of cystinotic patients and of $Ctns^{-/-}$ mice are lacking, it is conceivable that in cystinosis the efficacy of cysteamine may also be due, in addition to the lowering of intracellular levels of cystine, to an alternative anti-inflammatory mechanism of action. Cysteamine is further a potent inhibitor of apoptosis in cystinotic cells. This is mainly attributable to its cystine lowering effects [8]; however, its antioxidant and anti-inflammatory properties must play a role in this as well. These beneficial effects are certainly linked to the better preservation of kidney function and the delay of most complications in cystinosis patients on cysteamine therapy.

In contrast, cysteamine treatment had no significant effect on the lysosomal size and distribution or on the altered ultrastructure of the endosomal/lysosomal compartments in cystinosin-deficient cells, but it could partially improve the delayed lysosomal cargo processing in human PTECs [13]. Upon studying the effects of cysteamine therapy on the impaired proximal tubular endocytosis in cystinotic zebrafish, it could significantly increase the amount of low molecular weight dextran reabsorbed in the proximal tubules compared to the untreated group, which is in support of the human cell findings. However, defective megalin expression in cystinotic zebrafish was not restored after cysteamine treatment. Furthermore, both EEA1 (a tethering protein of early endosomes) and the small GTPase Rab11 associated with recycling endosomal trafficking to the plasma membrane were significantly less expressed in the proximal tubules of the cystinosis zebrafish larvae compared to the wild type. Cysteamine treatment did not restore the protein expression of either of them, denoting that cysteamine has a minimal effect on the defective endocytic machinery in cystinosis, which can partially explain its failure in preventing renal Fanconi syndrome [75,76]. Consistent with these observations, the treatment with cysteamine did not normalize the circulating MCP-1 levels that were found significantly increased in the sera of patients with cystinosis compared with healthy donors, which strongly suggests that the absence of cystinosin, rather than cystine accumulation, is responsible for MCP-1 increase in serum [21].

In short, cysteamine is a very beneficial drug for cystinosis patients. It significantly prolongs and improves the quality of their lives; however, it is far from a perfect drug or a cure for the disease. It is true that the majority of its beneficial effects are driven by its cystine-depleting capabilities, but its functional impact on the proximal tubular cells is limited, and its effects on the inflammation/autophagy/apoptosis axis signals in cystinotic cells are not yet fully clarified.

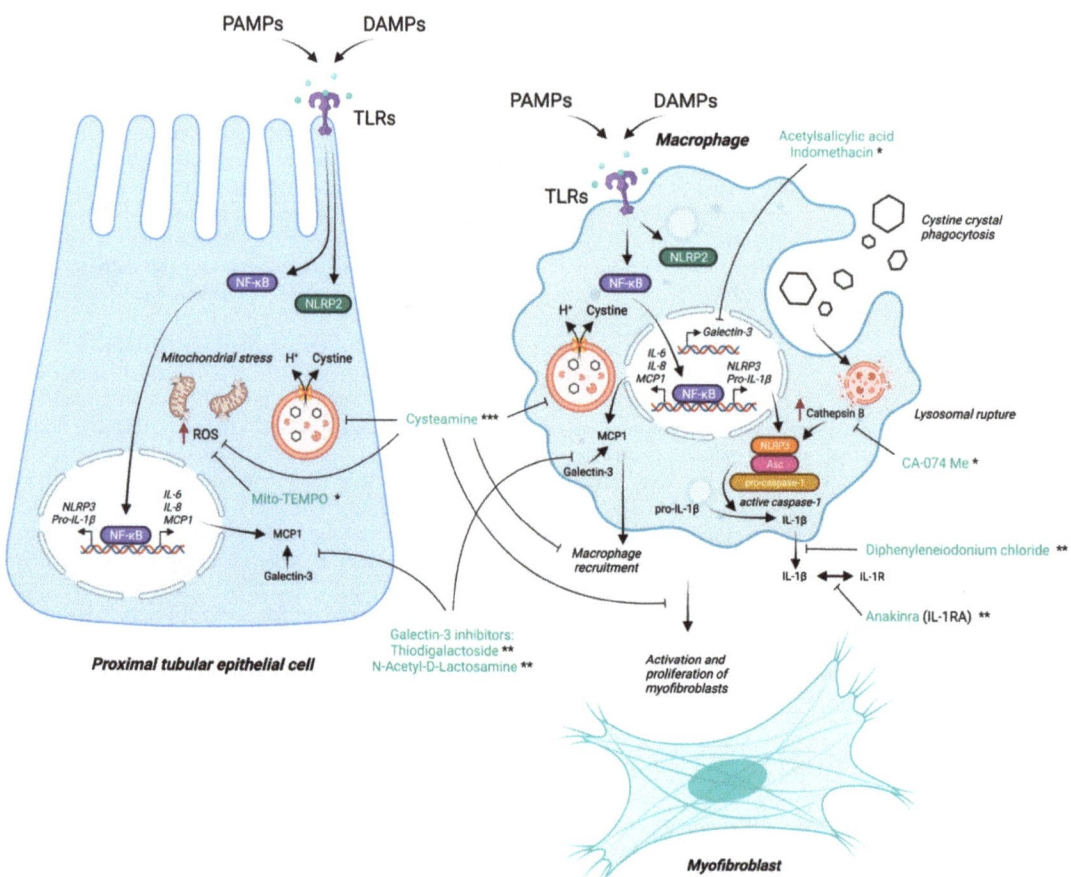

Figure 4. Inflammatory pathways in key cells involved in the pathophysiology of cystinosis and mechanisms of action of current and potential future therapeutic agents. Proximal tubular epithelial cells (PTECs), macrophages, and myofibroblasts are key cell players in the proximal tubular dysfunction and progressive chronic kidney disease, which characterizes cystinosis. Therapeutic agents are depicted with their specific mechanisms of action and classified according to the current evidence. * In vitro cellular models, **: in vivo animal models, ***: in vivo clinical-grade patient data. DAMPs, Damage-associated molecular patterns; IL, interleukin; MCP-1, monocytechemoattractant protein-1; NF-κB, nuclear factor kappa light chain enhancer of activated B cells; NLRP2, NLR family pyrin domain containing 2; PAMPs, pathogen-associated molecular patterns; ROS, reactive oxygen species; TLRs, Toll-like receptors.

6. Targeting Inflammation as a Potential Therapeutic Option in Cystinosis

With the recent perception that inflammatory processes are largely involved in many of the pathogenic aspects of cystinosis, and that inflammation is not only involved in facilitating the progression of the disease through the development of tissue fibrosis and damage, but also in contributing to the disruption of certain cellular functions—such as endocytosis in PTECs—it was logical to assume that targeting the inflammatory signals could be a novel potential therapeutic strategy complementing the conventional cystine-depleting therapies used in cystinosis.

Historically, indomethacin, the non-steroidal anti-inflammatory drug, has been proposed in the management of cystinosis patients. The drug caused clinical improvement by reducing polyuria and polydipsia, improved their general wellbeing, and partially normalized the electrolyte imbalance associated with the disease [77,78]. These beneficial effects are due to the inhibition of prostaglandin synthesis in the renal parenchyma and its partial restoration of the medullary blood flow, thereby enhancing salt reabsorption in the loop of Henle and the collecting tubules, and thus, partially compensating for the proximal tubular losses [78]. Although the studies reporting the use of indomethacin in cystinotic patients are scarce, several centers, particularly in Europe, widely use it in young cystinotic children to improve their renal Fanconi phenotype [78]. In a large multi-centre cohort of 453 cystinosis patients born between 1964 and 2016, the use of indomethacin was not associated with improved kidney function, and it cannot be excluded, though its direct anti-inflammatory effects were diluted in this large cohort, as the dose and the duration of treatment were not specified in this study [79]. In this regard, it is currently recommended to limit indomethacin to the first years of life, when renal water and salt losses are more severe, in order to avoid its potential long-term nephrotoxicity. To the best of our knowledge, the anti-inflammatory effects of indomethacin have never been evaluated at the cellular level either in in vitro or in vivo models of the disease.

Other, more recent studies have investigated the effects of other potential therapeutic agents on the inflammatory/oxidative stress axis, with the aim to alleviate some of the pathogenic processes of cystinosis in various cellular and animal models. Festa et al. incubated $Ctns^{-/-}$ PTECs with the mitochondria-localized-oxygen scavenger Mito-TEMPO. The blockage of the mitochondrial ROS/Gα12/Src signaling by this pharmacologic agent prevented the abnormal phosphorylation of ZO-1 and its lysosomal accumulation, which increased its abundance at cell boundaries and restored the differentiation and endocytic uptake of albumin in cystinotic cells [58]. Prencipe et al. targeted the activated NLRP3 inflammasome pathway in cystinosis through the cathepsin B inhibitors CA-074Me and diphenyleneiodonium chloride, which decreased the secretion of IL-1β induced by the cystine crystals in the peripheral blood monocytes and suppressing the inflammatory cascade that should follow, thereby paving the way for another mechanism that can be targeted in cystinosis patients [18]. Cheung et al. studied $Ctns^{-/-}$ mice for both the genetic deletion of $Il1b$ as well as treatment with the recombinant IL-1 receptor antagonist (IL-1ra) anakinra, which led to an attenuation of the cachexia phenotype in cystinotic mice, supporting the efficacy of the IL-1 anti-inflammatory-targeted therapy on adipose browning and muscle wasting in nephropathic cystinosis [41]. Adding to this effect, Gonzalez et al. demonstrated significant beneficial actions of the leptin receptor blockade, which is a well-known immunomodulatory cytokine and hormone on the cachexia phenotype in $Ctns^{-/-}$ mice. Inhibiting leptin action in these mice normalized their food intake and weight gain, increased fat and lean mass, decreased metabolic rate, and stabilized energy homeostasis in the adipose tissue and muscle [80]. However, further studies evaluating the efficacy of these drugs, alone and in combination with the available conventional therapies, in ameliorating kidney and other organ damage in cystinosis are needed.

Lobry et al. took advantage of cystinosin involvement in the regulation of the inflammatory mediator galectin-3. Galectin-3 inhibitors, such as thiodigalactoside and N-Acetyl-D-Lactosamine, decreased the interaction of Galectin-3 with MCP-1 in $Ctns^{-/-}$ mice and successfully limited macrophage recruitment and activation in mouse tissues [21]. Interestingly, non-steroidal anti-inflammatory drugs, such as aspirin and indomethacin, have been found to inhibit galectin-3 expression in human macrophages by inhibiting its transcription [81], which may be partially responsible for the beneficial effects seen with indomethacin in cystinosis patients.

In summary, the search for therapeutic agents that can interrupt the impact of the inflammation in cystinosis and restore, at least partially, the functionality of important cell types—such as PTECs—is currently a prime focus for cystinosis research. Although cysteamine has significant antioxidant and anti-inflammatory properties, they are clearly not enough in this regard. A complementary therapy, or therapies, that can efficiently suppress the inflammatory process in cystinosis still need to be validated in human individuals. Figure 4 summarizes the main targets of the potential new therapies aiming at suppressing the inflammatory signals in cystinosis.

7. Future Perspectives

Nephropathic cystinosis is a complex systemic disease with a lot of layers to its pathogenesis, risk assessment, and management strategy, and thus usually requires a multidisciplinary approach to properly care for the patient. Inflammation is certainly one of the pathogenic layers that has been documented repeatedly in different cellular and animal models of the disease, and in patients with cystinosis as well. However, this involvement in pathogenesis hasn't yet been translated to a validated aspect of the disease therapeutic strategy. This could be partially due to the recent discovery of the importance of inflammatory signals in cystinotic cell pathology, but it is also due to the fear of the potential kidney damaging effects of known anti-inflammatory agents, particularly when used for long periods in a disease that is originally harming the kidney. NSAIDs, for example, are famous for their counter vasodilatation effect through the inhibition of the cyclooxygenase enzyme, leading to a hemodynamically mediated acute and chronic kidney injury [82,83]. Corticosteroids, on the other hand, although already used for the treatment of many inflammatory kidney disorders, such as IgA nephropathy, lupus nephritis, and interstitial nephritis [84–86], are known for their long-term and severe side-effects, which impact the kidneys—among other organs—and may hinder their consideration as a lifelong treatment, even in low doses, for nephropathic cystinosis. To this date, no prospective therapeutic clinical trial has been conducted to address the inflammatory aspect of cystinosis in human patients.

Novel and experimental anti-inflammatory agents that do not target the cyclooxygenase/prostaglandins axis may provide a good alternative for classic NSAIDs in this regard, such as anakinra and N-Acetyl-D-Lactosamine, which block the biological activity of IL-1 and the binding of galectin-3 with MCP-1, respectively. Moreover, synthetic inhibitors of human chitinase enzymes, including chitotriosidase inhibitors, are currently being evaluated as potential therapeutic modalities in chronic inflammatory conditions, such as interstitial pulmonary fibrosis and inflammatory bowel disease [87,88]. Chitotriosidase plays an important role in abrogating the inflammatory loop in cystinotic tissue, especially through the recruitment and activation of multiple inflammatory cells [17,30,32]. The other active chitinase in human tissue is acidic mammalian chitinase (AMCase), which has also been implicated in the pathogenesis of bronchial asthma and other inflammatory conditions [89]; however, it has never been studied in cystinosis. The recent development of selective chitotriosidase and dual chitinase inhibitors with very good safety profiles [87,90] may provide further hope to address inflammatory disorders in a pathway that may not cause harm to the kidneys. It would be interesting to see the actions of such inhibitors in inflammation-associated conditions primarily affecting the kidney, such as cystinosis.

8. Conclusions

Altogether, inflammation is an important aspect of the pathogenesis of cystinosis that has been overlooked for a long time. Cysteamine is an excellent drug that can deplete cystine from the lysosomes and has some antioxidant and anti-inflammatory properties but cannot neutralize the inflammatory cascade in cystinotic cells and cannot restore some basic cellular functions in the kidney proximal tubules. It is time to address the enhanced inflammation in cystinosis with more specific and targeted therapies that can suppress the abnormal inflammatory signals. This may help to interrupt the cystine-induced cell damage/inflammatory cell recruitment cycle and correct, at least partially, some of the cellular abnormalities responsible for renal Fanconi syndrome and kidney failure down the road. It is definitely worth a try.

Author Contributions: Conceptualization, M.A.E.; data curation, M.A.E., G.P. and K.R.P.V.; writing—original draft preparation, M.A.E. and G.P.; writing—review and editing, M.A.E., G.P. and K.R.P.V.; supervision, M.A.E.; figures planning, M.A.E., G.P. and K.R.P.V.; figures execution, K.R.P.V. All authors have read and agreed to the published version of the manuscript.

Funding: This research received no external funding.

Institutional Review Board Statement: Not applicable.

Informed Consent Statement: Not applicable.

Data Availability Statement: No new data were created or analyzed in this study. Data sharing is not applicable to this article.

Acknowledgments: G.P. is supported by the Cystinosis Research Foundation (CRF).

Conflicts of Interest: The authors declare no conflict of interest.

References

1. Khan, S.R.; Canales, B.K.; Dominguez-Gutierrez, P.R. Randall's plaque and calcium oxalate stone formation: Role for immunity and inflammation. *Nat. Rev. Nephrol.* **2021**, *17*, 417–433. [CrossRef]
2. Mulay, S.R.; Anders, H.-J. Crystallopathies. *N. Engl. J. Med.* **2016**, *374*, 2465–2476. [CrossRef] [PubMed]
3. Ma, R.-H.; Luo, X.-B.; Li, Q.; Zhong, H.-Q. The systematic classification of urinary stones combine-using FTIR and SEM-EDAX. *Int. J. Surg.* **2017**, *41*, 150–161. [CrossRef]
4. Elmonem, M.A.; Veys, K.R.; Soliman, N.A.; van Dyck, M.; van den Heuvel, L.P.; Levtchenko, E. Cystinosis: A review. *Orphanet J. Rare Dis.* **2016**, *11*, 47. [CrossRef] [PubMed]
5. Nesterova, G.; Gahl, W.A. Cystinosis: The evolution of a treatable disease. *Pediatr. Nephrol.* **2013**, *28*, 51–59. [CrossRef]
6. David, D.; Berlingerio, S.P.; Elmonem, M.A.; Arcolino, F.O.; Soliman, N.; van den Heuvel, B.; Gijsbers, R.; Levtchenko, E. Molecular Basis of Cystinosis: Geographic Distribution, Functional Consequences of Mutations in the CTNS Gene, and Potential for Repair. *Nephron* **2019**, *141*, 133–146. [CrossRef]
7. Gahl, W.A.; Thoene, J.G.; Schneider, J.A. Cystinosis. *N. Engl. J. Med.* **2002**, *347*, 111–121. [CrossRef]
8. Park, M.A.; Pejovic, V.; Kerisit, K.G.; Junius, S.; Thoene, J.G. Increased Apoptosis in Cystinotic Fibroblasts and Renal Proximal Tubule Epithelial Cells Results from Cysteinylation of Protein Kinase Cδ. *J. Am. Soc. Nephrol.* **2006**, *17*, 3167–3175. [CrossRef] [PubMed]
9. Ivanova, E.A.; Arcolino, F.O.; Elmonem, M.A.; Rastaldi, M.P.; Giardino, L.; Cornelissen, E.M.; van den Heuvel, L.P.; Levtchenko, E.N. Cystinosin deficiency causes podocyte damage and loss associated with increased cell motility. *Kidney Int.* **2016**, *89*, 1037–1048. [CrossRef]
10. Wilmer, M.J.; van den Heuvel, L.P.; Levtchenko, E.N. The Use of CDME in Cystinosis Research. *Neurochem. Res.* **2008**, *33*, 2373–2374. [CrossRef] [PubMed]
11. Cherqui, S.; Courtoy, P.J. The renal Fanconi syndrome in cystinosis: Pathogenic insights and therapeutic perspectives. *Nat. Rev. Nephrol.* **2017**, *13*, 115–131. [CrossRef] [PubMed]
12. Bellomo, F.; Signorile, A.; Tamma, G.; Ranieri, M.; Emma, F.; De Rasmo, D. Impact of atypical mitochondrial cyclic-AMP level in nephropathic cystinosis. *Cell. Mol. Life Sci.* **2018**, *75*, 3411–3422. [CrossRef]
13. Ivanova, E.A.; De Leo, M.G.; van den Heuvel, L.; Pastore, A.; Dijkman, H.; De Matteis, M.A.; Levtchenko, E.N. Endo-Lysosomal Dysfunction in Human Proximal Tubular Epithelial Cells Deficient for Lysosomal Cystine Transporter Cystinosin. *PLoS ONE* **2015**, *10*, e0120998. [CrossRef]
14. Ivanova, E.A.; van den Heuvel, L.P.; Elmonem, M.; De Smedt, H.; Missiaen, L.; Pastore, A.; Mekahli, D.; Bultynck, G.; Levtchenko, E.N. Altered mTOR signalling in nephropathic cystinosis. *J. Inherit. Metab. Dis.* **2016**, *39*, 457–464. [CrossRef]
15. Rega, L.R.; Polishchuk, E.; Montefusco, S.; Napolitano, G.; Tozzi, G.; Zhang, J.; Bellomo, F.; Taranta, A.; Pastore, A.; Polishchuk, R.; et al. Activation of the transcription factor EB rescues lysosomal abnormalities in cystinotic kidney cells. *Kidney Int.* **2016**, *89*, 862–873. [CrossRef] [PubMed]
16. Settembre, C.; Fraldi, A.; Medina, D.L.; Ballabio, A. Signals from the lysosome: A control centre for cellular clearance and energy metabolism. *Nat. Rev. Mol. Cell Biol.* **2013**, *14*, 283–296. [CrossRef]
17. Elmonem, A.M.; Makar, S.H.; van den Heuvel, L.; Abdelaziz, H.; Abdelrahman, S.M.; Bossuyt, X.; Janssen, M.C.; Cornelissen, E.A.; Lefeber, D.J.; AB Joosten, L.; et al. Clinical utility of chitotriosidase enzyme activity in nephropathic cystinosis. *Orphanet J. Rare Dis.* **2014**, *9*, 155. [CrossRef] [PubMed]
18. Prencipe, G.; Caiello, I.; Cherqui, S.; Whisenant, T.; Petrini, S.; Emma, F.; De Benedetti, F. Inflammasome Activation by Cystine Crystals: Implications for the Pathogenesis of Cystinosis. *J. Am. Soc. Nephrol.* **2014**, *25*, 1163–1169. [CrossRef]
19. Stokes, M.; Jernigan, S.; D'Agati, V. Infantile nephropathic cystinosis. *Kidney Int.* **2008**, *73*, 782–786. [CrossRef]
20. Larsen, C.; Walker, P.D.; Thoene, J.G. The incidence of atubular glomeruli in nephropathic cystinosis renal biopsies. *Mol. Genet. Metab.* **2010**, *101*, 417–420. [CrossRef]

21. Lobry, T.; Miller, R.; Nevo, N.; Rocca, C.J.; Zhang, J.; Catz, S.D.; Moore, F.; Thomas, L.; Pouly, D.; Bailleux, A.; et al. Interaction between galectin-3 and cystinosin uncovers a pathogenic role of inflammation in kidney involvement of cystinosis. *Kidney Int.* **2019**, *96*, 350–362. [CrossRef] [PubMed]
22. Li, L.; Okusa, M.D. Macrophages, Dendritic Cells, and Kidney Ischemia-Reperfusion Injury. *Semin. Nephrol.* **2010**, *30*, 268–277. [CrossRef] [PubMed]
23. Das, A.; Sinha, M.; Datta, S.; Abas, M.; Chaffee, S.; Sen, C.K.; Roy, S. Monocyte and Macrophage Plasticity in Tissue Repair and Regeneration. *Am. J. Pathol.* **2015**, *185*, 2596–2606. [CrossRef]
24. Vannella, K.M.; Wynn, T.A. Mechanisms of Organ Injury and Repair by Macrophages. *Annu. Rev. Physiol.* **2017**, *79*, 593–617. [CrossRef] [PubMed]
25. Andrade-Oliveira, V.; Foresto-Neto, O.; Watanabe, I.K.M.; Zatz, R.; Câmara, N.O.S. Inflammation in Renal Diseases: New and Old Players. *Front. Pharmacol.* **2019**, *10*, 1192. [CrossRef]
26. Monier, L.; Mauvieux, L. Cystine crystals in bone marrow aspirate. *Blood* **2015**, *126*, 1515. [CrossRef] [PubMed]
27. Cherqui, S.; Sevin, C.; Hamard, G.; Kalatzis, V.; Sich, M.; Pequignot, M.O.; Gogat, K.; Abitbol, M.; Broyer, M.; Gubler, M.-C.; et al. Intralysosomal Cystine Accumulation in Mice Lacking Cystinosin, the Protein Defective in Cystinosis. *Mol. Cell. Biol.* **2002**, *22*, 7622–7632. [CrossRef]
28. Korn, D. Demonstration of Cystine Crystals in Peripheral White Blood Cells in a Patient with Cystinosis. *N. Engl. J. Med.* **1960**, *262*, 545–548. [CrossRef]
29. Lee, H.; Fessler, M.B.; Qu, P.; Heymann, J.; Kopp, J.B. Macrophage polarization in innate immune responses contributing to pathogenesis of chronic kidney disease. *BMC Nephrol.* **2020**, *21*, 270. [CrossRef]
30. Veys, K.R.; Elmonem, M.A.; van Dyck, M.; Janssen, M.C.; Cornelissen, E.A.; Hohenfellner, K.; Prencipe, G.; van den Heuvel, L.P.; Levtchenko, E. Chitotriosidase as a Novel Biomarker for Therapeutic Monitoring of Nephropathic Cystinosis. *J. Am. Soc. Nephrol.* **2020**, *31*, 1092–1106. [CrossRef]
31. Ries, M.; Schaefer, E.; Lührs, T.; Mani, L.; Kuhn, J.; Vanier, M.T.; Krummenauer, F.; Gal, A.; Beck, M.; Mengel, E. Critical assessment of chitotriosidase analysis in the rational laboratory diagnosis of children with Gaucher disease and Niemann–Pick disease type A/B and C. *J. Inherit. Metab. Dis.* **2006**, *29*, 647–652. [CrossRef]
32. Elmonem, M.A.; van den Heuvel, L.P.; Levtchenko, E.N. Immunomodulatory Effects of Chitotriosidase Enzyme. *Enzym. Res.* **2016**, *2016*, 2682680. [CrossRef]
33. Mulay, S.R.; Desai, J.; Kumar, S.V.; Eberhard, J.N.; Thomasova, D.; Romoli, S.; Grigorescu, M.; Kulkarni, O.P.; Popper, B.; Vielhauer, V.; et al. Cytotoxicity of crystals involves RIPK3-MLKL-mediated necroptosis. *Nat. Commun.* **2016**, *7*, 10274. [CrossRef] [PubMed]
34. Dolasia, K.; Bisht, M.K.; Pradhan, G.; Udgata, A.; Mukhopadhyay, S. TLRs/NLRs: Shaping the landscape of host immunity. *Int. Rev. Immunol.* **2018**, *37*, 3–19. [CrossRef]
35. Mulay, S.R.; Anders, H.-J. Crystal nephropathies: Mechanisms of crystal-induced kidney injury. *Nat. Rev. Nephrol.* **2017**, *13*, 226–240. [CrossRef]
36. Lamkanfi, M.; Dixit, V.M. Mechanisms and Functions of Inflammasomes. *Cell* **2014**, *157*, 1013–1022. [CrossRef]
37. Franklin, B.S.; Mangan, M.S.; Latz, E. Crystal Formation in Inflammation. *Annu. Rev. Immunol.* **2016**, *34*, 173–202. [CrossRef] [PubMed]
38. Nakayama, M. Macrophage Recognition of Crystals and Nanoparticles. *Front. Immunol.* **2018**, *9*, 103. [CrossRef] [PubMed]
39. Mulay, S.R.; Shi, C.; Ma, X.; Anders, H.J. Novel Insights into Crystal-Induced Kidney Injury. *Kidney Dis.* **2018**, *4*, 49–57. [CrossRef]
40. Paik, S.; Kim, J.K.; Silwal, P.; Sasakawa, C.; Jo, E.-K. An update on the regulatory mechanisms of NLRP3 inflammasome activation. *Cell. Mol. Immunol.* **2021**, *18*, 1141–1160. [CrossRef]
41. Cheung, W.W.; Hao, S.; Zheng, R.; Wang, Z.; Gonzalez, A.; Zhou, P.; Hoffman, H.M.; Mak, R.H. Targeting interleukin-1 for reversing fat browning and muscle wasting in infantile nephropathic cystinosis. *J. Cachexia Sarcopenia Muscle* **2021**, *12*, 1296–1311. [CrossRef]
42. Leemans, J.C.; Kors, L.; Anders, H.-J.; Florquin, S. Pattern recognition receptors and the inflammasome in kidney disease. *Nat. Rev. Nephrol.* **2014**, *10*, 398–414. [CrossRef]
43. Kim, S.-M.; Kim, Y.G.; Kim, D.-J.; Park, S.H.; Jeong, K.-H.; Lee, Y.H.; Lim, S.J.; Lee, S.-H.; Moon, J.-Y. Inflammasome-Independent Role of NLRP3 Mediates Mitochondrial Regulation in Renal Injury. *Front. Immunol.* **2018**, *9*, 2563. [CrossRef] [PubMed]
44. Ting, J.P.Y.; Duncan, J.A.; Lei, Y. How the Noninflammasome NLRs Function in the Innate Immune System. *Science* **2010**, *327*, 286–290. [CrossRef] [PubMed]
45. Rossi, M.N.; Pascarella, A.; Licursi, V.; Caiello, I.; Taranta, A.; Rega, L.R.; Levtchenko, E.; Emma, F.; De Benedetti, F.; Prencipe, G. NLRP2 Regulates Proinflammatory and Antiapoptotic Responses in Proximal Tubular Epithelial Cells. *Front. Cell Dev. Biol.* **2019**, *7*, 252. [CrossRef] [PubMed]
46. Sagoo, P.; Chan, G.; Larkin, D.F.P.; George, A.J.T. Inflammatory Cytokines Induce Apoptosis of Corneal Endothelium through Nitric Oxide. *Investig. Opthalmol. Vis. Sci.* **2004**, *45*, 3964–3973. [CrossRef] [PubMed]
47. Grunnet, L.G.; Aikin, R.; Tonnesen, M.F.; Paraskevas, S.; Blaabjerg, L.; Størling, J.; Rosenberg, L.; Billestrup, N.; Maysinger, D.; Mandrup-Poulsen, T. Proinflammatory Cytokines Activate the Intrinsic Apoptotic Pathway in β-Cells. *Diabetes* **2009**, *58*, 1807–1815. [CrossRef]

48. Jo, S.K.; Cha, D.R.; Cho, W.Y.; Kim, H.K.; Chang, K.H.; Yun, S.Y.; Won, N.H. Inflammatory Cytokines and Lipopolysaccharide Induce Fas-Mediated Apoptosis in Renal Tubular Cells. *Nephron* **2002**, *91*, 406–415. [CrossRef]
49. Collier, J.J.; Burke, S.J.; Eisenhauer, M.E.; Lu, D.; Sapp, R.C.; Frydman, C.J.; Campagna, S. Pancreatic β-Cell Death in Response to Pro-Inflammatory Cytokines Is Distinct from Genuine Apoptosis. *PLoS ONE* **2011**, *6*, e22485. [CrossRef]
50. Messer, J.S. The cellular autophagy/apoptosis checkpoint during inflammation. *Cell. Mol. Life Sci.* **2017**, *74*, 1281–1296. [CrossRef]
51. Wang, X.; Dai, Y.; Ding, Z.; Khaidakov, M.; Mercanti, F.; Mehta, J.L. Regulation of autophagy and apoptosis in response to angiotensin II in HL-1 cardiomyocytes. *Biochem. Biophys. Res. Commun.* **2013**, *440*, 696–700. [CrossRef] [PubMed]
52. Lambelet, M.; Terra, L.F.; Fukaya, M.; Meyerovich, K.; Labriola, L.; Cardozo, A.K.; Allagnat, F. Dysfunctional autophagy following exposure to pro-inflammatory cytokines contributes to pancreatic β-cell apoptosis. *Cell Death Dis.* **2018**, *9*, 92. [CrossRef]
53. Sansanwal, P.; Yen, B.; Gahl, W.A.; Ma, Y.; Ying, L.; Wong, L.-J.C.; Sarwal, M.M. Mitochondrial Autophagy Promotes Cellular Injury in Nephropathic Cystinosis. *J. Am. Soc. Nephrol.* **2010**, *21*, 272–283. [CrossRef] [PubMed]
54. Sansanwal, P.; Sarwal, M.M. Abnormal mitochondrial autophagy in nephropathic cystinosis. *Autophagy* **2010**, *6*, 971–973. [CrossRef]
55. Wei, H.; Kim, S.-J.; Zhang, Z.; Tsai, P.-C.; Wisniewski, K.E.; Mukherjee, A.B. ER and oxidative stresses are common mediators of apoptosis in both neurodegenerative and non-neurodegenerative lysosomal storage disorders and are alleviated by chemical chaperones. *Hum. Mol. Genet.* **2008**, *17*, 469–477. [CrossRef]
56. Chevronnay, H.P.G.; Janssens, V.; van der Smissen, P.; Liao, X.H.; Abid, Y.; Nevo, N.; Antignac, C.; Refetoff, S.; Cherqui, S.; Pierreux, C.; et al. A Mouse Model Suggests Two Mechanisms for Thyroid Alterations in Infantile Cystinosis: Decreased Thyroglobulin Synthesis Due to Endoplasmic Reticulum Stress/Unfolded Protein Response and Impaired Lysosomal Processing. *Endocrinology* **2015**, *156*, 2349–2364. [CrossRef]
57. Sansanwal, P.; Kambham, N.; Sarwal, M.M. Caspase-4 may play a role in loss of proximal tubules and renal injury in nephropathic cystinosis. *Pediatr. Nephrol.* **2010**, *25*, 105–109. [CrossRef]
58. Netea-Maier, R.T.; Plantinga, T.; van de Veerdonk, F.L.; Smit, J.W.; Netea, M.G. Modulation of inflammation by autophagy: Consequences for human disease. *Autophagy* **2016**, *12*, 245–260. [CrossRef] [PubMed]
59. Sukseree, S.; Bakiri, L.; Palomo-Irigoyen, M.; Uluçkan, Ö; Petzelbauer, P.; Wagner, E.F. Sequestosome 1/p62 enhances chronic skin inflammation. *J. Allergy Clin. Immunol.* **2021**, *147*, 2386–2393.e4. [CrossRef]
60. Lappas, M. The Adaptor Protein p62 Mediates Nuclear Factor κB Activation in Response to Inflammation and Facilitates the Formation of Prolabor Mediators in Human Myometrium. *Reprod. Sci.* **2017**, *24*, 762–772. [CrossRef]
61. Sansanwal, P.; Sarwal, M.M. p62/SQSTM1 prominently accumulates in renal proximal tubules in nephropathic cystinosis. *Pediatr. Nephrol.* **2012**, *27*, 2137–2144. [CrossRef]
62. Festa, B.P.; Chen, Z.; Berquez, M.; Debaix, H.; Tokonami, N.; Prange, J.A.; van de Hoek, G.; Alessio, C.; Raimondi, A.; Nevo, N.; et al. Impaired autophagy bridges lysosomal storage disease and epithelial dysfunction in the kidney. *Nat. Commun.* **2018**, *9*, 161. [CrossRef]
63. De Leo, E.; Elmonem, M.A.; Berlingerio, S.P.; Berquez, M.; Festa, B.P.; Raso, R.; Bellomo, F.; Starborg, T.; Janssen, M.J.; Abbaszadeh, Z.; et al. Cell-Based Phenotypic Drug Screening Identifies Luteolin as Candidate Therapeutic for Nephropathic Cystinosis. *J. Am. Soc. Nephrol.* **2020**, *31*, 1522–1537. [CrossRef]
64. Gump, J.M.; Thorburn, A. Autophagy and apoptosis: What is the connection? *Trends Cell Biol.* **2011**, *21*, 387–392. [CrossRef] [PubMed]
65. Moscat, J.; Diaz-Meco, M.T. p62 at the Crossroads of Autophagy, Apoptosis, and Cancer. *Cell* **2009**, *137*, 1001–1004. [CrossRef]
66. Rex, J.; Lutz, A.; Faletti, L.E.; Albrecht, U.; Thomas, M.; Bode, J.G.; Borner, C.; Sawodny, O.; Merfort, I. IL-1β and TNFα Differentially Influence NF-κB Activity and FasL-Induced Apoptosis in Primary Murine Hepatocytes During LPS-Induced Inflammation. *Front. Physiol.* **2019**, *10*, 117. [CrossRef] [PubMed]
67. Veys, K.R.; Elmonem, M.; Arcolino, F.O.; van den Heuvel, L.; Levtchenko, E. Nephropathic cystinosis: An update. *Curr. Opin. Pediatr.* **2017**, *29*, 168–178. [CrossRef]
68. Cherqui, S. Cysteamine therapy: A treatment for cystinosis, not a cure. *Kidney Int.* **2012**, *81*, 127–129. [CrossRef]
69. Gahl, W.A.; Balog, J.Z.; Kleta, R. Nephropathic Cystinosis in Adults: Natural History and Effects of Oral Cysteamine Therapy. *Ann. Intern. Med.* **2007**, *147*, 242–250. [CrossRef] [PubMed]
70. Van Stralen, K.J.; Emma, F.; Jager, K.J.; Verrina, E.E.; Schaefer, F.; Laube, G.F.; Lewis, M.A.; Levtchenko, E.N. Improvement in the Renal Prognosis in Nephropathic Cystinosis. *Clin. J. Am. Soc. Nephrol.* **2011**, *6*, 2485–2491. [CrossRef]
71. Okamura, D.M.; Bahrami, N.M.; Ren, S.; Pasichnyk, K.; Williams, J.M.; Gangoiti, J.A.; Lopez-Guisa, J.M.; Yamaguchi, I.; Barshop, B.A.; Duffield, J.S.; et al. Cysteamine Modulates Oxidative Stress and Blocks Myofibroblast Activity in CKD. *J. Am. Soc. Nephrol.* **2014**, *25*, 43–54. [CrossRef]
72. Revesz, L.; Modig, H. Cysteamine-induced Increase of Cellular Glutathione-level: A New Hypothesis of the Radioprotective Mechanism. *Nat. Cell Biol.* **1965**, *207*, 430–431. [CrossRef]
73. Besouw, M.; Masereeuw, R.; van den Heuvel, L.; Levtchenko, E. Cysteamine: An old drug with new potential. *Drug Discov. Today* **2013**, *18*, 785–792. [CrossRef] [PubMed]
74. Wilmer, M.J.; Kluijtmans, L.A.; van der Velden, T.J.; Willems, P.H.; Scheffer, P.G.; Masereeuw, R.; Monnens, L.A.; van den Heuvel, L.P.; Levtchenko, E.N. Cysteamine restores glutathione redox status in cultured cystinotic proximal tubular epithelial cells. *Biochim. Biophys. Acta (BBA) Mol. Basis Dis.* **2011**, *1812*, 643–651. [CrossRef]

75. Elmonem, M.; Khalil, R.; Khodaparast, L.; Khodaparast, L.; Arcolino, F.O.; Morgan, J.; Pastore, A.; Tylzanowski, P.; Ny, A.; Lowe, M.; et al. Cystinosis (ctns) zebrafish mutant shows pronephric glomerular and tubular dysfunction. *Sci. Rep.* **2017**, *7*, 42583. [CrossRef]
76. Elmonem, M.A.; Berlingerio, S.P.; Morgan, J.; Khodaparast, L.; Khodaparast, L.; Lowe, M.; van DenHeuvel, L.P.; Levtchenko, E. Cysteamine improves proximal tubular reabsorption of low molecular weight compounds in cystinotic zebrafish, but has no effect on the defective megalin expression. *Pediatr. Nephrol.* **2018**, *33*, 1821.
77. Haycock, G.B.; Al-Dahhan, J.; Mak, R.H.; Chantler, C. Effect of indomethacin on clinical progress and renal function in cystinosis. *Arch. Dis. Child.* **1982**, *57*, 934–939. [CrossRef]
78. Emma, F.; Nesterova, G.; Langman, C.; Labbé, A.; Cherqui, S.; Goodyer, P.; Janssen, M.C.; Greco, M.; Topaloglu, R.; Elenberg, E.; et al. Nephropathic cystinosis: An international consensus document. *Nephrol. Dial. Transplant.* **2014**, *429*, iv87–iv94. [CrossRef] [PubMed]
79. Emma, F.; Hoff, W.V.; Hohenfellner, K.; Topaloglu, R.; Greco, M.; Ariceta, G.; Bettini, C.; Bockenhauer, D.; Veys, K.; Pape, L.; et al. An international cohort study spanning five decades assessed outcomes of nephropathic cystinosis. *Kidney Int.* **2021**, *100*, 1112–1123. [CrossRef]
80. Gonzalez, A.; Cheung, W.W.; Perens, E.A.; Oliveira, E.A.; Gertler, A.; Mak, R.H. A Leptin Receptor Antagonist Attenuates Adipose Tissue Browning and Muscle Wasting in Infantile Nephropathic Cystinosis-Associated Cachexia. *Cells* **2021**, *10*, 1954. [CrossRef]
81. Dabelic, S.; Flogel, M.; Dumic, J. Effects of aspirin and indomethacin on galectin-3. *Croat. Chem. Acta* **2005**, *78*, 433–440.
82. Lucas, G.N.C.; Leitão, A.C.C.; Alencar, R.L.; Xavier, R.M.F.; Daher, E.D.F.; da Silva, G.B., Jr. Pathophysiological aspects of nephropathy caused by non-steroidal anti-inflammatory drugs. *Braz. J. Nephrol.* **2019**, *41*, 124–130. [CrossRef] [PubMed]
83. Nelson, D.A.; Marks, E.S.; Deuster, P.A.; O'Connor, F.G.; Kurina, L.M. Association of Nonsteroidal Anti-inflammatory Drug Prescriptions With Kidney Disease Among Active Young and Middle-aged Adults. *JAMA Netw. Open* **2019**, *2*, e187896. [CrossRef]
84. Coppo, R. Corticosteroids in IgA Nephropathy: Lessons from Recent Studies. *J. Am. Soc. Nephrol.* **2017**, *28*, 25–33. [CrossRef] [PubMed]
85. Mejía-Vilet, J.M.; Ayoub, I. The Use of Glucocorticoids in Lupus Nephritis: New Pathways for an Old Drug. *Front. Med.* **2021**, *8*, 622225. [CrossRef] [PubMed]
86. Prendecki, M.; Tanna, A.; Salama, A.D.; Tam, F.W.K.; Cairns, T.; Taube, D.; Cook, H.T.; Ashby, D.; Duncan, N.; Pusey, C.D. Long-term outcome in biopsy-proven acute interstitial nephritis treated with steroids. *Clin. Kidney J.* **2016**, *10*, 233–239. [CrossRef]
87. Koralewski, R.; Dymek, B.; Mazur, M.; Sklepkiewicz, P.; Olejniczak, S.; Czestkowski, W.; Matyszewski, K.; Andryianau, G.; Niedziejko, P.; Kowalski, M.; et al. Discovery of OATD-01, a First-in-Class Chitinase Inhibitor as Potential New Therapeutics for Idiopathic Pulmonary Fibrosis. *J. Med. Chem.* **2020**, *63*, 15527–15540. [CrossRef]
88. Mazur, M.; Zielińska, A.; Grzybowski, M.; Olczak, J.; Fichna, J. Chitinases and Chitinase-Like Proteins as Therapeutic Targets in Inflammatory Diseases, with a Special Focus on Inflammatory Bowel Diseases. *Int. J. Mol. Sci.* **2021**, *22*, 6966. [CrossRef] [PubMed]
89. Kim, L.K.; Morita, R.; Kobayashi, Y.; Eisenbarth, S.; Lee, C.G.; Elias, J.; Eynon, E.E.; Flavell, R.A. AMCase is a crucial regulator of type 2 immune responses to inhaled house dust mites. *Proc. Natl. Acad. Sci. USA* **2015**, *112*, E2891–E2899. [CrossRef]
90. Mazur, M.; Dymek, B.; Koralewski, R.; Sklepkiewicz, P.; Olejniczak, S.; Mazurkiewicz, M.; Piotrowicz, M.; Salamon, M.; Jędrzejczak, K.; Zagozdzon, A.; et al. Development of Dual Chitinase Inhibitors as Potential New Treatment for Respiratory System Diseases. *J. Med. Chem.* **2019**, *62*, 7126–7145. [CrossRef] [PubMed]

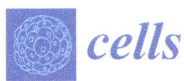

Review

Hematopoietic Stem Cell Gene Therapy for Cystinosis: From Bench-to-Bedside

Stephanie Cherqui

Department of Pediatrics, Division of Genetics, University of California, La Jolla, San Diego, CA 92093, USA; scherqui@ucsd.edu; Tel.: +1-858-822-1023, Fax: 858-246-1125

Abstract: Cystinosis is an autosomal recessive metabolic disease that belongs to the family of lysosomal storage disorders. The gene involved is the *CTNS* gene that encodes cystinosin, a seven-transmembrane domain lysosomal protein, which is a proton-driven cystine transporter. Cystinosis is characterized by the lysosomal accumulation of cystine, a dimer of cysteine, in all the cells of the body leading to multi-organ failure, including the failure of the kidney, eye, thyroid, muscle, and pancreas, and eventually causing premature death in early adulthood. The current treatment is the drug cysteamine, which is onerous and expensive, and only delays the progression of the disease. Employing the mouse model of cystinosis, using $Ctns^{-/-}$ mice, we first showed that the transplantation of syngeneic wild-type murine hematopoietic stem and progenitor cells (HSPCs) led to abundant tissue integration of bone marrow-derived cells, a significant decrease in tissue cystine accumulation, and long-term kidney, eye and thyroid preservation. To translate this result to a potential human therapeutic treatment, given the risks of mortality and morbidity associated with allogeneic HSPC transplantation, we developed an autologous transplantation approach of HSPCs modified ex vivo using a self-inactivated lentiviral vector to introduce a functional version of the *CTNS* cDNA, pCCL-CTNS, and showed its efficacy in $Ctns^{-/-}$ mice. Based on these promising results, we held a pre-IND meeting with the Food and Drug Administration (FDA) to carry out the FDA agreed-upon pharmacological and toxicological studies for our therapeutic candidate, manufacturing development, production of the GMP lentiviral vector, design Phase 1/2 of the clinical trial, and filing of an IND application. Our IND was cleared by the FDA on 19 December 2018, to proceed to the clinical trial using CD34+ HSPCs from the G-CSF/plerixafor-mobilized peripheral blood stem cells of patients with cystinosis, modified by ex vivo transduction using the pCCL-CTNS vector (investigational product name: CTNS-RD-04). The clinical trial evaluated the safety and efficacy of CTNS-RD-04 and takes place at the University of California, San Diego (UCSD) and will include up to six patients affected with cystinosis. Following leukapheresis and cell manufacturing, the subjects undergo myeloablation before HSPC infusion. Patients also undergo comprehensive assessments before and after treatment to evaluate the impact of CTNS-RD-04 on the clinical outcomes and cystine and cystine crystal levels in the blood and tissues for 2 years. If successful, this treatment could be a one-time therapy that may eliminate or reduce renal deterioration as well as the long-term complications associated with cystinosis. In this review, we will describe the long path from bench-to-bedside for autologous HSPC gene therapy used to treat cystinosis.

Keywords: cystinosis; CD34+ hematopoietic stem and progenitor cells; gene therapy; pre-clinical studies; investigational new drug application; clinical trial

Citation: Cherqui, S. Hematopoietic Stem Cell Gene Therapy for Cystinosis: From Bench-to-Bedside. *Cells* **2021**, *10*, 3273. https://doi.org/10.3390/cells10123273

Academic Editor: Elena N. Levtchenko

Received: 2 November 2021
Accepted: 19 November 2021
Published: 23 November 2021

Publisher's Note: MDPI stays neutral with regard to jurisdictional claims in published maps and institutional affiliations.

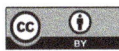

Copyright: © 2021 by the author. Licensee MDPI, Basel, Switzerland. This article is an open access article distributed under the terms and conditions of the Creative Commons Attribution (CC BY) license (https://creativecommons.org/licenses/by/4.0/).

1. Introduction

Cystinosis is an autosomal recessive disease that occurs in about 1 in 100,000–200,000 live births [1]. Cystinosis belongs to a family of lysosomal storage disorders and is characterized by the accumulation of cystine, the disulfide dimer of cysteine, within the lysosomes of all organs [2]. Three allelic forms of cystinosis exist. The most severe and the most common form of cystinosis is the infantile form of cystinosis (MIM #219800). The juvenile form

(MIM #219900) is characterized by an adolescent onset of photophobia and glomerular renal impairment that can progress to end-stage renal failure. The ocular form (MIM #219750) is characterized by an adult onset of photophobia. Children affected with infantile cystinosis, thereafter referred to as cystinosis, appear normal at birth, but at 6–18 months of age, present for medical attention with a failure to thrive, polyuria, polydipsia, glucosuria, proteinuria, and often rickets. All of these symptoms are caused by renal tubular dysfunction (renal Fanconi syndrome) [3]. Cystinosis is currently the leading cause of inherited renal Fanconi syndrome in children, representing up to 20% of patients with hereditary tubular disorders [4]. Non-renal complications of cystinosis may manifest clinically in these patients overtime, including impairment of the heart, thyroid, muscles, pancreas, eyes, and central nervous system [5]. The main ocular manifestation is the crystal deposition in the cornea, which begins in infancy, increases with age, and gradually leads to pain, photophobia, blepharospasm, and recurrent corneal erosions [6]. Retinopathy can also be seen as early as 5 weeks of age [7], sometimes causing blindness [8,9]. Patients have increased risks of cardiovascular complications [10], diabetes mellitus, and hypothyroidism, and in males, hypogonadism with infertility [11]. Cystinosis also causes bone deformities and fragility [12], attributed to massive urinary phosphate loss, defective vitamin D conversion, and cystine deposition in the bones, although pathophysiology is not fully understood [13]. Cystinotic patients later develop neuromuscular and brain complications including fine vision deficits, poor motor coordination, peripheral muscle weakness, and swallowing dysfunction [14–19]. Distal myopathy can result into chronic respiratory dysfunction, swallowing difficulties, and aspiration pneumonia, a major cause of death [20,21]. Central nervous system (CNS) complications can also involve mental deterioration, impaired cognitive function, cerebral atrophy, seizures, and ischemic lesions [18,22,23].

Mutations or deletions in the ubiquitous gene *CTNS* cause cystinosis [24]. This gene encodes cystinosin, a seven-transmembrane domain lysosomal protein, which is a proton-driven cystine transporter [25,26]. Lysosomal cystine accumulation leads to the formation of cystine crystals, pathognomonic of cystinosis. In addition to lysosomal cystine storage, cellular dysfunctions, such as abnormal vesicular trafficking, autophagy, apoptosis, and TFEB (Transcription Factor EB) signaling, have also been described as responsible for the pathogenesis of cystinosis [27–32].

Despite early advancements in available therapies to delay the progression of cystinosis, including dialysis, renal transplantation, and cysteamine therapy, a significant unmet medical need still exists for patients. While dialysis and renal transplantation have enabled the survival of many children with cystinosis into adulthood, they are associated with significant challenges including life-long immunosuppressant intake. The cystine reduction therapy, cysteamine, is requires dosing every 6 h or every 12 h [33,34]. Although cysteamine has been shown to decrease white blood cell cystine levels, patients receiving long-term cysteamine therapy may continue to develop late complications such as hypothyroidism, diabetes, myopathy (including difficulty swallowing), and neurologic defects [35–38]. In addition, while cysteamine can delay the onset of complications such as end-stage renal failure, many of these patients ultimately progress and require a kidney transplant. The average age of mortality, even with long-term (>2 years) use of cysteamine, has been reported to be as young as 28.5 years [37], and the prognosis is largely dependent upon how early in the disease course cysteamine therapy is initiated [35–37]. Cysteamine is also associated with substantial untoward side effects including gastrointestinal pain and sulphurous body and breath odor; the odor leads to significant issues with compliance, especially in adolescents and young adults. In addition, patients must take multiple pills, up to 60 pills per day, around the clock.

As most of the organs are affected by cystinosis, functional cystinosin expression has to be reinstituted in the whole body. Hematopoietic stem and progenitor cells (HSPCs) gene therapy have emerged as an efficient therapeutic technology for genetic disorders of the blood system but also for parenchymal diseases as they are able to travel and engraft into injured tissues [39–42]. In the context of cystinosis, *CTNS* gene-modified hematopoietic stem and progenitor cells (HSPCs), upon autologous transplantation, are intended to engraft into the bone marrow, divide, and differentiate, thus providing a population of corrected cells that can supply functional cystinosin in the diseased organs for the life of the patient. Preclinical studies have been conducted in the mouse model of cystinosis, the $Ctns^{-/-}$ mice [43,44]. The pre-clinical studies have shown the safety and efficacy of gene modified HSPCs for cystinosis leading to a clinical trial. If shown to be safe and effective for cystinosis, the one-time autologous transplantation of gene-modified HSPCs would represent a life-long therapy that has the potential to prevent kidney transplantation and long-term complications associated with cystinosis. Therefore, a Phase 1/2 study is currently being conducted at the University of California San Diego (UC San Diego) to evaluate the safety and efficacy of a single transplantation of autologous $CD34^+$ enriched cell fractions transduced with a lentiviral vector containing the complementary deoxyribonucleic acid sequence that encodes for human cystinosin, the lysosomal cystine transporter protein (product name CTNS-RD-04), in patients with cystinosis. The path to go from bench-to-bedside is a colossal task that requires numerous people with regulatory, manufacturing, toxicology, and clinical expertise, as well as important funding support. Here, we review the path from the pre-clinical studies to the clinical trial for the hematopoietic stem cell gene therapy strategy for cystinosis.

2. Preclinical Proof of Concept and Mechanism of Action for Using HSPC for Cystinosis

As a preclinical proof of concept, we used the mouse model of cystinosis, using $Ctns^{-/-}$ mice, a relevant model that recapitulates most of the main characteristics of the disease found in human cystinosis patients, such as mild renal Fanconi syndrome, chronic kidney disease, eye anomalies, and thyroid dysfunction [43–47]. As the source of HSPCs, we used the analogous murine stem cells antigen-1 ($Sca1^+$) cells to the human $CD34^+$ cells [48]. We showed that the transplantation of HSPCs expressing a functional *Ctns* gene isolated from congenic wild-type mice resulted in abundant tissue integration of bone marrow-derived cells, the significant decrease of cystine accumulation (up to 97% clearance), and long-term kidney preservation [49,50]. Indeed, while non-treated $Ctns^{-/-}$ mice, or $Ctns^{-/-}$ mice transplanted with $Ctns^{-/-}$ mHSPCs, progressed to end-stage renal failure, age-matched $Ctns^{-/-}$ mice transplanted with wild-type HSPCs maintained normal renal function and only focal histological kidney anomalies after more than a year post-transplant [50]. However, effective therapy depends on achieving a relatively high level of donor-derived *Ctns*-expressing cell engraftment (>50%). Finally, few to no cystine crystals were observed in the kidneys of treated mice, in contrast to non-treated $Ctns^{-/-}$ mice, in which abundant cystine crystals were consistently observed in the kidney. We also demonstrated that HSPC transplantation was able to prevent eye defects in the $Ctns^{-/-}$ mice [51]. $Ctns^{-/-}$ mice with high engraftment levels (>50%) exhibited a dramatic reduction in crystal counts from the epithelial layer to the middle stroma (100% to 72% reduction, respectively), as well as normal corneal thickness and intraocular pressure as opposed to $Ctns^{-/-}$ mice controls. This work was the first to demonstrate that transplanted HSPCs could rescue corneal defects and bring a new perspective to ocular regenerative medicine. The impact of transplanted HSPCs on the thyroid gland has been studied in collaboration with Dr. Pierre Courtoy (de Duve Institute, Belgium). $Ctns^{-/-}$ mice present with sustained TSH activation combined with thyrocyte hypertrophy, hyperplasia, and vascular proliferation [52]. In contrast, $Ctns^{-/-}$ mice treated with transplanted HSPCs exhibited normalization of cystine and TSH values and normal histology [53].

The extent of transplanted HSPC efficacy in cystinosis was surprising, especially considering that cystinosin is a transmembrane lysosomal protein as opposed to a secreted enzyme that can be recaptured by adjacent diseased cells [54–56]. In order to identify the cellular mechanism of action of this approach, we demonstrated for the first time that transplanted HSPCs, after differentiating into macrophages, transferred cystinosin-bearing lysosomes to the adjacent endogenous host cells via tunneling nanotubes (TNTs) [57]. We also demonstrated in vitro that Ctns-deficient cells exploited the same route to retrogradely transfer cystine-loaded lysosomes to macrophages, providing a bidirectional correction mechanism. This bidirectional exchange, allowing the clearance of the lysosomal cystine load in both cell types, probably accounts for the robust decrease in cystine levels observed in all tissues in the HSPC-transplanted $Ctns^{-/-}$ mice [49]. TNT formation was enhanced by the presence of diseased cells [57,58]. In vivo macrophage-derived tubular extensions penetrated the dense tubular basement membrane and directly delivered cystinosin-containing vesicles into the epithelia in $Ctns^{-/-}$ mice, preventing proximal tubular cell degeneration [57]. Macrophages were also observed in the cornea (and retina) as the primary differentiated cells from the transplanted HSPCs and transferred cystinosin-bearing lysosomes via TNTs to keratocytes [51]. TNTs were also observed in the transplanted HSPC-derived cells engrafted in the thyroid [53]. This was the first proof of concept of a genetic lysosomal defect correction by bidirectional vesicular exchange via TNTs, suggesting broader potential for HSPC transplantation for the treatment of other disorders due to defective vesicular proteins.

3. Ex Vivo Gene Modified Cell Therapy: A Safer Approach Than Allogeneic Transplantation

Given the considerable risk of morbidity and mortality associated with allogeneic HSPC transplantation, it remains an uncertain therapeutic choice for many diseases after the consideration of the risk/benefit ratio. The major complication is graft-versus-host disease (GVHD) [59,60]. Acute GVHD grade II-IV occurred in 20% to 32% of patients and chronic GVHD in 16% to 59%, both significantly impacting the survival of the recipients [61–63]. Allogeneic hematopoietic stem cell transplantation (HSCT) has been performed on one patient affected with cystinosis [64]. The patient was a 16-year-old Caucasian male, who was diagnosed with cystinosis at the age of 2.7 years and immediately treated with cysteamine. The patient underwent allogeneic HSCT from a full HLA-matched unrelated donor. Cysteamine treatment was discontinued 2 months prior to transplantation. For post-transplant immunosuppression, tacrolimus, mycophenolate mofetil, methotrexate, and prednisolone were used. Acute GVHD and adenovirus reactivation developed during the third week following HSPC transplantation, presenting with fever and profound diarrhea. Due to partial graft failure, a second HSPC infusion from the same donor was administered 15 months after the first HSCT, resulting in a higher yield of engraftment. However, a severe therapy-resistant chronic cutaneous, gastro-intestinal, and liver GVHD developed, for which several immunosuppressive agents were applied, including prednisolone, azathioprine, cyclosporine, ATG, and sirolimus. The patient died 35 months after transplantation from severe pneumonia due to a multi-resistant Pseudomonas infection. Despite GVHD and other severe adverse events due to the allogenic transplant, efficacy of HSPC transplantation on cystinosis was demonstrated. During the first few months post-HSPC transplant, kidney function stabilized, and polyuria decreased. Patient's photophobia score improved from grade 5 to no photophobia. Stomach biopsies, taken after transplantation, showed a significant decrease in cystine crystal accumulation. The cDNA derived from patient's tubular epithelial cells collected from urine and liver biopsy taken at 24 months post-HSC transplantation showed donor HSPC-derived tissue engraftment of 22% and 40%, respectively. This dramatic case report underlines that HSPC transplantation holds the potential for therapeutic benefits for cystinosis with the restoration of *CTNS* expression in tissues, a decrease in cystine crystal accumulation, and the improvement of polyuria and photophobia. However, this case also strongly highlights the high risks associated allogeneic HSC transplantation with a potentially lethal outcome.

In contrast, autologous HSPC gene therapy morbidity is substantially lower because it abrogates the risk of GVHD and immune rejection. Another key advantage of this approach is that no immunosuppressants are necessary after transplantation. For HSPC gene therapy, the patients' own HSPCs are ex vivo gene-modified to correct the gene defect. Patients still require myeloablation conditioning but at a reduced intensity. Inherent risks in this approach reside in the use of retroviral vectors to bring the normal copy of the gene and these vectors will integrate within the genome. Cases of leukemogenic complications were reported in clinical trials for severe combined immunodeficiency-X1 (SCID-X1) using autologous HSPCs and the murine leukemia virus (MLV) vector [65]. Extensive investigation of this issue revealed that MLV vector was preferentially integrated near cancer-implicated genes such as CCND2 and HMGA2, and the long terminal repeats (LTR) of the vectors contained strong enhancer/promoters that triggered the distant enhancer activation of these genes [66]. Since then, MLV vectors have been supplanted by a lentiviral vector (LV) for ex vivo gene modification of HSPCs because of their safety. The third generation of LV, self-inactivated (SIN)-lentiviral vectors, have engineered LTRs which removes their very strong promoter/enhancer activity. Therefore, an internal promoter is added in order to drive the therapeutic gene (transgene). These promoters are far less potent which reduces the potential risk of interactions with nearby cellular genes and thus, enhances safety [67,68]. Moreover, in contrast to the MLV, lentiviral vectors are not associated with oncogenesis and therefore may represent a safety advantage over oncoretroviral gene therapy vectors. In the last 12 years, 400–500 patients have been treated with lentiviral ex vivo gene therapy, including three regulatory approved products in Europe for thalassemia, metachromatic leukodystrophy, and cerebral-adrenoleukodystrophy (C-ALD) [56,69–74]. Thousands more oncology patients have been treated with lentiviral-transduced T cells, known as CARTs. All these patients are closely followed up. There have been no reported cases of oncogenesis until two recent cases. Both were in a Bluebird Bio C-ALD clinical trial. The two patients developed dominant clonal expansions within a year of gene therapy infusion, with persistent thrombocytopenia and dysplastic (abnormal) megakaryocytes. A diagnosis of myelodysplastic syndrome of single lineage dysplasia (MDS-SLD) was made. This type of MDS is not common, and seldom, if ever, progresses to acute myeloid leukemia. Patients often live a long time even without treatment. The root cause of the MDS-SLDs is at present unknown and under investigation. As a result of the many differences between all the lentiviral ex vivo gene therapies, the two cases of MDS-SLD are considered specific to this clinical trial. Overall, lentiviral vectors continue to demonstrate a significant safety advantage over gamma-retroviral vectors.

4. Preclinical Studies for the Autologous Gene-Modified Hematopoietic Stem Cell Approach for Cystinosis

The lentiviral vector backbone we used for cystinosis is pCCL-EFS-X-WPRE [75], which was provided by Dr. Donald Kohn who used the same vector for the (ADA)-Deficient Severe Combined Immunodeficiency (SCID) clinical trial [76]. This is a third generation self-inactivating (SIN)-lentiviral vector. A central polypurine tract (cPPT) fragment that increases the nuclear import of viral DNA was added to the CCL vector backbone [77]. A woodchuck hepatitis virus posttranslational regulatory element (WPRE) is present to boost titer and gene expression. However, its open-reading frame was eliminated [78], as it overlapped with the woodchuck hepatitis virus X protein, a transcriptional activator involved in the development of liver tumors [79]. The transgene expression is driven by the ubiquitously expressed short intron-less human Elongation Factor 1 alpha promoter (EFS, 242 bp) [80]. The EFS promoter, which lacks the intron and enhancers of the larger elements used in many expression plasmids, has been shown to direct high level transcription of reporter genes in murine HSCs and to have significantly reduced *trans*-activation potential compared to γ-retroviral LTR [81]. We subcloned the human *CTNS* complementary deoxyribonucleic acid (cDNA) from the starting codon (ATG) to the stop codon (TAG) in the pCCL-EFS-X-WPRE lentiviral vector (pCCL-CTNS).

We performed the first proof-of-concept in the mouse model of cystinosis, the $Ctns^{-/-}$ mice, believing that autologous gene-modified HSC transplantation using a SIN-LV could work. We worked with the human *CTNS* gene and the vector backbone (pCCL-CTNS) to create the preclinical proof-of-concept for a human trial. The analogous cells of the human CD34$^+$ HSPCs are the murine Sca1$^+$ HSPCs. We used freshly isolated Sca1$^+$ HSPCs from $Ctns^{-/-}$ mice [82]. We optimized an efficient transduction protocol for the murine HSPCs that could achieve >80% of transduced cells and showed that pCCL-CTNS-transduced HSPCs kept their capacity to engraft efficiently into all organs with a long-term expression of the transgene [82]. Then, we showed that transduced cells were capable of decreasing cystine content in all tissues and improving kidney function in the $Ctns^{-/-}$ mice [82].

5. Investigational New Drug-Enabling Studies

Based on our preclinical results, we submitted a pre-investigational new drug (IND) application regarding the gene-modified HSPCs for cystinosis in March 2013 and had the first teleconference with the Food and Drug Administration (FDA) one month later. We proposed a plan for the pharmacology/toxicology, manufacturing development, and clinical design for the future clinical trial; these three categories composing the IND application (Figure 1). Based on FDA feedback, we designed the studies necessary for inclusion in an IND.

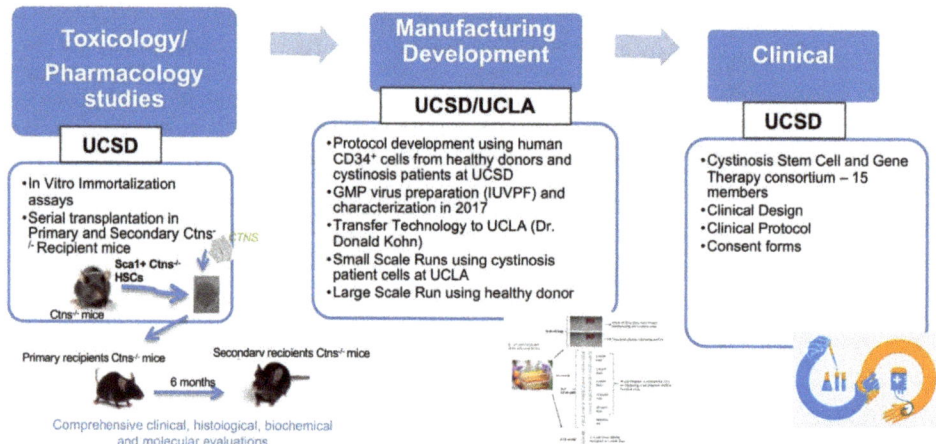

Figure 1. The investigational new drug application for cystinosis. The investigational new drug application contains three main categories, the toxicology/pharmacology studies, the manufacturing development, and the clinical design. The main studies performed in each category are listed in the figure.

5.1. Pharmacology/Toxicology Studies

CTNS-RD-04 consists of CD34$^+$ enriched HSPCs that underwent ex vivo transduction using the pCCL-CTNS that carries the full-sequence, human cystinosis gene (*CTNS*) cDNA. As the use of human HSPCs for nonclinical experimentation is not feasible in the $Ctns^{-/-}$ mouse disease model, due to xenogeneic reaction towards human stem cells, the in vivo characterization of pCCL-CTNS construct functionality was performed and the murine analogous cells Sca1$^+$ HSPCs were isolated from the $Ctns^{-/-}$ mice. Studies were designed as a serial transplantation study, with either pCCL-CTNS-transduced (test article) or mock-transduced (control article) murine $Ctns^{-/-}$ Sca1$^+$ HSPCs transplanted into primary recipient $Ctns^{-/-}$ mice; then, at 6 months post-transplant, bone marrow from the primary recipients was transplanted into secondary recipient $Ctns^{-/-}$ mice. We conducted the pharmacology/toxicology studies for the autologous transplantation of HSPCs ex vivo gene-modified with pCCL-CTNS using a batch of pCCL-CTNS lentiviral vector preparation produced under comparable good manufacturing practice (GMPc). Toxicity was determined by comprehensive clinical and histological tissue analyses and the determination of vector copy number (VCN) in blood, bone marrow, and hematopoietic lineage cells; VCN representing the average of vector copies per cell. Treated mice exhibited normal kidney function, and no indications of toxicity or histological anomalies attributable to the transplanted pCCL-CTNS-transduced HSPCs. Sustained multilineage hematopoietic cell transduction was obtained, and *CTNS* expression was detected in all tissues tested in primary test male and female mice. Finally, tissue cystine levels were reduced in most of the tissues in the primary test male and female mice compared to control male and female mice, demonstrating test article efficacy. Persistence of gene marking and *CTNS* expression in the secondary transplanted mice showed the capacity of the pCCL-CTNS vector in transducing primitive repopulating murine HSPCs. In addition, a vector integration site (VIS) analysis was performed by Dr. Frederic Bushman at the University of Pennsylvania and did not detect enrichment of integration events near oncogenes; the frequency of integration sites near oncogenes in bone marrow cells in the recipient mice was generally less than that of mice in a previously published thalassemia mouse study from which no adverse events have been reported [83]. Lastly, the potential genotoxicity associated with the pCCL-CTNS lentiviral vector was analyzed by two in vitro immortalization assay (IVIM) analyses performed in two independent laboratories, which detected transformed clones of murine bone marrow cells by insertional mutagenesis arising after multiple plating of the cells [84]. These assays demonstrated that the lentiviral vector, pCCL-CTNS, did not show growth of insertional mutants, suggesting the absence of vector associated genotoxicity, even at high vector copies per cell (up to VCN 16.9), and does not possess significant transforming capability in this in vitro assay. Altogether, the nonclinical data (pharmacology, distribution, and toxicology) collected in the $Ctns^{-/-}$ mice, indicate that CTNS-RD-04 was expected to be safe when administered in human subjects and has the potential to improve patients' welfare.

5.2. Manufacturing Development

We optimized a protocol to transduce human $CD34^+$ hematopoietic stem cells with our lentiviral vector to obtain a VCN included between one and five. We performed colony forming unit (CFU) assays using human $CD34^+$ peripheral blood stem cells (PBSC) isolated from five healthy donors and four cystinotic patients. No aberrant proliferation or differentiation potential with the lentivirus compared to negative controls was observed in any of these assays. Moreover, vector integration site (VIS) analysis in the patient's cells showed no enrichment of the integration sites near proto-oncogene 5′ ends. The clinical grade pCCL-CTNS virus preparation was produced as a ~60 L full-scale preparation at the Gene Therapy Resources Program (GTRP), Clinical Grade Lentivirus Vector Core (Indiana University National Gene Vector Laboratory) directed by Dr. Kenneth Cornetta who also prepared the good manufacturing practice (GMP)-comparable virus used for the toxicology studies. Technology transfer, small-scale runs, and large-scale runs using the GMP pCCL-CTNS lentiviral vector preparation were then performed at the GMP Human Gene and Cell Therapy Facility (HGCTF) at the University of California, Los Angeles (UCLA) directed by Dr. Donald Kohn where the manufacturing of the patients' cell product is currently taking place. Stability of the GMP pCCL-CTNS virus vector and investigational product have been established.

5.3. Clinical Design

The clinical protocol was designed by the Cystinosis Stem Cell Gene Therapy Consortium composed of 15 members including 13 clinicians in the field of bone marrow transplant, nephrology, metabolic, gastroenterology, neurology, ophthalmology, and dermatology.

The toxicology/pharmacology studies, manufacturing development, and clinical design have been reported in an IND application that was submitted to FDA on 19 November 2018, and we received clearance to proceed to a phase 1/2 clinical trial in 19 December 2018. A Data Safety Monitoring Board was established to review the protocol and provide subsequent trial oversight.

6. Autologous Gene-Modified HSPC Clinical Trial for Cystinosis

The phase 1/2 open-label, first-in-human clinical trial started in July 2019 after receiving funding from the California Institute of Regenerative Medicine (CIRM), the Cystinosis Research Foundation, and the National Institute of Health (NIH). The investigational product CTNS-RD-04 consists of the gene-modified $CD34^+$ enriched HSPCs. A target of six patients will be enrolled staggered by cohort of two patients; the two first cohorts include adult male, or females and the third cohort may include adolescents. The primary objective is to assess the clinical tolerability and safety of the treatment of CTNS-RD-04. The secondary objective is to evaluate the impact of treatment with CTNS-RD-04 on cystine levels and cystine crystal counts in the intestinal mucosa and skin, cystine crystal counts in the cornea and cystine level on white blood cells and to evaluate the effect of treatment on clinical disease outcomes, including kidney function, vision, muscle strength, respiratory function, bone density, muscle mass, endocrine function, and quality of life. As a non-invasive way to image and quantify cystine crystals in the skin, we developed and optimized a new method using intradermal confocal microscopy and an advanced imaging software [85]. The inclusion criteria include a diagnosis of infantile cystinosis, a glomerular filtration rate (GFR) > 15 mL/min/1.73 m^2, adequate thyroid function (TSH: 0.27–4.2 mIU/L, and T4 < 2 × ULN mcg/dL), and adequate respiratory function (FEV1 > 50%). For patients who underwent a kidney transplant, one-year post-transplant is required for enrolling. After provision of informed consent, subjects undergo screening and baseline clinical, histological and biochemical evaluations to determine health status, study eligibility, and blood and tissue cystine levels. The use of oral cysteamine is interrupted 2 weeks before baseline assessments and subsequently resumed. Eligible subjects undergo granulocyte colony stimulating factor (G-CSF) and plerixafor-mediated peripheral blood stem cell (PBSC) mobilization, and apheresis. Plerixafor is a small-molecule antagonist of CXCR4 and CXCL12-mediated chemotaxis, and the combination G-CSF/plerixafor has been shown to improve mobilization and the cells display a more primitive stem cell phenotype [86]. One apheresis bag is kept at UC San Diego as backup, and one bag is transported via a certified carrier to HGCTF at UCLA (Figure 2). $CD34^+$ cells are isolated, transduced using the pCCL-CTNS lentiviral vector, and cryopreserved while the cellular investigational product is being characterized (Figure 2). Once the investigational product meets release criteria, subjects discontinue oral cysteamine therapy 2 weeks prior to reduced intensity myeloablation conditioning because the impact of cysteamine on conditioning and bone marrow reconstitution is unknown. The dosing for myeloablation of the clinical trial is completed using busulfan, which is not nephrotoxic so is particularly important in the case of patients with cystinosis. CTNS-RD-04 is infused once intravenously, at the minimal dose of 3×10^6 $CD34^+$ cells/kg (Figure 2). Subjects discontinue cysteamine eye drops 1-month post-infusion. Follow-up visits for clinical, histological, and biochemical evaluations occur at approximately 3-, 6-, 12-, 18-, and 24-month post-transplant. CTNS-RD-04 will engraft into the bone marrow, divide, and differentiate, thus providing a population of corrected circulating cells with normal *CTNS* encoding cystinosin. Corrected cells are expected to engraft in cystinosis-mediated injured tissues, and the production of the normal protein is expected to cross-correct other cells in the body via tunnelling nanotubes. By allowing restoration of functional cystinosin, it is anticipated that cell survival will improve and ultimately lead to reduction in morbidity and early mortality in cystinosis patients. Three patients affected with cystinosis have been infused so far, the first patient was transplanted on 7 October 2019. Assessment of the outcomes are currently being evaluated. A partnership has been established with the ex vivo gene therapy biotech company, AVROBIO, Inc, that is currently planning to conduct a phase 3 clinical trial.

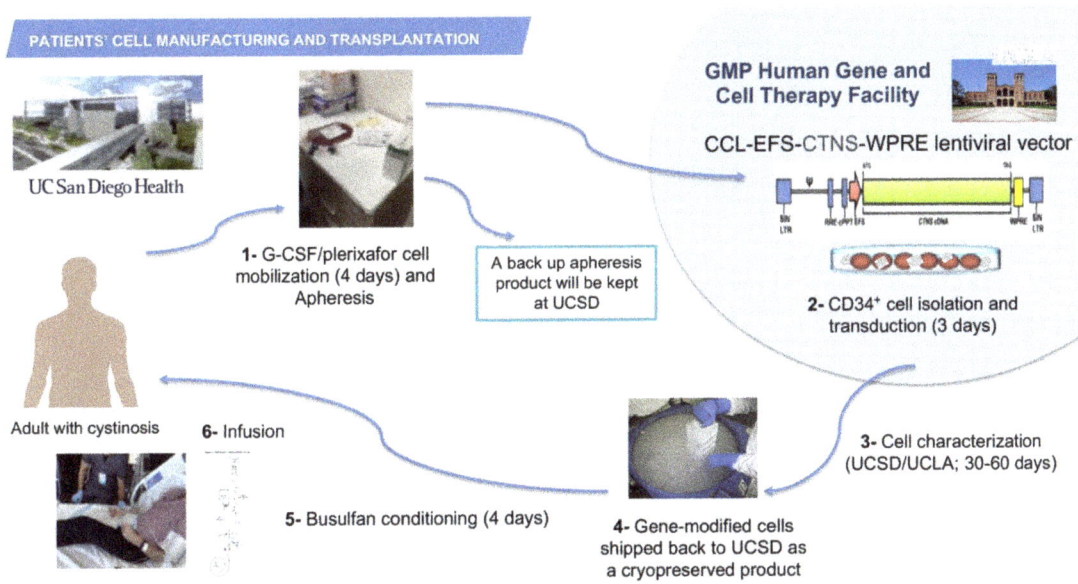

Figure 2. Manufacturing and infusion of the investigational product CTNS-RD-004. Patients with cystinosis undergo G-CSF/plerixafor stem cell mobilization in the peripheral blood, and then apheresis. One bag of apheresis is kept at UC San Diego and one bag is shipped to the HGCTF at UCLA, where the $CD34^+$ cells are isolated and transduced with the GMP pCCL-CTNS virus preparation. The cell product is then cryopreserved and characterized. If the product meets the release criteria, it is shipped to UC San Diego where it is infused to the patient.

7. Conclusions

Significant medical unmet needs still exist for patients with cystinosis. Autologous hematopoietic stem cell gene therapy represents a promising new therapeutic approach for the treatment of cystinosis that may have the potential to address most of the complications associated with this disease, and the current clinical trial will assess its potential in patients. The path from bench-to-bedside took a village, high financial support, and many years. Alongside this, the presence of the Cystinosis Research Foundation advocacy group has been instrumental in the successful clinical translation of this project.

Funding: This research was funded by the Cystinosis Research Foundation, the National Institute of Health (NIH) RO1-DK090058 and R01-NS108965, and the California Institute of Regenerative Medicine (CIRM, CLIN-09230 and CLIN2-11478).

Acknowledgments: The author acknowledges all the personnel who participated to these studies and who allowed this project to move to clinical trial, all the patient volunteers to the clinical trial, and the funding agencies.

Conflicts of Interest: Stephanie Cherqui is co-inventor on a patent entitled "Methods of treating lysosomal disorders" (#20378-101530), and is a cofounder, shareholder and a member of both the Scientific Board and board of directors of Papillon Therapeutics Inc. Stephanie Cherqui serves as a consultant for AVROBIO, Inc. and receives compensation for these services. Stephanie Cherqui also serves as a member of the Scientific Review Board and Board of Trustees of the Cystinosis Research Foundation. The terms of this arrangement have been reviewed and approved by the University of California San Diego in accordance with its conflict-of-interest policies.

References

1. Levy, M.; Feingold, J. Estimating prevalence in single-gene kidney diseases progressing to renal failure. *Kidney Int.* **2000**, *58*, 925–943. [CrossRef] [PubMed]
2. Gahl, W.A.; Thoene, J.G.; Schneider, J.A. Cystinosis. *N. Engl. J. Med.* **2002**, *347*, 111–121. [CrossRef]
3. Cherqui, S.; Courtoy, P.J. The renal Fanconi syndrome in cystinosis: Pathogenic insights and therapeutic perspectives. *Nat. Rev. Nephrol.* **2017**, *13*, 115–131. [CrossRef] [PubMed]
4. Haffner, D.; Weinfurth, A.; Manz, F.; Schmidt, H.; Bremer, H.J.; Mehls, O.; Scharer, K. Long-term outcome of paediatric patients with hereditary tubular disorders. *Nephron* **1999**, *83*, 250–260. [CrossRef] [PubMed]
5. Nesterova, G.; Gahl, W. Nephropathic cystinosis: Late complications of a multisystemic disease. *Pediatr. Nephrol.* **2008**, *23*, 863–878. [CrossRef]
6. Gahl, W.A.; Kuehl, E.M.; Iwata, F.; Lindblad, A.; Kaiser-Kupfer, M.I. Corneal crystals in nephropathic cystinosis: Natural history and treatment with cysteamine eyedrops. *Mol. Genet. Metab.* **2000**, *71*, 100–120. [CrossRef] [PubMed]
7. Schneider, J.A.; Wong, V.; Seegmiller, J.E. The early diagnosis of cystinosis. *J. Pediatr.* **1969**, *74*, 114–116. [CrossRef]
8. Dufier, J.L.; Dhermy, P.; Gubler, M.C.; Gagnadoux, M.F.; Broyer, M. Ocular changes in long-term evolution of infantile cystinosis. *Ophthalmic Paediatr. Genet.* **1987**, *8*, 131–137. [CrossRef]
9. Tsilou, E.; Zhou, M.; Gahl, W.; Sieving, P.C.; Chan, C.C. Ophthalmic manifestations and histopathology of infantile nephropathic cystinosis: Report of a case and review of the literature. *Surv. Ophthalmol.* **2007**, *52*, 97–105. [CrossRef]
10. Ueda, M.; O'Brien, K.; Rosing, D.R.; Ling, A.; Kleta, R.; McAreavey, D.; Bernardini, I.; Gahl, W.A. Coronary artery and other vascular calcifications in patients with cystinosis after kidney transplantation. *Clin. J. Am. Soc. Nephrol.* **2006**, *1*, 555–562. [CrossRef] [PubMed]
11. Keser, A.G.; Topaloglu, R.; Bilginer, Y.; Besbas, N. Long-term endocrinologic complications of cystinosis. *Minerva Pediatr.* **2014**, *66*, 123–130.
12. Klusmann, M.; Van't Hoff, W.; Monsell, F.; Offiah, A.C. Progressive destructive bone changes in patients with cystinosis. *Skeletal Radiol.* **2013**, *43*, 387–391. [CrossRef]
13. Bacchetta, J.; Greco, M.; Bertholet-Thomas, A.; Nobili, F.; Zustin, J.; Cochat, P.; Emma, F.; Boivin, G. Skeletal implications and management of cystinosis: Three case reports and literature review. *Bonekey Rep.* **2016**, *5*, 828. [CrossRef]
14. Ballantyne, A.O.; Trauner, D.A. Neurobehavioral consequences of a genetic metabolic disorder: Visual processing deficits in infantile nephropathic cystinosis. *Neuropsychiatry Neuropsychol. Behav. Neurol.* **2000**, *13*, 254–263.
15. Scarvie, K.M.; Ballantyne, A.O.; Trauner, D.A. Visuomotor performance in children with infantile nephropathic cystinosis. *Percep. Mot. Skills* **1996**, *82*, 67–75. [CrossRef]
16. Trauner, D.A.; Chase, C.; Scheller, J.; Katz, B.; Schneider, J.A. Neurologic and cognitive deficits in children with cystinosis. *J. Pediatr.* **1988**, *112*, 912–914. [CrossRef]
17. Trauner, D.A.; Spilkin, A.M.; Williams, J.; Babchuck, L. Specific cognitive deficits in young children with cystinosis: Evidence for an early effect of the cystinosin gene on neural function. *J. Pediatr.* **2007**, *151*, 192–196. [CrossRef] [PubMed]
18. Trauner, D.A.; Williams, J.; Ballantyne, A.O.; Spilkin, A.M.; Crowhurst, J.; Hesselink, J. Neurological impairment in nephropathic cystinosis: Motor coordination deficits. *Pediatr. Nephrol.* **2010**, *25*, 2061–2066. [CrossRef] [PubMed]
19. Viltz, L.; Trauner, D.A. Effect of age at treatment on cognitive performance in patients with cystinosis. *J. Pediatr.* **2013**, *163*, 489–492. [CrossRef]
20. Anikster, Y.; Lacbawan, F.; Brantly, M.; Gochuico, B.L.; Avila, N.A.; Travis, W.; Gahl, W.A. Pulmonary dysfunction in adults with nephropathic cystinosis. *Chest* **2001**, *119*, 394–401. [CrossRef]
21. Sonies, B.C.; Almajid, P.; Kleta, R.; Bernardini, I.; Gahl, W.A. Swallowing dysfunction in 101 patients with nephropathic cystinosis: Benefit of long-term cysteamine therapy. *Medicine* **2005**, *84*, 137–146. [CrossRef]
22. Berger, J.R.; Dillon, D.A.; Young, B.A.; Goldstein, S.J.; Nelson, P. Cystinosis of the brain and spinal cord with associated vasculopathy. *J. Neurol. Sci.* **2009**, *184*, 182–185. [CrossRef] [PubMed]
23. Trauner, D.A.; Fahmy, R.F.; Mishler, D.A. Oral motor dysfunction and feeding difficulties in nephropathic cystinosis. *Pediatr. Neurol.* **2001**, *24*, 365–368. [CrossRef]
24. Town, M.; Jean, G.; Cherqui, S.; Attard, M.; Forestier, L.; Whitmore, S.A.; Callen, D.F.; Gribouval, O.; Broyer, M.; Bates, G.P.; et al. A novel gene encoding an integral membrane protein is mutated in nephropathic cystinosis. *Nat. Genet.* **1998**, *18*, 319–324. [CrossRef]
25. Kalatzis, V.; Cherqui, S.; Antignac, C.; Gasnier, B. Cystinosin, the protein defective in cystinosis, is a H(+)-driven lysosomal cystine transporter. *EMBO J.* **2001**, *20*, 5940–5949. [CrossRef]
26. Cherqui, S.; Kalatzis, V.; Trugnan, G.; Antignac, C. The targeting of cystinosin to the lysosomal membrane requires a tyrosine-based signal and a novel sorting motif. *J. Biol. Chem.* **2001**, *276*, 13314–13321. [CrossRef] [PubMed]
27. Andrzejewska, Z.; Nevo, N.; Thomas, L.; Chhuon, C.; Bailleux, A.; Chauvet, V.; Courtoy, P.; Chol, M.; Guerrera, I.C.; Antignac, C. Cystinosin is a Component of the Vacuolar H+-ATPase-Ragulator-Rag Complex Controlling Mammalian Target of Rapamycin Complex 1 Signaling. *J. Am. Soc. Nephrol.* **2016**, *27*, 1678–1688. [CrossRef]
28. Johnson, J.L.; Napolitano, G.; Monfregola, J.; Rocca, C.J.; Cherqui, S.; Catz, S.D. Upregulation of the Rab27a-Dependent Trafficking and Secretory Mechanisms Improves Lysosomal Transport, Alleviates Endoplasmic Reticulum Stress, and Reduces Lysosome Overload in Cystinosis. *Mol. Cell. Biol.* **2013**, *33*, 2950–2962. [CrossRef]

29. Napolitano, G.; Johnson, J.L.; He, J.; Rocca, C.J.; Monfregola, J.; Pestonjamasp, K.; Cherqui, S.; Catz, S.D. Impairment of chaperone-mediated autophagy leads to selective lysosomal degradation defects in the lysosomal storage disease cystinosis. *EMBO Mol. Med.* **2015**, *7*, 158–174. [CrossRef] [PubMed]
30. Rega, L.R.; Polishchuk, E.; Montefusco, S.; Napolitano, G.; Tozzi, G.; Zhang, J.; Bellomo, F.; Taranta, A.; Pastore, A.; Polishchuk, R.; et al. Activation of the transcription factor EB rescues lysosomal abnormalities in cystinotic kidney cells. *Kidney Int.* **2016**, *89*, 862–873. [CrossRef] [PubMed]
31. Park, M.A.; Pejovic, V.; Kerisit, K.G.; Junius, S.; Thoene, J.G. Increased apoptosis in cystinotic fibroblasts and renal proximal tubule epithelial cells results from cysteinylation of protein kinase Cdelta. *J. Am. Soc. Nephrol.* **2006**, *17*, 3167–3175. [CrossRef] [PubMed]
32. Sansanwal, P.; Kambham, N.; Sarwal, M.M. Caspase-4 may play a role in loss of proximal tubules and renal injury in nephropathic cystinosis. *Pediatr. Nephrol.* **2010**, *25*, 105–109. [CrossRef]
33. Dohil, R.; Fidler, M.; Gangoiti, J.A.; Kaskel, F.; Schneider, J.A.; Barshop, B.A. Twice-daily cysteamine bitartrate therapy for children with cystinosis. *J. Pediatr.* **2010**, *156*, 71–75.e3. [CrossRef] [PubMed]
34. Schneider, J.A. Approval of cysteamine for patients with cystinosis. *Pediatr. Nephrol.* **1995**, *9*, 254. [CrossRef] [PubMed]
35. Brodin-Sartorius, A.; Tete, M.J.; Niaudet, P.; Antignac, C.; Guest, G.; Ottolenghi, C.; Charbit, M.; Moyse, D.; Legendre, C.; Lesavre, P.; et al. Cysteamine therapy delays the progression of nephropathic cystinosis in late adolescents and adults. *Kidney Int.* **2012**, *81*, 179–189. [CrossRef]
36. Emma, F.; Hoff, W.V.; Hohenfellner, K.; Topaloglu, R.; Greco, M.; Ariceta, G.; Bettini, C.; Bockenhauer, D.; Veys, K.; Pape, L.; et al. An international cohort study spanning five decades assessed outcomes of nephropathic cystinosis. *Kidney Int.* **2021**, *100*, 1112–1123. [CrossRef] [PubMed]
37. Gahl, W.A.; Balog, J.Z.; Kleta, R. Nephropathic cystinosis in adults: Natural history and effects of oral cysteamine therapy. *Ann. Intern. Med.* **2007**, *147*, 242–250. [CrossRef] [PubMed]
38. Cherqui, S. Cysteamine therapy: A treatment for cystinosis, not a cure. *Kidney Int.* **2012**, *81*, 127–129. [CrossRef] [PubMed]
39. Cartier, N.; Hacein-Bey-Abina, S.; Bartholomae, C.C.; Bougneres, P.; Schmidt, M.; Kalle, C.V.; Fischer, A.; Cavazzana-Calvo, M.; Aubourg, P. Lentiviral hematopoietic cell gene therapy for X-linked adrenoleukodystrophy. *Methods Enzymol.* **2012**, *507*, 187–198. [PubMed]
40. Biffi, A.; Montini, E.; Lorioli, L.; Cesani, M.; Fumagalli, F.; Plati, T.; Baldoli, C.; Martino, S.; Calabria, A.; Canale, S.; et al. Lentiviral hematopoietic stem cell gene therapy benefits metachromatic leukodystrophy. *Science* **2013**, *341*, 1233158. [CrossRef] [PubMed]
41. Gentner, B.; Bernardo, M.E.M.E.; Tucci, F.; Zonari, E.; Fumagalli, F.; Pontesilli, S.; Acquati, S.; Silvani, P.; Ciceri, F.; Rovelli, A.; et al. Extensive Metabolic Correction of Hurler Disease by Hematopoietic Stem Cell-Based Gene Therapy: Preliminary Results from a Phase I/II Trial. *Blood* **2019**, *134*, 607. [CrossRef]
42. Visigalli, I.; Delai, S.; Politi, L.S.; di Domenico, C.; Cerri, F.; Mrak, E.; D'Isa, R.; Ungaro, D.; Stok, M.; Sanvito, F.; et al. Gene therapy augments the efficacy of hematopoietic cell transplantation and fully corrects mucopolysaccharidosis type I phenotype in the mouse model. *Blood* **2010**, *116*, 5130–5139. [CrossRef] [PubMed]
43. Cherqui, S.; Sevin, C.; Hamard, G.; Kalatzis, V.; Sich, M.; Pequignot, M.O.; Gogat, K.; Abitbol, M.; Broyer, M.; Gubler, M.C.; et al. Intralysosomal cystine accumulation in mice lacking cystinosin, the protein defective in cystinosis. *Mol. Cell. Biol.* **2002**, *22*, 7622–7632. [CrossRef] [PubMed]
44. Nevo, N.; Chol, M.; Bailleux, A.; Kalatzis, V.; Morisset, L.; Devuyst, O.; Gubler, M.C.; Antignac, C. Renal phenotype of the cystinosis mouse model is dependent upon genetic background. *Nephrol. Dial. Transpl.* **2010**, *25*, 1059–1066. [CrossRef] [PubMed]
45. Chevronnay, H.P.G.; Janssens, V.; van der Smissen, P.; N'Kuli, F.; Nevo, N.; Guiot, Y.; Levtchenko, E.; Marbaix, E.; Pierreux, C.E.; Cherqui, S.; et al. Time course of pathogenic and adaptation mechanisms in cystinotic mouse kidneys. *J. Am. Soc. Nephrol.* **2014**, *25*, 1256–1269. [CrossRef] [PubMed]
46. Kalatzis, V.; Serratrice, N.; Hippert, C.; Payet, O.; Arndt, C.; Cazevieille, C.; Maurice, T.; Hamel, C.; Malecaze, F.; Antignac, C.; et al. The ocular anomalies in a cystinosis animal model mimic disease pathogenesis. *Pediatr. Res.* **2007**, *62*, 156–162. [CrossRef]
47. Simpson, J.; Nien, C.J.; Flynn, K.; Jester, B.; Cherqui, S.; Jester, J. Quantitative in vivo and ex vivo confocal microscopy analysis of corneal cystine crystals in the Ctns knockout mouse. *Mol. Vis.* **2011**, *17*, 2212–2220.
48. Challen, G.A.; Boles, N.; Lin, K.K.; Goodell, M.A. Mouse hematopoietic stem cell identification and analysis. *Cytometry A* **2009**, *75*, 14–24. [CrossRef]
49. Syres, K.; Harrison, F.; Tadlock, M.; Jester, J.V.; Simpson, J.; Roy, S.; Salomon, D.R.; Cherqui, S. Successful treatment of the murine model of cystinosis using bone marrow cell transplantation. *Blood* **2009**, *114*, 2542–2552. [CrossRef]
50. Yeagy, B.A.; Harrison, F.; Gubler, M.C.; Koziol, J.A.; Salomon, D.R.; Cherqui, S. Kidney preservation by bone marrow cell transplantation in hereditary nephropathy. *Kidney Int.* **2011**, *79*, 1198–1206. [CrossRef]
51. Rocca, C.J.; Kreymerman, A.; Ur, S.N.; Frizzi, K.E.; Naphade, S.; Lau, A.; Tran, T.; Calcutt, N.A.; Goldberg, J.L.; Cherqui, S. Treatment of Inherited Eye Defects by Systemic Hematopoietic Stem Cell Transplantation. *Investig. Ophthalmol. Vis. Sci.* **2015**, *56*, 7214–7223. [CrossRef]
52. Chevronnay, H.P.G.; Janssens, V.; van der Smissen, P.; Liao, X.H.; Abid, Y.; Nevo, N.; Antignac, C.; Refetoff, S.; Cherqui, S.; Pierreux, C.E.; et al. A mouse model suggests two mechanisms for thyroid alterations in infantile cystinosis: Decreased thyroglobulin synthesis due to endoplasmic reticulum stress/unfolded protein response and impaired lysosomal processing. *Endocrinology* **2015**, *156*, 2349–2364. [CrossRef]

53. Chevronnay, H.P.G.; Jansen, V.; van der Smissen, P.; Rocca, C.J.; Liao, X.H.; Refetoff, S.; Pierreux, C.E.; Cherqui, S.; Courtoy, P. Hematopoietic stem cell transplantation can normalize thyroid function in a cystinosis mouse model. *Endocrinology* **2016**, *157*, 1363–1371. [CrossRef]
54. Biffi, A.; de Palma, M.; Quattrini, A.; del Carro, U.; Amadio, S.; Visigalli, I.; Sessa, M.; Fasano, S.; Brambilla, R.; Marchesini, S.; et al. Correction of metachromatic leukodystrophy in the mouse model by transplantation of genetically modified hematopoietic stem cells. *J. Clin. Investig.* **2004**, *113*, 1118–1129. [CrossRef] [PubMed]
55. di Domenico, C.; Villani, G.R.; di Napoli, D.; Reyero, E.G.; Lombardo, A.; Naldini, L.; di Natale, P. Gene therapy for a mucopolysaccharidosis type I murine model with lentiviral-IDUA vector. *Hum. Gene Ther.* **2005**, *16*, 81–90. [CrossRef]
56. Massaro, G.; Geard, A.F.; Liu, W.; Coombe-Tennant, O.; Waddington, S.N.; Baruteau, J.; Gissen, P.; Rahim, A.A. Gene Therapy for Lysosomal Storage Disorders: Ongoing Studies and Clinical Development. *Biomolecules* **2021**, *11*, 611. [CrossRef]
57. Naphade, S.; Sharma, J.; Chevronnay, H.P.G.; Shook, M.A.; Yeagy, B.A.; Rocca, C.J.; Ur, S.N.; Lau, A.J.; Courtoy, P.J.; Cherqui, S. Brief reports: Lysosomal cross-correction by hematopoietic stem cell-derived macrophages via tunneling nanotubes. *Stem Cells* **2015**, *33*, 301–309. [CrossRef]
58. Goodman, S.; Naphade, S.; Khan, M.; Sharma, J.; Cherqui, S. Macrophage polarization impacts tunneling nanotube formation and intercellular organelle trafficking. *Sci. Rep.* **2019**, *9*, 14529. [CrossRef] [PubMed]
59. Johnston, L. Acute graft-versus-host disease: Differing risk with differing graft sources and conditioning intensity. *Best Pract. Res. Clin. Haematol.* **2008**, *21*, 177–192. [CrossRef]
60. Pallera, A.M.; Schwartzberg, L.S. Managing the toxicity of hematopoietic stem cell transplant. *J. Support Oncol.* **2004**, *2*, 223–237; discussion 237–228, 241, 246–227.
61. Cutler, C.; Li, S.; Ho, V.T.; Koreth, J.; Alyea, E.; Soiffer, R.J.; Antin, J.H. Extended follow-up of methotrexate-free immunosuppression using sirolimus and tacrolimus in related and unrelated donor peripheral blood stem cell transplantation. *Blood* **2007**, *109*, 3108–3114. [CrossRef]
62. Geyer, M.B.; Jacobson, J.S.; Freedman, J.; George, D.; Moore, V.; van de Ven, C.; Satwani, P.; Bhatia, M.; Garvin, J.H.; Bradley, M.B.; et al. A comparison of immune reconstitution and graft-versus-host disease following myeloablative conditioning versus reduced toxicity conditioning and umbilical cord blood transplantation in paediatric recipients. *Br. J. Haematol.* **2011**, *155*, 218–234. [CrossRef]
63. Schleuning, M.; Judith, D.; Jedlickova, Z.; Stubig, T.; Heshmat, M.; Baurmann, H.; Schwerdtfeger, R. Calcineurin inhibitor-free GVHD prophylaxis with sirolimus, mycophenolate mofetil and ATG in Allo-SCT for leukemia patients with high relapse risk: An observational cohort study. *Bone Marrow. Transpl.* **2009**, *43*, 717–723. [CrossRef] [PubMed]
64. Elmonem, M.A.; Veys, A.; Arcolino, F.O.; van Dyck, M.; Benedetti, M.C.; Diomedi-Camassei, F.; de Hertogh, G.; van den Heuvel, L.P.; Renard, M.; Levtchenko, E. Allogeneic HSCT transfers wild-type cystinosin to nonhematological epithelial cells in cystinosis: First human report. *Am. J. Transpl.* **2018**, *18*, 2823–2828. [CrossRef]
65. Hacein-Bey-Abina, S.; Garrigue, A.; Wang, G.P.; Soulier, J.; Lim, A.; Morillon, E.; Clappier, E.; Caccavelli, L.; Delabesse, E.; Beldjord, K.; et al. Insertional oncogenesis in 4 patients after retrovirus-mediated gene therapy of SCID-X1. *J. Clin. Investig.* **2008**, *118*, 3132–3142. [CrossRef] [PubMed]
66. Wang, G.P.; Berry, C.C.; Malani, N.; Leboulch, P.; Fischer, A.; Hacein-Bey-Abina, S.; Cavazzana-Calvo, M.; Bushman, F.D. Dynamics of gene-modified progenitor cells analyzed by tracking retroviral integration sites in a human SCID-X1 gene therapy trial. *Blood* **2010**, *115*, 4356–4366. [CrossRef]
67. Modlich, U.; Bohne, J.; Schmidt, M.; von Kalle, C.; Knoss, S.; Schambach, A.; Baum, C. Cell-culture assays reveal the importance of retroviral vector design for insertional genotoxicity. *Blood* **2006**, *108*, 2545–2553. [CrossRef]
68. Montini, E.; Cesana, D.; Schmidt, M.; Sanvito, F.; Bartholomae, C.C.; Ranzani, M.; Benedicenti, F.; Sergi, L.S.; Ambrosi, A.; Ponzoni, M.; et al. The genotoxic potential of retroviral vectors is strongly modulated by vector design and integration site selection in a mouse model of HSC gene therapy. *J. Clin. Investig.* **2009**, *119*, 964–975. [CrossRef]
69. Tucci, F.; Scaramuzza, S.; Aiuti, A.; Mortellaro, A. Update on Clinical Ex Vivo Hematopoietic Stem Cell Gene Therapy for Inherited Monogenic Diseases. *Mol. Ther.* **2021**, *29*, 489–504. [CrossRef]
70. DiGiusto, D.L.; Stan, R.; Krishnan, A.; Li, H.; Rossi, J.J.; Zaia, J.A. Development of hematopoietic stem cell based gene therapy for HIV-1 infection: Considerations for proof of concept studies and translation to standard medical practice. *Viruses* **2013**, *5*, 2898–2919. [CrossRef]
71. Drakopoulou, E.; Papanikolaou, E.; Georgomanoli, M.; Anagnou, N.P. Towards more successful gene therapy clinical trials for beta-thalassemia. *Curr. Mol. Med.* **2013**, *13*, 1314–1330. [CrossRef]
72. Eichler, F.; Duncan, C.; Musolino, P.L.; Orchard, P.J.; de Oliveira, S.; Thrasher, A.J.; Armant, M.; Dansereau, C.; Lund, T.C.; Miller, W.P.; et al. Hematopoietic Stem-Cell Gene Therapy for Cerebral Adrenoleukodystrophy. *N. Engl. J. Med.* **2017**, *377*, 1630–1638. [CrossRef] [PubMed]
73. Porter, D.L.; Levine, B.L.; Kalos, M.; Bagg, A.; June, C.H. Chimeric antigen receptor-modified T cells in chronic lymphoid leukemia. *N. Engl. J. Med.* **2011**, *365*, 725–733. [CrossRef]
74. Zhang, L.; Thrasher, A.J.; Gaspar, H.B. Current progress on gene therapy for primary immunodeficiencies. *Gene Ther.* **2013**, *20*, 963–969. [CrossRef]
75. Zufferey, R.; Dull, T.; Mandel, R.J.; Bukovsky, A.; Quiroz, D.; Naldini, L.; Trono, D. Self-inactivating lentivirus vector for safe and efficient in vivo gene delivery. *J. Virol.* **1998**, *72*, 9873–9880. [CrossRef] [PubMed]

76. Kohn, D.B.; Booth, C.; Shaw, K.L.; Xu-Bayford, J.; Garabedian, E.; Trevisan, V.; Carbonaro-Sarracino, D.A.; Soni, K.; Terrazas, D.; Snell, K.; et al. Autologous Ex Vivo Lentiviral Gene Therapy for Adenosine Deaminase Deficiency. *N. Engl. J. Med.* **2021**, *384*, 2002–2013. [CrossRef]
77. Demaison, C.; Parsley, K.; Brouns, G.; Scherr, M.; Battmer, K.; Kinnon, C.; Grez, M.; Thrasher, A.J. High-level transduction and gene expression in hematopoietic repopulating cells using a human immunodeficiency [correction of imunodeficiency] virus type 1-based lentiviral vector containing an internal spleen focus forming virus promoter. *Hum. Gene Ther.* **2002**, *13*, 803–813. [CrossRef]
78. Zanta-Boussif, M.A.; Charrier, S.; Brice-Ouzet, A.; Martin, S.; Opolon, P.; Thrasher, A.J.; Hope, T.J.; Galy, A. Validation of a mutated PRE sequence allowing high and sustained transgene expression while abrogating WHV-X protein synthesis: Application to the gene therapy of WAS. *Gene Ther.* **2009**, *16*, 605–619. [CrossRef]
79. Kingsman, S.M.; Mitrophanous, K.; Olsen, J.C. Potential oncogene activity of the woodchuck hepatitis post-transcriptional regulatory element (WPRE). *Gene Ther.* **2005**, *12*, 3–4. [CrossRef]
80. Wakabayashi-Ito, N.; Nagata, S. Characterization of the regulatory elements in the promoter of the human elongation factor-1 alpha gene. *J. Biol. Chem.* **1994**, *269*, 29831–29837. [CrossRef]
81. Zychlinski, D.; Schambach, A.; Modlich, U.; Maetzig, T.; Meyer, J.; Grassman, E.; Mishra, A.; Baum, C. Physiological Promoters Reduce the Genotoxic Risk of Integrating Gene Vectors. *Mol. Ther.* **2008**, *16*, 718–725. [CrossRef] [PubMed]
82. Harrison, F.; Yeagy, B.A.; Rocca, C.J.; Kohn, D.B.; Salomon, D.R.; Cherqui, S. Hematopoietic stem cell gene therapy for the multisystemic lysosomal storage disorder cystinosis. *Mol. Ther.* **2013**, *21*, 433–444. [CrossRef]
83. Ronen, K.; Negre, O.; Roth, S.; Colomb, C.; Malani, N.; Denaro, M.; Brady, T.; Fusil, F.; Gillet-Legrand, B.; Hehir, K.; et al. Distribution of lentiviral vector integration sites in mice following therapeutic gene transfer to treat beta-thalassemia. *Mol. Ther.* **2011**, *19*, 1273–1286. [CrossRef] [PubMed]
84. Arumugam, P.I.; Higashimoto, T.; Urbinati, F.; Modlich, U.; Nestheide, S.; Xia, P.; Fox, C.; Corsinotti, A.; Baum, C.; Malik, P. Genotoxic potential of lineage-specific lentivirus vectors carrying the beta-globin locus control region. *Mol. Ther.* **2009**, *17*, 1929–1937. [CrossRef] [PubMed]
85. Bengali, M.; Goodman, S.; Sun, X.; Dohil, M.A.; Dohil, R.; Newbury, R.; Lobry, T.; Hernandez, L.; Antignac, C.; Jain, S.; et al. Non-invasive intradermal imaging of cystine crystals in cystinosis. *PLoS ONE* **2021**, *16*, e0247846. [CrossRef] [PubMed]
86. Yannaki, E.; Karponi, G.; Zervou, F.; Constantinou, V.; Bouinta, A.; Tachynopoulou, V.; Kotta, K.; Jonlin, E.; Papayannopoulou, T.; Anagnostopoulos, A.; et al. Hematopoietic stem cell mobilization for gene therapy: Superior mobilization by the combination of granulocyte-colony stimulating factor plus plerixafor in patients with beta-thalassemia major. *Hum. Gene Ther.* **2013**, *24*, 852–860. [CrossRef]

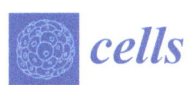

Article

Response to Cysteamine in Osteoclasts Obtained from Patients with Nephropathic Cystinosis: A Genotype/Phenotype Correlation

Thomas Quinaux [1,2], Aurélia Bertholet-Thomas [1,2], Aude Servais [3], Olivia Boyer [4], Isabelle Vrillon [5], Julien Hogan [6], Sandrine Lemoine [7,8], Ségolène Gaillard [9], Candide Alioli [2], Sophie Vasseur [10], Cécile Acquaviva [10], Olivier Peyruchaud [2], Irma Machuca-Gayet [2,†] and Justine Bacchetta [1,2,8,*,†]

1. Centre de Référence des Maladies Rénales Rares, Centre de Référence des Maladies Rares du Calcium et du Phosphore, Filières de Santé Maladies Rares OSCAR, ORKID et ERK-Net, Hôpital Femme Mère Enfant, 69500 Bron, France; itommy640@gmail.com (T.Q.); aurelia.bertholet-thomas@chu-lyon.fr (A.B.-T.)
2. INSERM 1033 Research Unit, 69008 Lyon, France; candide.alioli@inserm.fr (C.A.); olivier.peyruchaud@inserm.fr (O.P.); irma.machuca-gayet@inserm.fr (I.M.-G.)
3. Service de Néphrologie, Hôpital Necker, 75015 Paris, France; aude.servais@aphp.fr
4. Service de Néphrologie Pédiatrique, Centre de Référence des Maladies Rénales Héréditaires de l'Enfant et de l'Adulte, Hôpital Necker-Enfants Malades, AP-HP, 75015 Paris, France; olivia.boyer@aphp.fr
5. Service de Néphrologie Dialyse et Transplantation Pédiatriques, Hôpital d'Enfants, CHRU de Nancy, 54000 Nancy, France; i.vrillon@chru-nancy.fr
6. Service de Néphrologie Pédiatrique, APHP, Hôpital Robert Debré, 75019 Paris, France; julien.hogan@aphp.fr
7. Service de Néphrologie, Dialyse et Hypertension Artérielle, Hôpital Edouard Herriot, 69008 Lyon, France; sandrine.lemoine01@chu-lyon.fr
8. Faculté de Médecine Lyon Est, Université de Lyon, 69008 Lyon, France
9. EPICIME-CIC 1407, Département d'Epidémiologie Clinique, Groupement Hospitalier Est, Hospices Civils de Lyon, 69500 Bron, France; segolene.gaillard@chu-lyon.fr
10. Service de Biochimie et Biologie Moléculaire, Unité Maladies Héréditaires du Métabolisme, Groupement Hospitalier Est, Hospices Civils de Lyon, 69500 Bron, France; sophie.vasseur@chu-lyon.fr (S.V.); cecile.acquaviva-bourdain@chu-lyon.fr (C.A.)

* Correspondence: justine.bacchetta@chu-lyon.fr
† These authors equally contributed to the manuscript.

Abstract: Bone complications of cystinosis have been recently described. The main objectives of this paper were to determine in vitro the impact of CTNS mutations and cysteamine therapy on human osteoclasts and to carry out a genotype-phenotype analysis related to osteoclastic differentiation. Human osteoclasts were differentiated from peripheral blood mononuclear cells (PBMCs) and were treated with increasing doses of cysteamine (0, 50, 200 µM) and then assessed for osteoclastic differentiation. Results are presented as median (min-max). A total of 17 patients (mainly pediatric) were included, at a median age of 14 (2–61) years, and a eGFR of 64 (23–149) mL/min/1.73 m^2. Most patients (71%) were under conservative kidney management (CKM). The others were kidney transplant recipients. Three functional groups were distinguished for CTNS mutations: cystinosin variant with residual cystin efflux activity (RA, residual activity), inactive cystinosin variant (IP, inactive protein), and absent protein (AP). PBMCs from patients with residual cystinosin activity generate significantly less osteoclasts than those obtained from patients of the other groups. In all groups, cysteamine exerts an inhibitory effect on osteoclastic differentiation at high doses. This study highlights a link between genotype and osteoclastic differentiation, as well as a significant impact of cysteamine therapy on this process in humans.

Keywords: cystinosis; cysteamine; bone; osteoclast; genotype

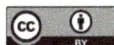

1. Introduction

Nephropathic cystinosis (NC; 1/200,000 live births) is a monogenic autosomal recessive lysosomal storage disease caused by a bi-allelic mutation of the *CTNS* gene (17p13.2), consisting of 12 exons [1]. This gene encodes cystinosin, a lysosomal seven-transmembrane domain cystine transporter of 367 amino acids. So far, over 140 pathogenic mutations have been reported in the *CTNS* gene [2], the most frequent one being a large deletion of 57 kb involving the promoter region and the first 9 exons and part of exon 10. This deletion represents approximately 50% of mutant alleles in patients of North European and North American origin [2].

Cystinosin deficiency causes an accumulation of cystine in all organs and tissues, making cystinosis a systemic disease [3,4]. Early clinical manifestations are related to complete proximal tubulopathy and therefore include polyuric-polydipsic syndrome, growth retardation, and hypophosphatemic rickets. The natural history of this disorder is marked by chronic interstitial nephritis, leading to end stage renal disease during the second decade of life. In this regard, the beneficial role of cysteamine therapy in NC has been well known for nearly four decades: Although it does not prevent nor improve tubulopathy, it considerably slows the progression of renal lesions [4,5], delays the need for transplantation [6], and prevents late complications [7].

Since patient survival has improved considerably with cysteamine therapy, late onset complications have emerged, notably bone involvement. Indeed, the concept of "cystinosis metabolic bone disease" (CMBD) is currently emerging [8]. We were the first to show in a pilot study on 10 teenagers and young adults, at a median age of 23 (range 10–35) years, that 70% of patients complained of a bone symptom (past of fracture, bone deformations, and/or bone pain), with a tendency toward low PTH and low FGF23 levels [9]. At the same time, an American study in 30 patients displayed similar results [10]. Physicians are currently aware of this specific "novel" complication of NC, and international guidelines on the diagnosis and management of CMBD were published in 2019 [8].

Even though its exact underlying pathophysiology remains unclear, at least five distinct but complementary entities can explain CMBD in addition to the classical mineral and bone disorders associated with CKD and post-transplant [8,11]: long-term consequences of hypophosphatemic rickets and renal Fanconi syndrome; deficiency in nutrition and micro-nutrition, and notably copper deficiency; hormonal disturbances such as hypothyroidism, hypogonadism, hypoparathyroidism and resistance to growth hormone and IGF1; myopathy; and intrinsic and iatrogenic bone lesions such as direct bone effects of *CTNS* mutation on osteoblasts and osteoclasts, both in murine models of cystinosis and cystinosis patients [11]. Recent experimental data corroborate clinical observations suggesting a toxicity of high-dose cysteamine on bone cells [12–14]. We previously showed that if monocytes derived from NC patients PBMCs were more prone to differentiate into osteoclasts than healthy donor monocytes, they displayed less efficient resorption activity. However, intriguingly enough, cysteamine treatment did not revert this tendency nor did it revert the deficient resorption activity in vitro of NC patients-derived osteoclasts [14]. These findings suggested that cystinosin might be a negative regulator of osteoclast differentiation but also that cystine efflux is not essential to osteoclastogenesis.

Thus, the objectives of the present study are to determine in vitro the impact of *CTNS* mutations and cysteamine therapy on human osteoclasts derived from peripheral blood mononuclear cells (PBMCs), and to carry out a genotype-phenotype analysis in terms of osteoclastic differentiation and response to cysteamine therapy, to better decipher the functional role of cystinosin in osteoclasts.

2. Materials and Methods

2.1. Clinical Study

The CYSTEABONE study (NCT03919981) was a prospective multicenter clinical study. The main objective of this clinical study was to evaluate the impact of cysteamine on osteoclastic differentiation in patients with NC, depending on the underlying genotype. Inclusion criteria were the following: patients older than 2 years of age, confirmed diagnosis of NC, and ongoing oral cysteamine therapy at inclusion. In addition to the routine biological follow-up, we obtained a sample of total blood in order to conduct osteoclastic differentiation analyses.

Clinical data were recorded: current age; age at diagnosis; renal status (conservative kidney management, CKM, dialysis, renal transplant); date(s) of dialysis initiation/renal transplantation(s); body weight and height; daily dose of cysteamine (keeping in mind that it is usually admitted that the daily dose with delayed-release (DR) cysteamine is around 75% of that using short-acting(SA) cysteamine) [15]; current treatment with growth hormone (rhGH); type of immunosuppression if any; and characterization of genetic mutation(s) and clinical bone symptoms, i.e., history of fracture(s), bone pain, bone deformities, and details concerning orthopedic surgery. Routine biological data were also recorded: plasma creatinine and estimated glomerular filtration rate (eGFR) using the 2009 Schwartz formula [16], calcium, phosphate (expressed as SDS for age) [17], and total alkaline phosphatase (ALP) expressed as xx-fold the upper normal limit of ALP for age and gender [18], parathyroid hormone (PTH) and 25-hydroxyvitamin D levels, as well as an average concentration of white blood cell hemicystin concentration in the past year. Since techniques for hemicystin were different among centers, we presented the results from the two different assays separately.

2.2. Primary Cultures of Human Osteoclasts

Blood samples were drawn fasting before the administration of cysteamine, whose plasmatic concentration was therefore residual in patients receiving maintenance cysteamine therapy. As previously published [14,19], mononuclear cells were purified from peripheral blood, loaded onto a lymphocyte separation medium (Eurobio, Courtaboeuf, France), fractionated in a density gradient in order to purify peripheral blood mononuclear cells (PBMCs) and then seeded in 96-wells plates. Osteoclasts were obtained by incubating PBMCs with M-CSF at 20 ng/mL (PeproTech, Rocky Hill, NJ, USA) and RANKL at 40 ng/mL (PeproTech) from day 1 to terminal differentiation. By day 3, osteoclast precursors were treated with increasing doses of cysteamine during differentiation: 0 (baseline conditions), 50, and 200 µM. At the end of the osteoclastic differentiation protocol, cells were collected in Trizol reagent (Invitrogen, Thermo Fisher Scientific, Waltham, MA, USA) for real-time PCR analysis or fixed with 4% paraformaldehyde (PFA) and submitted to histochemical staining using a TRAP staining kit, in accordance with the manufacturer's instructions (Sigma-Aldrich, St. Louis, MO, USA). Positively labeled cells with over three nuclei were then counted to assess in vitro osteoclastic differentiation of PBMCs.

2.3. Statistical Analyses

Clinical and biological data in patients are presented as median (min-max). Comparison between groups was performed using a Chi-square test or non-parametric Mann–Whitney tests. Data concerning osteoclastic differentiation are presented as mean number of osteoclasts per well ± standard error of the mean (SEM). Values collected under different cell culture conditions were compared using one-way analysis of variance (ANOVA) followed by Bonferroni's post hoc test for multiple comparisons. Data regarding osteoclastic differentiation of mononuclear progenitors according to their genotype, at various cysteamine concentrations, were compared using the Mann–Whitney test. A result with $p < 0.05$ was considered significant. Analyses were performed using the PRISM 5 software.

2.4. Ethical Considerations

The CYSTEABONE study was approved by the *Comité de Protection des Personnes Sud-Méditerranée IV* (2019-A00166-51). All patients and/or parents gave informed oral consent (*Jardé type 3 protocol* by French law).

3. Results

3.1. Patients' Clinical Characteristics

Seventeen patients suffering from NC, of which nine females, were included in this study, from different tertiary centres in France (four pediatric and two adult units). Most subjects were pediatric patients, with a median age of 14 (2–61) years, and eGFR of 64 (23–149) mL/min per 1.73 m^2. Most patients (71%) were undergoing CKM, and five of them had received a kidney transplant (29%). Baseline characteristics of the patients, including details regarding mutations in the *CTNS* gene and involved exons, are summarized in Table 1.

In total, 47% of patients displayed bone symptoms, and 17% had to undergo orthopedic surgery. Patient 6 presented a spontaneous fracture of the metatarsal bone at the age of 16, and patient 15 presented a trauma fracture of the metacarpal bone at the age of 58. Among the seven patients who displayed bone deformations, there were three scoliosis/kyphosis, two pectus carinatum, and six genu valgum/varum. Surgery was performed in 38% of patients presenting with overt bone symptoms. Therapeutic compliance was rather satisfactory in the cohort, since only five patients out of 17 displayed hemicystin levels above the local target. As expected, the median daily doses of cysteamine were lower in patients receiving DR cysteamine as compared to the ones receiving SA cysteamine: 1012(368–1902) and 1632(1236–3607) mg/m^2 (p = 0.003). Table 2 compares these two-subgroups, the only significant difference being the proportion of patients within the target for LHL.

We also distinguished patients according to their renal status: CKM or renal transplant, as illustrated in Table 3. Patients receiving CKM were significantly younger than transplant recipients. In these young patients, bone symptoms of any kind were significantly less common than in older transplant patients but already present (33% versus 80% respectively, p = 0.04), although eGFR did not differ significantly. The number of osteoclasts obtained at the end of the differentiation process did not differ among the two groups.

3.2. High Dose Cysteamine Decreases the Propensity of Patients-Derived Mononuclear Progenitors to Generate Osteoclasts

Results of in vitro osteoclastic differentiation with different cysteamine concentrations for each patient are summarized in Table 4: Except for two patients, a decreased number of TRAP positive multinucleated cells was observed with high doses of cysteamine (200 µM), as compared to baseline conditions and low doses of cysteamine (50 µM). This decrease was overall significant, as illustrated in Figure 1. Importantly, all osteoclastic cultures were generated from the same number of monocyte progenitors at the beginning of the experiment. Thus, these findings indicate that, at high concentrations, cysteamine decreases the propensity of patients-derived mononuclear progenitors to generate osteoclasts.

Table 1. Baseline characteristics of patients.

Pt	Age at Diag (Years)	Renal Status	Age at Eval (Years)	Sex	DNA Mutation	Protein Predicted Effect	Affected Exons	GFR	Cysteamine Daily Dose (mg/m²)	Type of Cysteamine	LHL < 1	LHL < 2	rhGH	Past of Fracture	BD	BP	Any Bone Symptoms	Orthopedic Surgery
1	1.3	C	4	M	c.922G > A/c.922G > A	RA	11/11	34	564	DR	0.7		No	No	No	No	No	No
2	2.5	T	30	F	c.1015G > A/del 57 kb	RA	12/1 to 10	62	1632	SA		2.1	No	No	Yes	No	Yes	No
3	1.7	C	15	F	c.829dupA/c.829dupA	IP	10/10	38	1630	SA		1.9	Yes	No	Yes	Yes	Yes	No
4	0.9	C	5	F	c.1-? 61 + ?del	AP	1 to 10/1 to 10	71	954	DR	1		No	No	No	No	No	No
5	1.0	C	7	F	del 57 kb/c.1-?_61 + ?del	RA	1 to 10/3	79	580	DR	0.2		No	No	No	No	No	No
6	5.5	T	17	M	c.314_317del/c.314_317del	IP	6/6	112	986	DR	0.7		No	Yes	Yes	Yes	Yes	No
7	0.8	C	16	M	del 57 kb/c.873C > G	AP	1 to 10/1 to 10	23	1236	SA		3.7	Yes	No	Yes	Yes	Yes	Yes
8	1.2	C	3	F	del 57 kb/c.873C > G	IP	1 to 10/11	149	2505	SA		1.8	No	No	No	No	No	No
9	0.1	C	2	F	del 57 kb/c.873C > G	IP	1 to 10/11	105	3607	SA		2.2	No	No	No	No	No	No
10	4.0	T	18	F	del 57 kb/c.62-?_225 + ?del	AP	1 to 10/4 and 5	105	1457	SA	0.2		No	No	Yes	No	Yes	No
11	1.0	C	14	F	del 57 kb/c.62-?_225 + ?del	AP	1 to 10/4 and 5	64	1761	SA	1.1		Yes	No	No	No	No	No
12	2.0	C	9	M	del 57 kb/del 57 kb	AP	1 to 10/1 to 10	84	1420	DR	0.8		Yes	No	No	No	No	No
13	5.3	C	8	M	c.198_218del/c.559_561 + 24del	RA	5/8	62	1111	DR		1.4	Yes	No	Yes	No	Yes	No
14	1.3	C	15	M	del 57 kb/del 57 kb	AP	1 to 10/1 to 10	127	1232	DR	1		Yes	No	No	No	No	No
15	1.1	T	61	F	del 57 kb/c.923G > T	RA			368 (theory) but 0 in reality				No	Yes	No	No	Yes	No
16	6.5	T	18	M	Del exons 1-2/del exons 1-2	AP	1 and 2	59	1039	DR	0.7	3.3	No	No	Yes	Yes	Yes	Yes
17	2.0	C	14	M	Del exons 1-2/del exons 1-2	AP	1 and 2	28	1902	DR		1.2	No	No	Yes	No	Yes	Yes

PN, patient number; GFR, glomerular filtration rate (mL/min/1.73 m²); rhGH, recombinant human growth hormone; LHL, leukocyte hemicystin levels (µmol/g of proteins), obtained from two different labs and as such presented in different columns with the target value for each lab displayed on top of the table; BD, bone deformation; BP, bone pain; C, conservative kidney management; T, kidney transplant; M, male; F, female; RA, residual activity; IP, inactive protein; AP, absent protein; DR: delayed release cysteamine (PROCYSBI®); SA: short acting cysteamine (CYSTAGON®); diag: diagnosis; eval: evaluation.

Table 2. Patients' characteristics according to the type of cysteamine.

Nephropathic Cystinosis Patients	Short Acting Cysteamine	Delayed Release Cysteamine
Number of patients	7	10
Age (y/o)	15 (2–30)	12 (4–61)
Cysteamine daily dose (mg/m^2) *	1632 (1236–3607)	1012 (368–1902)
Patients in the target for LHL *	3 (43%)	9 (90%)
GFR (mL/min per 1.73 m^2)	46 (16–149)	65 (33–84)
Calcium (mmol/L)	2.27 (2.11–2.50)	2.42 (2.23–2.92)
Phosphate (standard deviation for age)	−1.8 (−4.2;1.7)	−1.5 (−3.6;2.4)
PTH (ng/L)	34 (18–127)	20 (5–90)
25-D (ng/mL)	28 (10–42)	26 (21–49)
Total ALP (times the upper physiological value for gender and age)	0.87 (0.41–4.29)	0.74 (0.28–1.19)
Any bone symptoms (%)	3 (43%)	5 (50%)
Number of osteoclasts obtained at the end of the differentiation process	168 (97–187)	162 (111–203)

Results are presented as median (min-max) and percentage. * $p < 0.05$; LHL, leukocyte hemicystin levels; GFR: glomerular filtration rate; PTH: parathyroid hormone; 25-D: 25 hydroxy vitamin D; ALP: alkaline phosphatase.

Table 3. Patients' characteristics according to renal management modality.

Nephropathic Cystinosis Patients	Conservative Management	Renal Transplantation
Number of patients	12	5
Patients receiving SA cysteamine	5	2
Age (y/o) *	9 (2–16)	18 (17–61)
Cysteamine daily dose (mg/m^2)	1328 (564–3607)	1039 (368–1632)
Patients in the target for LHL	9 (75%)	3 (60%)
GFR (mL/min per 1.73 m^2)	65 (16–149)	56 (45–76)
Calcium (mmol/L)	2.40 (2.23–2.92)	2.42 (2.11–2.57)
Phosphate (standard deviation for age)	−1.6 (−4.2;2.4)	−1.4 (−2.8;−0.5)
PTH (ng/L)	21 (8–90)	32 (5–127)
25-D (ng/mL)	28 (10–49)	26 (22–26)
Total ALP (times the upper physiological value for gender and age)	0.9 (0.3–4.2)	0.5 (0.4–0.8)
Any bone symptoms (%) *	33	80
Number of osteoclasts obtained at the end of the differentiation process	159 (94–203)	165 (105–181)

Results are presented as median(min-max) and percentage. * $p < 0.05$; SA: short-acting; LHL, leukocyte hemicystin levels; GFR: glomerular filtration rate; PTH: parathyroid hormone; 25-D: 25 hydroxy vitamin D; ALP: alkaline phosphatase.

Table 4. Osteoclastic differentiation outcomes in each patient.

Patient Number	Protein Functionality	Cysteamine Concentration		
		0 µM	50 µM	200 µM
1	RA	203 ± 41	185 ± 44	147 ± 31
2	RA	105 ± 11	122 ± 13	67 ± 6
5	RA	111 ± 12	121 ± 19	97 ± 14
13	RA	117 ± 7	125 ± 12	107 ± 9
15	RA	197 ± 9	210 ± 20	178 ± 8
3	IP	44 ± 4	36 ± 5	29 ± 3
6	IP	181 ± 14	183 ± 23	147 ± 14
8	IP	171 ± 16	180 ± 13	160 ± 13
9	IP	187 ± 19	206 ± 22	205 ± 25
4	AP	65 ± 7	75 ± 6	52 ± 7
7	AP	94 ± 11	90 ± 6	100 ± 6
10	AP	168 ± 14	173 ± 17	127 ± 5
11	*AP*	*48 ± 3*	*48 ± 4*	*42 ± 5*
12	AP	148 ± 9	115 ± 9	87 ± 6
14	*AP*	*44 ± 5*	*48 ± 4*	*39 ± 3*
16	AP	162 ± 16	129 ± 17	114 ± 14
17	AP	172 ± 20	121 ± 14	105 ± 10

Multinucleated TRAP-positive cells (over three nuclei) were generated from PBMCs with increasing doses of cysteamine (untreated, 50 and 200 µM) and counted. RA, Residual Activity; IP, Inactive Protein; AP, Absent Protein; The results are presented as means for 7 to 8 wells ± SEM (standard error of the mean). In italics, the results of differentiation were not taken into account for Figures 1 and 3, and Tables 2 and 3, because of the low number of obtained cells that may impact the global results.

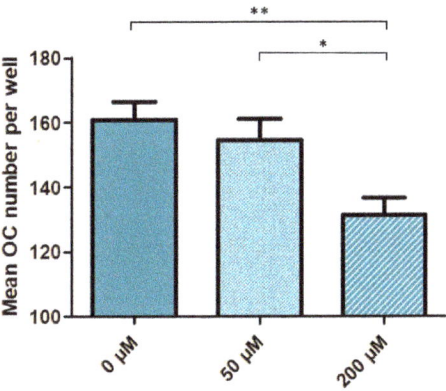

Figure 1. Impact of cysteamine treatment on osteoclast differentiation in patients with nephropathic cystinosis. Osteoclasts (TRAP-positive cells with over three nuclei) were generated from PBMCs of NC patients and treated with increasing doses of cysteamine (untreated, 50 and 200 µM). Results in terms of osteoclasts number are presented as means for seven to eight wells, with SEM. A total of 13 patients were included in the analysis, as results of cell cultures were not satisfactory for the remaining four patients. OC, osteoclasts; TRAP, Tartrate-Resistant Acid Phosphatase; PBMC, Peripheral Blood Mononuclear Cells; SEM, Standard Error of the Mean. * $p < 0.05$, and ** $p < 0.01$ compared between indicated groups by Anova followed by Bonferroni.

3.3. Inactive or Absent Cystinosin in Monocyte-Macrophage Precursors Favor Osteoclast Formation Whereas Cysteamine Treatment Impairs It Independently of the Genotype

Patients were divided into three groups according to the impact of their mutations on the translated cystinosin. Indeed, we distinguished three functional groups: those that led to the synthesis of a cystinosin variant with residual cystin efflux activity (RA, residual activity), those that led to the synthesis of an inactive cystinosin variant (IP, inactive protein), and those that did not allow for the protein to be translated and present at the lysosome membrane (AP, absent protein). The justification of mutations classification is proposed in Table 5 [2,20–24]. The localization of the different mutations is illustrated in Figure 2 [1,2,20,23,25,26].

Table 5. Justification of the classification of the mutations.

	DNA Mutation	Protein Mutation	Protein Predicted Effect	Justification Based on Experimental Data and Clinical Phenotype
1	c.922G > A/ c.922G > A	p.G308R/p.G308R	RA	Clinically quite severe (advanced CKD at 4 years of age) despite early diagnosis and satisfactory compliance, quite low and stable cysteamine doses with LHL within the target, in experimental models prediction of abolished transport [20].
2	c.1015G > A/ del 57 kb	p.G339R/p.?	RA	Heterozygous form of the large deletion of CTNS + point mutation on the last exon. Transplantation at the age of 11 years in 2000 (median age at that time for transplantation in historical cohorts), standard cysteamine daily dose, and prediction of severe impact (but no functional analysis of transport) [21]. Point mutation in the last transmembrane domain in the C-terminal part may be important for protein–protein interaction.
3	c.829dupA/ c.829dupA	p.T277NfsX19/ p.T277NfsX19	IP	Premature stop [21]
4	del 57 kb/ del 57 kb	p.?/p.?	AP	Homozygous form of the large deletion of CTNS
5	del 57 kb/ c.1-?_61 + ?del	p.?/p.?	RA	Heterozygous form of the large deletion of CTNS + deletion exon 3 (first coding exon). This second mutation was never described. Is there an alternative start? Clinically stable, satisfactory compliance, and quite low and stable cysteamine doses with LHL within the target.
6	c.314_317del/ c.314_317del	p.H105PfsX12/ p.H105PfsX12	IP	Stop in exon 6, this second mutation was not described.
7	del 57 kb/ del 57 kb	p.?/p.?	AP	Homozygous form of the large deletion of CTNS
8	del 57 kb/ c.873C > G	p.?/p.Tyr291X	IP	Heterozygous form of the large deletion of CTNS + early stop in exon 11. Severe clinical phenotype.
9	del 57 kb/ c.873C > G	p.?/p.Tyr291X	IP	Heterozygous form of the large deletion of CTNS + early stop in exon 11. Severe clinical phenotype.
10	del 57 kb/ c.62-?_225 + ?del	p.?/p.?	AP	Heterozygous form of the large deletion of CTNS + exons 4 and 5 missing at the beginning of the protein. This second mutation was never described.

Table 5. Cont.

	DNA Mutation	Protein Mutation	Protein Predicted Effect	Justification Based on Experimental Data and Clinical Phenotype
11	del 57 kb/ c.62-?_225 + ?del	p.?/p.?	AP	Heterozygous form of the large deletion of CTNS + exons 4 and 5 missing at the beginning of the protein. This second mutation was never described.
12	del 57 kb/ del 57 kb	p.?/p.?	AP	Homozygous form of the large deletion of CTNS.
13	c.198_218del/ c.559_561 + 24del	p.Ile67_Pro73del/ splicing	RA	Clinically stable, satisfactory compliance, and quite low and stable cysteamine doses with LHL within the target. The first mutation is described with residual activity [22]. The second mutation induces a splicing and leads to a truncated protein [24].
14	del 57 kb/ del 57 kb	p.?/p.?	AP	Homozygous form of the large deletion of CTNS.
15	del 57 kb/ c.923G > T	p.?/p.G308V	RA	Diagnosis at 13 months, ESRD 14 years, transplantation 18 years, still on the first graft, bad compliance, two pregnancies. Initiation of CYSTAGON at 37 years of age, switch to PROCYSBI at the age of 60 years. Very atypical clinical course with mild phenotype. Moreover, the described functional impact of the second mutation favors the existence of residual activity [23].
16	Del exons 1–2/ del exons 1–2	p.?/p.?	AP	Severe clinical phenotype with muscular impairment. Likely corresponds to the homozygous form of the large CTNS deletion. Could correspond to a contiguous gene syndrome.
17	Del exons 1–2/ del exons 1–2	p.?/p.?	AP	Severe clinical phenotype. Likely corresponds to the homozygous form of the large CTNS deletion. Could correspond to a contiguous gene syndrome.

Protein mutation "p.?", protein variant of undetermined structure; fs frameshift; del: deletion; LHL, leukocyte hemicystin levels, CKD: chronic kidney disease.

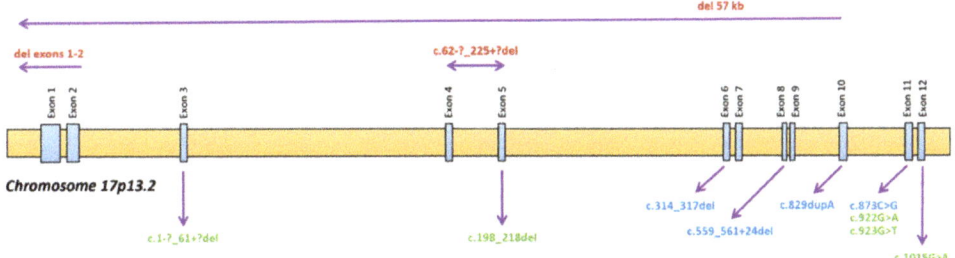

Figure 2. Topography of the mutations in the CTNS gene in this cohort. Schematic illustration of the CTNS gene with display of the mutations' genomic location within our cohort. Exonic mutations are displayed in the bottom area of the figure. Large deletions are displayed in the top area. Green: residual activity (RA); Blue: inactive protein (IP); Red: absent protein (AP).

Sub-group analyses depending on the expected cystinosin functionality were also performed from a clinical and biochemical point of view, as illustrated in Table 6: Even though statistical significance was not obtained, the AP sub-group seemed to be less well controlled in terms of hemicystin levels, and the RA sub-group appeared to be older than the other sub-groups. However, Spearman bivariate analyses showed no significant association between age and the number of obtained osteoclasts at the end of the differentiation process ($-R = -0.424$, $p = NS$).

Table 6. Patients' characteristics according to the underlying genotype.

Nephropathic Cystinosis Patients	RA	IP	AP
Number of patients	5	4	8
Age (y/o)	22 (4;61)	9 (2;17)	14 (5;18)
CKM/ Tx (N/N)	3/2	3/1	6/2
Past of rhGH therapy (N)	1	1	4
Cysteamine daily dose (mg/m^2) *	777 (0;1632)	1932 (986;3607)	1375 (954;1902)
Number of patients receiving SA cysteamine	1 (20%)	3 (75%)	3 (38%)
Proportion of patients in the target for LHL	4 (80%)	3 (75%)	5 (62%)
Number of patients with past of rhGH	1	1	4
GFR (ml/min per 1.73 m^2)	57 (34;79)	101 (38;149)	70 (23;127)
Calcium (mmol/L)	2.5 (2.1;2.9)	2.5 (2.4;2.5)	2.3 (2.2;2.6)
Phosphate (standard deviation for age)	−1.4 (−3.6;2.4)	−1.9 (−2.9;−1.2)	−1.3 (−4.2;1.7)
PTH (ng/L)	35 (8;127)	22 (18;37)	36 (5;90)
25-D (ng/mL)	28 (22;35)	30 (26;39)	28 (10;49)
Total ALP (times the upper physiological value for gender and age)	0.7 (0.3;1.2)	0.7 (0.4;0.9)	1.5 (0.4;4.3)
Any bone symptoms	60%	50%	38%

Results are presented as median (min-max) and percentage; * $p < 0.05$; CKM: conservative kidney management/Tx: past of renal transplantation; SA: short-acting; LHL, leukocyte hemicystin levels; GFR: glomerular filtration rate; PTH: parathyroid hormone; 25-D: 25 hydroxy vitamin D; ALP: alkaline phosphatase.

We therefore performed a genotype/phenotype analysis, the read-out being osteoclastic differentiation of monocyte progenitors from patients with nephropathic cystinosis depending on the underlying genotype, as illustrated in Figure 3a. At baseline, the number of osteoclasts was significantly higher in the IP and AP groups than it was in the RA group. In these two later groups (IP and AP), the number of osteoclasts obtained in cultures dropped alongside with the increase in cysteamine concentration, in a dose-dependent manner, although it was only statistically significant at high doses. In the RA group, there was no difference in the mean osteoclast number per well without and with 50 µM of cysteamine, in contrast with a significant decrease at 200 µM (as compared to 50 µM but not with absence of cysteamine). Overall for each of the three groups, treatment with a moderate dose of cysteamine (50µM) had no or mild effect, indicating that cystine efflux is likely not involved in the process of osteoclast formation. On the other hand, the decrease in osteoclast number at 200 µM of cysteamine appeared less pronounced in the RA group when compared to pooled IP and AP results as shown in Figure 3b.

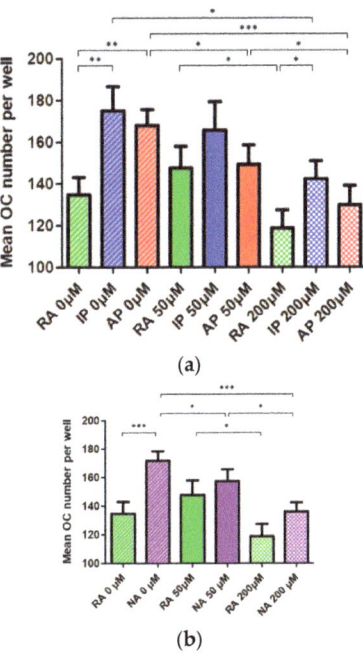

Figure 3. Impact of genotype and cysteamine treatment on osteoclast differentiation in patients with nephropathic cystinosis, (**a**) when analyzing the three genotypes independently, and (**b**) when combining the inactive and absent protein. Osteoclasts (TRAP-positive cells with over three nuclei) were generated from PBMCs of cystinotic patients, and treated with increasing doses of cysteamine (untreated, 50 and 200 µM). Results in terms of osteoclasts number are presented as means for seven to eight wells, with SEM. A total of 11 patients were included in the analysis, as data on genotype were not available for two of the 13 patients whose cultures developed properly. RA, residual activity; IP, inactive protein; AP, absent protein; NA: inactive or absent protein. OC, osteoclasts; TRAP, Tartrate-Resistant Acid Phosphatase; PBMC, Peripheral Blood Mononuclear Cells; SEM, Standard Error of the Mean. * $p < 0.05$, ** $p < 0.01$ and *** $p < 0.001$ compared between indicated groups.

4. Discussion

Mineral and bone homeostasis disorders displayed by CKD patients increase as kidney function declines. It results in a high number fractures and ectopic vascular calcifications as a consequence of impaired mineral metabolism. In nephropathic cystinosis, these aspecific mineral and bone disorders are worsened by what is now called CMBD [8]. From a clinical point of view, we here confirm that bone involvement is a late complication of cystinosis occurring in teenagers and young adults. Indeed, transplant patients were significantly older than patients under conservative management, and they also presented a higher frequency of bone symptoms. Interestingly, even though the study was not designed for this aim, we here show that the only significant difference between patients receiving SA or DR cysteamine is the proportion of patients within the target for LHL. Additionally, the fact that the ratio DR/SA is 0.62, as opposed to 0.75 in previous publications [15], likely reflects a better compliance in patients receiving DR cysteamine, as expected [27]. This is an indirect plea in "real life" for using DR whenever possible, to optimize the control of LHL, even though there were no differences in term of osteoclastic differentiation in these two sub-groups.

The underlying pathophysiology of CMBD nevertheless remains complex and multi-factorial, but cellular defects have been well documented at the cellular level, both in osteoblasts and osteoclasts, in terms of differentiation and specific activity [12–14]. However, cystinosin function in bone cells, and particularly in osteoclasts, remains unclear. Here, we focused on osteoclasts in order to better explain the altered bone phenotype of patients with nephropathic cystinosis. The main strength of this study is the protocol implemented to obtain human bone cells directly from patients presenting an orphan disease. It is an innovative, minimally invasive but time-consuming technique that allows direct access to osteoclasts from a small sample of total blood sample.

Thus, we extend the results of our previous work on cystinosin-induced osteoclastic dysfunction, in which we showed that cystinosin is required for proper osteoclastic differentiation with a peak of expression on day 6 of the differentiation process following the same pattern as cathepsin K transcripts [14]. We also showed that cysteamine has anti-resorptive effects in vitro on osteoclasts derived both from controls and patients [14].

Herein, we have classified cystinosin-identified mutations in three groups corresponding to its predicted in vivo activity, in an attempt to assign a phenotype to a genotype. The main findings of the present study are therefore the following: cells with residual cystinosin activity generate less osteoclasts as opposed to inactive or absent protein, indicating that cystinosin might be a negative modulator of osteoclast formation; moderate doses of cysteamine have no effect on either of the three groups, that is to say that in the RA, IP, or AP group, cysteamine treatment did not increase nor further reduce the number of osteoclasts; osteoclast formation remained of the same order of magnitude, supporting our previous results showing no evidence of a significant effect of cysteamine on osteoclastic differentiation at low doses [14]. In contrast, we here demonstrate a significant inhibitory effect of cysteamine on osteoclastic differentiation at higher doses. These apparent discrepancies with our previous results may be explained by an increased number of patients in this study (17 versus 7), but also by the different clinical profiles of the patients, our previous cases being older (median age 31 years), at different stages of kidney disease (transplantation, $N = 5$, hemodialysis, $N = 2$, no conservative management) [14]. Anyway, this inhibitory effect of cysteamine on osteoclastic differentiation appeared to be dose-dependent in the pooled IP and AP groups whereas the response profile to cysteamine appeared to be different in the RA group, as the number of osteoclasts at low doses of cysteamine remained comparable to the number of osteoclasts at baseline.

The genotype/phenotype analysis that we propose hinges on the first rational classification of mutations in the *CTNS* gene and is based on the functional consequences of these mutations on the structure of cystinosin. The justification of mutations classification is based on a multi-disciplinary approach taking into account both published experimental data and patients' clinical phenotype, with a discussion involving physicians, biochemists, geneticists, and basic scientists [2,20–23]. In light of the results, this classification appears relevant since it makes it possible to predict a response profile to cysteamine as a function of the patient's underlying genotype. These findings may be of clinical interest for the management of cysteamine therapy, which should reconcile, especially in patients most at risk of toxicity, effectiveness in reducing lysosomal cystine concentrations and preservation of bone capital. Without cysteamine, the number of osteoclasts was higher in cultures from subjects in whom cystinosin was inactive or absent, as compared to subjects in whom cystinosin retained residual activity. One may argue that a potential bias in the interpretation of these results may be induced by the different number of osteoclasts obtained depending on age, since younger healthy donors are more prone to produce more cells, but there was no significant association between age and osteoclastic number at the end of the differentiation process in the cells obtained from these peculiar patients. The fact that all but one patient received maintenance cysteamine therapy may also influence the results of subsequent cell culture experiments, but it would not be ethical to propose a wash-out period in these patients.

Mechanistically, this observation of a different profile of osteoclastogenesis depending on the underlying cystinosin functionality may be explained by the role that the mammalian target of rapamycin complex 1 (mTORC1) and its interaction with the Ragulator–Rag complex play during osteoclastogenesis, as discussed thoroughly in a recent review on the topic [11]. Indeed, it has been established that mTORC1 activity is down-regulated during osteoclastic differentiation through the negative regulator TSC1, whose absence impairs RANKL-dependent osteoclastogenesis. Furthermore, Andrzejewska et al. showed that the mTORC1 pathway is downregulated in proximal tubular cell lines derived from Ctns$^{-/-}$ mice [28]. A similar down-regulation in human osteoclastic progenitors might account for the overall increased osteoclastogenesis that we observe in NC patients, as compared to controls. Andrzejewska et al. also demonstrated that cystinosin is a component of the vacuolar H + -ATPase–Ragulator–Rag complex, which controls mTORC1 localization to lysosomes and thus, mTORC1 signaling [28].

DNA mutations in the *CTNS* gene have various functional consequences linked to their structural impact on cystinosin. Extensive deletions (such as the 57-kb deletion) cause the absence of protein, while severe truncating mutations lead to the synthesis of an inactive variant. Both these situations amount to a loss of cystinosin efflux function. In contrast, milder mutations allow the synthesized cystinosin variant to retain residual activity. It is interesting to hypothesize that, as well as canceling cystinosin efflux function, severe *CTNS* mutations impair the interaction between the Ragulator–Rag complex (of which cystinosin is a component) and mTORC1, preventing its activation. On the other hand, mutations of more limited structural impact might allow, to some extent, to maintain an efflux activity as well as the interaction between mTORC1 and the lysosomal membrane-attached Ragulator–Rag complex. This hypothesis would explain the correlation we observed at baseline between the severity of the mutation, its impact on cystinosin efflux function, and the outcome in terms of osteoclastogenesis (increased osteoclast number in the AP and IP groups, compared to the RA group). It could be argued that the downregulation of mTORC1 is due to the accumulation of cystine, which would logically be greater in the AP and IP groups. However, as shown in the Andrzejewska et al. study, decrease of lysosomal cystine levels by cysteamine did not rescue mTORC1 activation in proximal tubular cells, thus suggesting that the downregulation of mTORC1 is due to the absence of cystinosin rather than to the accumulation of cystine [28].

5. Conclusions

Bone involvement is a late complication of nephropathic cystinosis, whose recent description is linked to the considerable improvement in patients' survival under cysteamine therapy. In regards to its clinical importance and deleterious effects on patients' quality of life, recent international guidelines on evaluation and management of NC bone disease have been published, but its exact underlying pathophysiology remains to be fully determined.

In addition to its beneficial effects in terms of renal survival and overall morbidity and mortality, cysteamine has a direct effect on bone metabolism, which depends on the concentration at which it is administered. Here, the differences observed in terms of osteoclastic outcomes between the different genotypes confirm that cystinosin has a modulating role on osteoclastogenesis.

Author Contributions: Conceptualization, I.M.-G., O.P. and J.B.; methodology, I.M.-G., J.B. and S.G.; validation, I.M.-G. and J.B.; experiments, T.Q., I.M.-G. and C.A. (Candide Alioli); formal analysis, T.Q., I.M.-G., A.B.-T., C.A. (Cécile Acquaviva) and J.B.; investigation, T.Q.; patients' recruitment, A.S., O.B., A.B.-T., S.L., I.V., J.H.; software, S.V.; writing—original draft preparation, T.Q.; writing—review and editing, A.B.-T., C.A. (Cécile Acquaviva), I.M.-G. and J.B.; supervision, I.M.-G. and J.B.; funding acquisition, I.M.-G. and J.B. All authors have read and agreed to the published version of the manuscript.

Funding: J.B. and I.M.-G. received a research grant from the Cystinosis Research Foundation for the CYSTEA-BONE project. T.Q. received a personal grant from the *Agence Régionale de Santé Grand Est* (*Année Recherche* Fellowship). The funders had no role in the design of the study; in the collection, analyses, or interpretation of data; in the writing of the manuscript, or in the decision to publish the results.

Institutional Review Board Statement: The CYSTEABONE study was approved by the *Comité de Protection des Personnes Sud-Méditerranée IV* (2019-A00166-51).

Informed Consent Statement: All patients and/or parents gave informed oral consent (*Jardé type 3 protocol* by French law).

Data Availability Statement: Datasets analyzed during the current study are not publicly available but are available from the corresponding author on reasonable request.

Acknowledgments: The authors would like to thank Diane Platel (lab tech, INSERM 1033) for her daily help in the lab, and all patients who agreed to participate to this study.

Conflicts of Interest: T.Q., I.V., S.G., C.Al., S.V., O.P., I.M.-G. and J.B. declare no conflict of interest in association with this manuscript. A.B.-T. received speaker fees from Chiesi, A.S. received speaker fees from Chiesi and Recordati Rare Diseases, O.B. received a travel grant from Chiesi, J.H. received speaker fees from Recordati Rare Diseases, S.L. received consulting fees from Chiesi, and C.Ac. received consulting and travel fees from Chiesi.

References

1. Town, M.; Jean, G.; Cherqui, S.; Attard, M.; Forestier, L.; Whitmore, S.A.; Callen, D.F.; Gribouval, O.; Broyer, M.; Bates, G.P.; et al. A novel gene encoding an integral membrane protein is mutated in nephropathic cystinosis. *Nat. Genet.* **1998**, *18*, 319–324. [CrossRef]
2. David, D.; Princiero Berlingerio, S.; Elmonem, M.A.; Oliveira Arcolino, F.; Soliman, N.; van den Heuvel, B.; Gijsbers, R.; Levtchenko, E. Molecular Basis of Cystinosis: Geographic Distribution, Functional Consequences of Mutations in the CTNS Gene, and Potential for Repair. *Nephron* **2019**, *141*, 133–146. [CrossRef] [PubMed]
3. Gahl, W.A.; Thoene, J.G.; Schneider, J.A. Cystinosis. *N. Engl. J. Med.* **2002**, *347*, 111–121. [CrossRef] [PubMed]
4. Emma, F.; Nesterova, G.; Langman, C.; Labbé, A.; Cherqui, S.; Goodyer, P.; Janssen, M.C.; Greco, M.; Topaloglu, R.; Elenberg, E.; et al. Nephropathic cystinosis: An international consensus document. *Nephrol. Dial. Transplant.* **2014**, *29* (Suppl. 4), iv87–iv94. [CrossRef] [PubMed]
5. Markello, T.C.; Bernardini, I.M.; Gahl, W.A. Improved renal function in children with cystinosis treated with cysteamine. *N. Engl. J. Med.* **1993**, *328*, 1157–1162. [CrossRef]
6. Brodin-Sartorius, A.; Tête, M.-J.; Niaudet, P.; Antignac, C.; Guest, G.; Ottolenghi, C.; Charbit, M.; Moyse, D.; Legendre, C.; Lesavre, P.; et al. Cysteamine therapy delays the progression of nephropathic cystinosis in late adolescents and adults. *Kidney Int.* **2012**, *81*, 179–189. [CrossRef]
7. Gahl, W.A.; Balog, J.Z.; Kleta, R. Nephropathic cystinosis in adults: Natural history and effects of oral cysteamine therapy. *Ann. Intern. Med.* **2007**, *147*, 242–250. [CrossRef]
8. Hohenfellner, K.; Rauch, F.; Ariceta, G.; Awan, A.; Bacchetta, J.; Bergmann, C.; Bechtold, S.; Cassidy, N.; Deschenes, G.; Elenberg, E.; et al. Management of bone disease in cystinosis: Statement from an international conference. *J. Inherit. Metab. Dis.* **2019**, *42*, 1019–1029. [CrossRef]
9. Bertholet-Thomas, A.; Claramunt-Taberner, D.; Gaillard, S.; Deschênes, G.; Sornay-Rendu, E.; Szulc, P.; Cohen-Solal, M.; Pelletier, S.; Carlier, M.-C.; Cochat, P.; et al. Teenagers and young adults with nephropathic cystinosis display significant bone disease and cortical impairment. *Pediatr. Nephrol.* **2018**, *33*, 1165–1172. [CrossRef]
10. Florenzano, P.; Ferreira, C.; Nesterova, G.; Roberts, M.S.; Tella, S.H.; de Castro, L.F.; Brown, S.M.; Whitaker, A.; Pereira, R.C.; Bulas, D.; et al. Skeletal Consequences of Nephropathic Cystinosis. *J. Bone Miner. Res.* **2018**, *33*, 1870–1880. [CrossRef]
11. Machuca-Gayet, I.; Quinaux, T.; Bertholet-Thomas, A.; Gaillard, S.; Claramunt-Taberner, D.; Acquaviva-Bourdain, C.; Bacchetta, J. Bone Disease in Nephropathic Cystinosis: Beyond Renal Osteodystrophy. *Int. J. Mol. Sci.* **2020**, *21*, 3109. [CrossRef] [PubMed]
12. Conforti, A.; Taranta, A.; Biagini, S.; Starc, N.; Pitisci, A.; Bellomo, F.; Cirillo, V.; Locatelli, F.; Bernardo, M.E.; Emma, F. Cysteamine treatment restores the in vitro ability to differentiate along the osteoblastic lineage of mesenchymal stromal cells isolated from bone marrow of a cystinotic patient. *J. Transl. Med.* **2015**, *13*, 143. [CrossRef] [PubMed]
13. Battafarano, G.; Rossi, M.; Rega, L.R.; Di Giovamberardino, G.; Pastore, A.; D'Agostini, M.; Porzio, O.; Nevo, N.; Emma, F.; Taranta, A.; et al. Intrinsic Bone Defects in Cystinotic Mice. *Am. J. Pathol.* **2019**, *189*, 1053–1064. [CrossRef] [PubMed]
14. Claramunt-Taberner, D.; Flammier, S.; Gaillard, S.; Cochat, P.; Peyruchaud, O.; Machuca-Gayet, I.; Bacchetta, J. Bone disease in nephropathic cystinosis is related to cystinosin-induced osteoclastic dysfunction. *Nephrol. Dial. Transplant.* **2017**, *33*, 1525–1532. [CrossRef] [PubMed]
15. Ahlenstiel-Grunow, T.; Kanzelmeyer, N.K.; Froede, K.; Kreuzer, M.; Drube, J.; Lerch, C.; Pape, L. Switching from immediate- to extended-release cysteamine in nephropathic cystinosis patients: A retrospective real-life single-center study. *Pediatr. Nephrol.* **2017**, *32*, 91–97. [CrossRef] [PubMed]
16. Schwartz, G.J.; Work, D.F. Measurement and estimation of GFR in children and adolescents. *Clin. J. Am. Soc. Nephrol.* **2009**, *4*, 1832–1843. [CrossRef]
17. Ardeshirpour, L.; Cole, D.E.C.; Carpenter, T.O. Evaluation of bone and mineral disorders. *Pediatr. Endocrinol Rev.* **2007**, *5* (Suppl. 1), 584–598.

18. Shaw, J.L.V.; Cohen, A.; Konforte, D.; Binesh-Marvasti, T.; Colantonio, D.A.; Adeli, K. Validity of establishing pediatric reference intervals based on hospital patient data: A comparison of the modified Hoffmann approach to CALIPER reference intervals obtained in healthy children. *Clin. Biochem.* **2014**, *47*, 166–172. [CrossRef]
19. Bernardor, J.; Flammier, S.; Ranchin, B.; Gaillard, S.; Platel, D.; Peyruchaud, O.; Machuca-Gayet, I.; Bacchetta, J. Inhibition of osteoclast differentiation by 1.25-D and the calcimimetic KP2326 reveals 1.25-D resistance in advanced CKD. *J. Bone Miner. Res.* **2020**, *35*, 2265–2274. [CrossRef]
20. Kalatzis, V.; Nevo, N.; Cherqui, S.; Gasnier, B.; Antignac, C. Molecular pathogenesis of cystinosis: Effect of CTNS mutations on the transport activity and subcellular localization of cystinosin. *Hum. Mol. Genet.* **2004**, *13*, 1361–1371. [CrossRef]
21. Topaloglu, R.; Gulhan, B.; İnözü, M.; Canpolat, N.; Yilmaz, A.; Noyan, A.; Dursun, İ.; Gökçe, İ.; Gürgöze, M.K.; Akinci, N.; et al. The Clinical and Mutational Spectrum of Turkish Patients with Cystinosis. *Clin. J. Am. Soc. Nephrol.* **2017**, *12*, 1634–1641. [CrossRef]
22. Servais, A.; Morinière, V.; Grünfeld, J.-P.; Noël, L.-H.; Goujon, J.-M.; Chadefaux-Vekemans, B.; Antignac, C. Late-onset nephropathic cystinosis: Clinical presentation, outcome, and genotyping. *Clin. J. Am. Soc. Nephrol.* **2008**, *3*, 27–35. [CrossRef] [PubMed]
23. Kiehntopf, M.; Schickel, J.; von der Gönne, B.; Koch, H.G.; Superti-Furga, A.; Steinmann, B.; Deufel, T.; Harms, E. Analysis of the CTNS gene in patients of German and Swiss origin with nephropathic cystinosis. *Hum. Mutat.* **2002**, *20*, 237. [CrossRef] [PubMed]
24. Kalatzis, V.; Cherqui, S.; Jean, G.; Cordier, B.; Cochat, P.; Broyer, M.; Antignac, C. Characterization of a putative founder mutation that accounts for the high incidence of cystinosis in Brittany. *J. Am. Soc. Nephrol.* **2001**, *12*, 2170–2174. [CrossRef] [PubMed]
25. Soliman, N.A.; Elmonem, M.A.; van den Heuvel, L.; Abdel Hamid, R.H.; Gamal, M.; Bongaers, I.; Marie, S.; Levtchenko, E. Mutational Spectrum of the CTNS Gene in Egyptian Patients with Nephropathic Cystinosis. *JIMD Rep.* **2014**, *14*, 87–97. [CrossRef] [PubMed]
26. Shotelersuk, V.; Larson, D.; Anikster, Y.; McDowell, G.; Lemons, R.; Bernardini, I.; Guo, J.; Thoene, J.; Gahl, W.A. CTNS mutations in an American-based population of cystinosis patients. *Am. J. Hum. Genet.* **1998**, *63*, 1352–1362. [CrossRef]
27. Gaillard, S.; Roche, L.; Lemoine, S.; Deschênes, G.; Morin, D.; Vianey-Saban, C.; Acquaviva-Bourdain, C.; Ranchin, B.; Bacchetta, J.; Kassai, B.; et al. Adherence to cysteamine in nephropathic cystinosis: A unique electronic monitoring experience for a better understanding. A prospective cohort study: CrYSTobs. *Pediatr. Nephrol.* **2021**, *36*, 581–589. [CrossRef]
28. Andrzejewska, Z.; Nevo, N.; Thomas, L.; Chhuon, C.; Bailleux, A.; Chauvet, V.; Courtoy, P.J.; Chol, M.; Guerrera, I.C.; Antignac, C. Cystinosin is a Component of the Vacuolar H+-ATPase-Ragulator-Rag Complex Controlling Mammalian Target of Rapamycin Complex 1 Signaling. *J. Am. Soc. Nephrol.* **2016**, *27*, 1678–1688. [CrossRef]

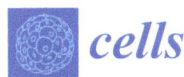

Article

Benefits and Toxicity of Disulfiram in Preclinical Models of Nephropathic Cystinosis

Anna Taranta [1,*], Mohamed A. Elmonem [2,3], Francesco Bellomo [1], Ester De Leo [1], Sara Boenzi [4], Manoe J. Janssen [5], Amer Jamalpoor [5], Sara Cairoli [4], Anna Pastore [6], Cristiano De Stefanis [7], Manuela Colucci [1], Laura R. Rega [1], Isabella Giovannoni [8], Paola Francalanci [8], Lambertus P. van den Heuvel [3,9], Carlo Dionisi-Vici [4], Bianca M. Goffredo [4], Rosalinde Masereeuw [5], Elena Levtchenko [3,10] and Francesco Emma [1,11]

1. Renal Diseases Research Unit, Genetics and Rare Diseases Research Division, Bambino Gesù Children's Hospital, IRCCS, 00165 Rome, Italy; francesco.bellomo@opbg.net (F.B.); ester.deleo@opbg.net (E.D.L.); manuela.colucci@opbg.net (M.C.); laurarita.rega@opbg.net (L.R.R.); francesco.emma@opbg.net (F.E.)
2. Department of Clinical and Chemical Pathology, Faculty of Medicine, Cairo University, Cairo 11956, Egypt; mohamed.abdelmonem@kasralainy.edu.eg
3. Laboratory of Pediatric Nephrology, Department of Development and Regeneration, KU Leuven, 3000 Leuven, Belgium; Bert.vandenHeuvel@radboudumc.nl (L.P.v.d.H.); elena.levtchenko@uzleuven.be (E.L.)
4. Laboratory of Metabolic Biochemistry Unit, Department of Pediatric Medicine, Bambino Gesù Children's Hospital, IRCCS, 00165 Rome, Italy; sara.boenzi@opbg.net (S.B.); sara.cairoli@opbg.net (S.C.); carlo.dionisivici@opbg.net (C.D.-V.); bianca.goffredo@opbg.net (B.M.G.)
5. Division of Pharmacology, Utrecht Institute for Pharmaceutical Sciences, Utrecht University, 3584 CG Utrecht, The Netherlands; m.j.janssen1@uu.nl (M.J.J.); a.jamalpoor@uu.nl (A.J.); r.masereeuw@uu.nl (R.M.)
6. Genetics and Rare Diseases Research Division, Bambino Gesù Children's Hospital, IRCCS, 00165 Rome, Italy; anna.pastore@opbg.net
7. Histology-Core Facility, Bambino Gesù Children's Hospital, IRCCS, 00165 Rome, Italy; cristiano.destefanis@opbg.net
8. Department of Pathology, Bambino Gesù Children's Hospital, IRCCS, 00165 Rome, Italy; isabella.giovannoni@opbg.net (I.G.); paola.francalanci@opbg.net (P.F.)
9. Department of Pediatric Nephrology, Radboud University Medical Center, 6525 GA Nijmegen, The Netherlands
10. Division of Pediatric Nephrology, Department of Pediatrics, University Hospitals Leuven, 3000 Leuven, Belgium
11. Division of Nephrology, Department of Pediatric Subspecialities, Bambino Gesù Children's Hospital, IRCSS, 00165 Rome, Italy
* Correspondence: anna.taranta@opbg.net; Tel.: +39-06-6859-2997

Abstract: Nephropathic cystinosis is a rare disease caused by mutations of the CTNS gene that encodes for cystinosin, a lysosomal cystine/H+ symporter. The disease is characterized by early-onset chronic kidney failure and progressive development of extra-renal complications related to cystine accumulation in all tissues. At the cellular level, several alterations have been demonstrated, including enhanced apoptosis, altered autophagy, defective intracellular trafficking, and cell oxidation, among others. Current therapy with cysteamine only partially reverts some of these changes, highlighting the need to develop additional treatments. Among compounds that were identified in a previous drug-repositioning study, disulfiram (DSF) was selected for in vivo studies. The cystine depleting and anti-apoptotic properties of DSF were confirmed by secondary in vitro assays and after treating $Ctns^{-/-}$ mice with 200 mg/kg/day of DSF for 3 months. However, at this dosage, growth impairment was observed. Long-term treatment with a lower dose (100 mg/kg/day) did not inhibit growth, but failed to reduce cystine accumulation, caused premature death, and did not prevent the development of renal lesions. In addition, DSF also caused adverse effects in cystinotic zebrafish larvae. DSF toxicity was significantly more pronounced in $Ctns^{-/-}$ mice and zebrafish compared to wild-type animals, suggesting higher cell toxicity of DSF in cystinotic cells.

Keywords: cystinosis; disulfiram; mice; zebrafish

1. Introduction

Nephropathic cystinosis (NC) is an inherited metabolic disease secondary to mutations in the CTNS gene, which encodes for cystinosin, a cystine proton symporter allowing efflux of cystine from lysosomes [1]. In patients with NC, cystine progressively accumulates in nearly all tissues. Symptoms begin with renal Fanconi syndrome in the first year of life, followed by cystine crystal depositions in the cornea [2]. In time, patients develop other symptoms, including hypothyroidism, pancreatic insufficiency, gonadal failure, poor growth, myopathy, cholestatic liver disease, and central and peripheral nervous system involvement [3]. Kidney damage is characterized in part by increased apoptosis of proximal tubular cells in mice [4], confirming previous in vitro studies showing that cystinotic cells are more sensitive to apoptotic stimuli [5,6].

Cysteamine was approved for the treatment of NC in the 1990s, and allows cystine clearance from lysosomes through the formation of a mixed cysteine–cysteamine disulfide that can exit lysosomes through the PQLC2 transporter [7]. Cysteamine significantly improves NC, but does not cure the disease. Despite adequate treatment, the majority of patients progress to end-stage kidney disease in the second or third decade of life [8].

In order to identify new molecules that can improve the treatment of patients with NC, two drug screenings were performed using conditionally immortalized human cystinotic proximal tubule cells [9]. A high throughput screening based on cell cystine concentration identified 24 compounds that reduced cystine content by >50%. Similarly, a high content screening identified 27 compounds that decreased apoptosis (caspase-3/7 positivity) by >40% [9]. We combined results from these two screenings, and identified disulfiram (DSF) as a potential treatment for cystinosis. Herein, we report the results of in vitro and in vivo studies assessing the efficacy of DSF in cystinotic human proximal tubule epithelial cells, mice, and zebrafish. Our results confirm the cystine-depleting and anti-apoptotic effects of DSF, but show significant toxicity that is enhanced in cystinotic animal models.

2. Materials and Methods

2.1. Cell Culture

In vitro assays were performed using conditionally immortalized proximal tubule epithelial cells (ciPTECs) obtained from the urine of a patient with nephropathic cystinosis or from healthy controls that have been described elsewhere [10] and were provided to us by Radboud University Medical Center (Nijmegen, The Netherlands). Growth media included DMEM-F12 medium supplemented with 10% FBS, Penicillin (100 U/mL)/Streptomycin (0.1 mg/mL), ITS (5 µg/mL Insulin, 5 µg/mL Transferrin, 5 ng/mL Selenium), hydrocortisone (36 ng/mL), EGF (10 ng/mL), and tri-iodothyronine (40 pg/mL). Cells were grown at 33 °C for proliferation and 37 °C for 7 days to allow differentiation. Medium, FBS and Penicillin/Streptomycin were supplied by Gibco (Thermo Fisher Scientific, Waltham, MA, USA). All other reagents were from Sigma-Aldrich (Merck, Darmstadt, Germany).

2.2. Quantitative Determination of Cystine in Cells

Cystinotic ciPTECs were seeded at a density of 5×10^4 cells/well in 48-well plates. After 48 h, cells grown at 33 °C were treated with different concentrations of DSF (from 0.1 to 100 µM) and cysteamine. After 24 h, cells were washed twice in PBS and lysed in 75 µL of 10 mM N-ethylmaleimide (NEM) with five freezing/thawing cycles. Cell lysates were precipitated with 75 µL of 10% 5-sulfosalicylic acid (SSA) and left overnight at 4 °C. Plates were then centrifuged at $3900 \times g$ for 15 min at 4 °C. Supernatant (25 µL) was analyzed by reverse-phase high-performance liquid chromatography and fluorescence detection (HPLC-FLD) for thiol measurements [11]. The remaining samples were used to measure protein content after adding 50 µL of 0.1 M NaOH and BCA reagent (Bio Rad Laboratories, Hercules, CA, USA).

2.3. Measurement of Apoptosis in Cells

Cystinotic ciPTECs were seeded at a density of 4×10^3 cells/well in 384-well plates coated with poly-D-lysine (Perkin Elmer, Waltham, MA, USA). After 48 h, cells were pre-treated with different concentrations of DSF for one hour and apoptosis was induced with Fas-ligand (0.5 µg/mL) and cycloheximide (10 µg/ml) for 5 h. ciPTECs were then incubated with 4 µM of cellEvent probe (Invitrogen life technologies, Carlsbad, CA, USA) for 30 min. This reagent is a cell permeant dye that emits fluorescence when cleaved by caspases-3/7. For the analysis, cells were fixed in 4% paraformaldehyde and nuclei were stained with Hoechst 33258. Cells were imaged with the automated Opera system (Perkin Elmer, Beaconsfield, UK). Apoptotic cells were quantified as positive nuclei/total number of cells. We performed 16 replicas per each treatment; 250 cells/well were analyzed.

2.4. Cell Viability Assay

Cystinotic and wild-type ciPTECs were seeded at a density of 55×10^3 cells/cm^2 and grown at 33 °C for 24 h and 37 °C for 7 days. Cells were then treated for 24 h with L-cysteine (1.8 mM), N-acetyl cysteine (1.8 mM), DSF (different concentrations; see below), or a combination of the above. Cell viability was evaluated using the PrestoBlue Cell Viability Reagent (Thermo Fisher Scientific) according to the manufacturer's instructions.

2.5. Redox Status

Cystinotic ciPTECs were seeded and grown as described above. After treatment with 10 µM DSF, cells were incubated with CellROX Green Reagent (Thermo Fisher Scientific) for 30 min at room temperature and reactive oxygen species (ROS) were measured by live cell flow cytometry. GSH and GSSG levels were analyzed as described by Jamalpoor et al., who have performed extensive metabolomic investigations in the same cell conditions [12].

2.6. Tandem Mass Spectrometry

L-cystine (416 µM at pH 7.4) and DSF (200 µM in DMSO) were stirred overnight at RT. Tandem mass spectrometry analyses were carried out on a 4000-QTRAP mass spectrometer (ABSciex, Toronto, ON, Canada), equipped with a Turbo Ion Spray Source operating in positive ion mode with a needle potential of 5500 V. The flow rate of mobile phase was set at 150 µL/min and infused into the spectrometer using an Agilent 1290 infinity pump (Agilent Technologies Inc., Wilmington, DE, USA). Instrument setting and calibration were performed with 10 µM DSF and 10 µM cystine solutions. The analysis was conducted to evaluate the formation of hybrid disulfide molecule of 269 m/z.

2.7. Studies on Cystinotic Mice

Ctns knockout mice (C57BL/6 background) were kindly provided by Dr. Corinne Antignac [13]. Animal care and experimental procedures were conducted in accordance with the European 2010/63/EU directive on the protection of animals used for scientific purposes, and authorized by the Italian Ministry of Health (authorization number 230/2015-PR).

Drugs were mixed with standard 4RF21 diet and prepared in pellets (Mucedola, Settimo Milanese, Italy). Concentrations of drug in pellets were calculated based on the average daily food intake (approximately 3 g/day) and body weight (approximately 22 g) of female mice, to administer estimated doses of 50, 100, and 200 mg/kg of body weight/day of DSF. Female mice started treatment at 2 months of age. Animal length and weight were measured monthly. Every two months, mice were acclimatized in metabolic cages for 24 h, and their urine was collected for 24 h. Blood samples were collected at sacrifice. Analyzed parameters included urine volume, electrolytes, glucose, proteins, BUN, and creatinine. Measurements were performed by the Appia Laboratory (Rome, Italy). In addition, low-molecular weight proteinuria was estimated using the Clara cell 16 protein (CC16) as a marker (Biomatik Corporation, Kitchener, ON, Canada). Power analysis was performed to calculate the minimum number of mice per treatment arm.

2.8. Quantitative Determination of Diethyldithiocarbamate (DDC) and Cystine in Tissues

For DDC quantitative determination, 10 mg of tissue samples were sonicated in 100 µL NaCl 0.9% solution. The supernatant (50 µL) was extracted with 200 µL of acetonitrile, vortexed and centrifuged at 18,000× g for 9 min. A solution of DDC was prepared by dissolving in methanol to make up a standard solution of 1 mg/mL.

For cystine quantitative determination, tissue samples were sonicated in the presence of 10 mM NEM. Homogenates were centrifuged at 1000× g for 5 min and supernatants were mixed with 10% SSA (3:1 volume ratio), incubated at 4 °C for 60 min, and centrifuged at 20,000× g for 15 min. The supernatants (50 µL) were spiked with 50 µL of the internal standard solution (Cystine d6). The mixture was then extracted with 200 µL of acetonitrile, vortexed and centrifuged at 18,000× g for 9 min. Protein concentrations were measured on the first supernatant using Bio-Rad Protein Assay Reagent Kit (Bio-Rad Laboratories Inc.), following the manufacturer's protocol. All chemicals were of analytical grade and were obtained from Sigma-Aldrich (St. Louis, MO, USA).

Liquid chromatography/mass spectrometry analysis was performed using a UHPLC Agilent 1290 Infinity II 6470 (Agilent Technologies Inc.) equipped with an ESI-JET-STREAM source operating in positive ion (ESI+) mode. The MassHunter Workstation software (Agilent Technologies Inc.) was used for data analysis. InfinityLab Poroshell 120 HILIC 1.9 µm 100 × 2.1 mm (Agilent Technologies Inc.) were used as separation columns. A full validation assay was performed, including selectivity, specificity, linearity, limits of quantification, accuracy, precision, matrix effects, recovery, and stability.

2.9. Measurement of Apoptosis in Tissue

Immunohistochemistry was performed on 2 µm thick sections obtained from formalin-fixed tissue embedded in paraffin. After dewaxing and rehydrating, heat-induced epitope retrieval was performed by boiling the slides with sodium citrate (pH 6) (Dako, Glostrup, Denmark). Endogenous peroxidase was blocked with 3% hydrogen peroxide and then with 5% BSA. Sections were incubated overnight at 4 °C with rabbit monoclonal (9661S) to Cleaved Caspase-3 (Cell Signaling Technology, Danvers, MA, USA), diluted 1:400. Detection of the primary antibody was performed by using the appropriate secondary biotinylated antibody (K8024) (ready to use) (Dako, Carpinteria, CA, USA) and the peroxidase DAB kit (Dako, Carpinteria, CA, USA). Counterstaining was performed with hematoxylin solution Gill2.

2.10. Zebrafish Assays

Experiments were performed on wild-type and cystinotic zebrafish larvae that have already been characterized [14]. Adult fish were raised at 28.5 °C, on a 14/10 h light/dark cycle under standard aquaculture conditions [15]. Fertilized wild-type or cystinotic embryos (20–30 per well) were transferred to 6-well plates containing 5 mL of clean egg water (Instant Ocean Sea Salts 60 µg/mL + methylene blue 0.5 ppm). DSF was dissolved directly in the egg water at the specified concentrations. Embryos were incubated at 28.5 °C in the dark and the medium was refreshed daily. Wells were cleaned from debris daily and dead embryos were removed and counted. Larvae viability was monitored for the first 96 h post-fertilization (hpf). Hatching rates were calculated in surviving embryos at 48, 72, and 96 hpf. Final deformity rates were evaluated at 96 hpf. Animal care and experimental procedures were conducted in accordance with the ethical committee guidelines for laboratory animal experimentation at KU Leuven, in accordance with the European 2010/63/EU directive on the protection of animals used for scientific purposes.

For cystine quantitative determination, homogenates of surviving zebrafish larvae were assessed using liquid chromatography tandem mass spectrometry. Groups of 30–60 larvae for each condition were homogenized by sonication in 200 µL of 5 mM NEM in 0.1 M PBS. Then, 100 µL of 12% SSA was added to each homogenate and samples were centrifuged for 10 min at 4 °C at 12,000× g. Supernatants were used for cystine measurements and stored at

−80 °C. Pellets for protein measurements were dissolved overnight at 4 °C in 300 μL of 0.1 M NaOH, and stored at −80 °C.

2.11. Statistical Analysis

Categorical data are represented as counts and percentages. Continuous normal data are expressed as mean ± standard error of the mean. Continuous data that do not follow a normal distribution are expressed as median value and interquartile range. Normality of data was tested with the D'Agostino–Pearson test. The Chi-squared test was used to compare hatching and deformity rates. Student's *t*-test, ANOVA followed by Bonferroni's post-hoc correction, and the Mann–Whitney U-test were used as appropriate. Survival was estimated by the Kaplan–Meier method and assessed by the Log-Rank test. All *p*-values are two-sided and considered significant for $p < 0.05$. Statistical analyses were performed using the GraphPad Prism 6 software (San Diego, CA, USA).

3. Results

3.1. In Vitro DSF Studies

At the end of two drug screenings [9] that used cystine accumulation and apoptosis as read-outs, we identified six compounds that showed positive effects in both assays. Among these, we selected DSF for future tests, based on its pharmacological properties and known safety profile.

Unlike cysteamine, which is the current standard of care for cystinosis, DSF is a disulfide compound composed of two S-methyl-N,N-diethyldithiocarbamate (DDC), lacking free sulfhydryl residues (Figure 1A,B).

We hypothesized that under physiologic conditions, cystine and DSF are in equilibrium with their reduced form, allowing the formation of mixed disulfides. To this end, we co-incubated liquid solutions of DSF and cystine for 14 h at room temperature and analyzed them by tandem mass spectrometry. As illustrated in Figure 1C, several mixed disulfides formed, indicating that the cystine-lowering effect of DSF is likely mediated by the formation of mixed disulfides that can bypass the non-functioning cystinosin transporter, similarly to what has been described for cysteamine.

We then performed dose-response experiments to identify the lowest concentration of DSF that prevented cystine accumulation and apoptosis in cystinotic ciPTEC and compared the effect with cysteamine. As shown in Figure 2A, DSF lowered cystine slightly better (IC50: 9 μM) than cysteamine (IC50: 22 μM). DSF also prevented apoptosis at concentrations ≥2.5 μM (Figure 2B).

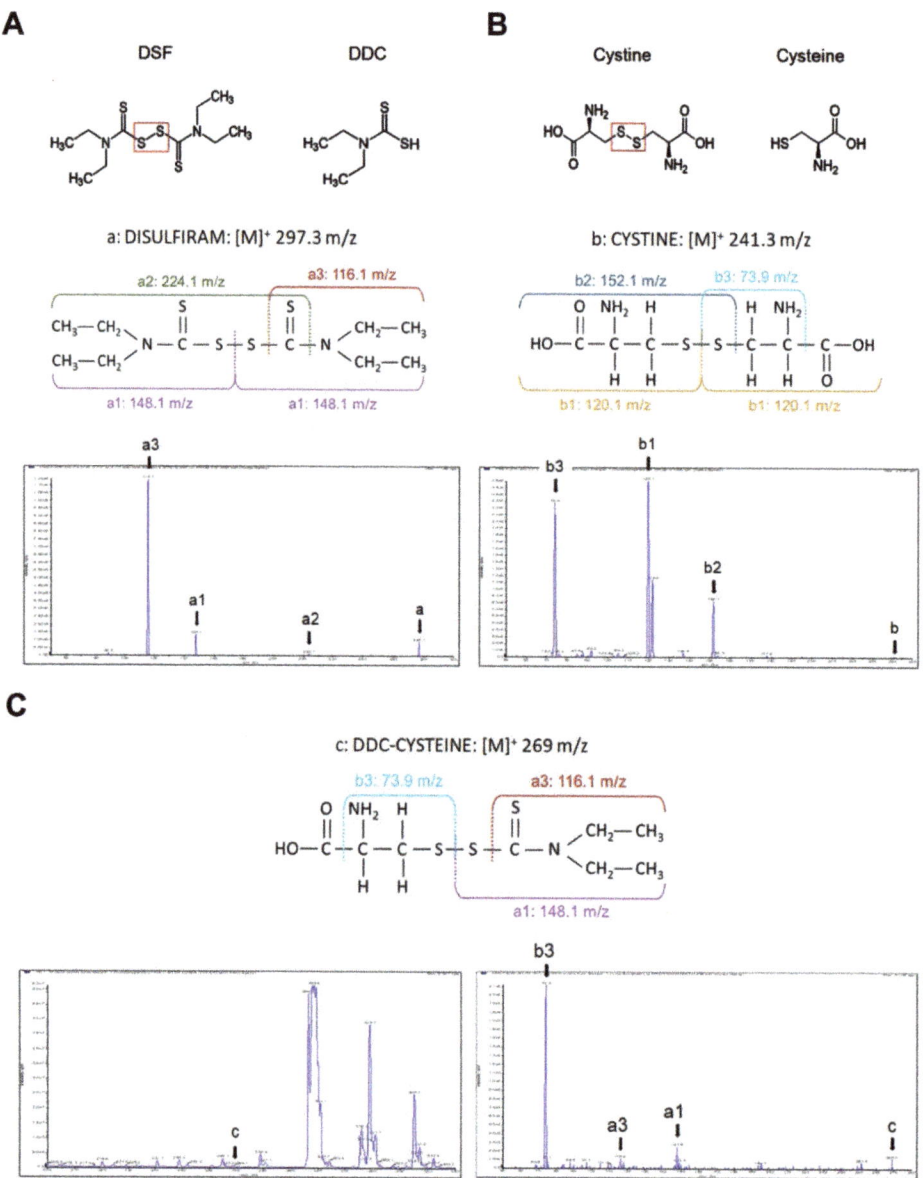

Figure 1. MS/MS determination of DSF, cystine and mixed-disulfides. (**A**) Chemical structures of DSF and diethyldithiocarbamate (DDC). The chromatogram shows peaks corresponding to DSF (a), half molecule of DSF (a1) and two molecules obtained by breaking the carbon-sulfur bond (a2 and a3). (**B**) Chemical structures of cystine and cysteine. The chromatogram shows peaks corresponding to cystine (b), half molecule of cystine (b1), and fragments obtained after breaking carbon-sulfur (b2) and carbon–carbon bonds (b3). (**C**) Mixed disulfides. The chromatogram on the left panel shows a peak indicating the formation of a mixed-disulfide with a calculated mass–charge ratio (m/z) of 269 (c). The right panel shows the product ion scan for the 269 m/z peak, identifying three fragments: the 148 m/z peak corresponds to half molecules of DSF (a1), the 116 m/z peak is produced by thiol-ester bond cleavage of DSF (a3), and the 74 m/z peak corresponds to cystine (b3).

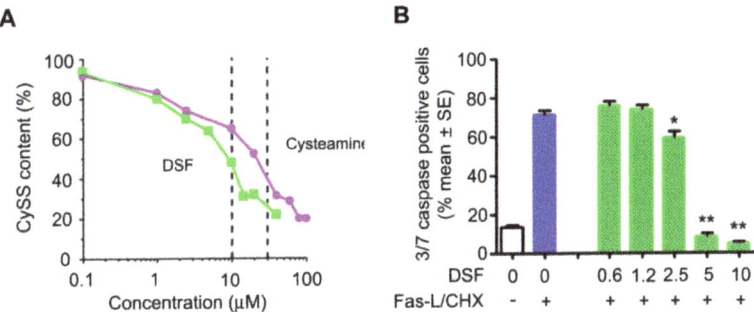

Figure 2. Cystine-depleting and anti-apoptotic proprieties of DSF. (**A**) Comparison of dose–response curves. Cystine (CySS) accumulation was measured after treatment for 24 h with the indicated concentrations of DSF and cysteamine in cystinotic ciPTECs. Vertical dashed lines indicate IC50 for DSF (9 µM) and cysteamine (22 µM). Data represent 4 independent experiments. (**B**) Anti-apoptotic dose response of DSF. The white and blue columns indicate spontaneous or induced apoptosis with Fas-Ligand (Fas-L) and cycloheximide (CHX) in cystinotic ciPTECs, respectively. The green columns indicate the treatment with DSF (0.6–10 µM) in cells exposed to apoptotic stimuli. Data represent 3 independent experiments. * $p < 0.005$ and ** $p < 0.0005$ vs. blue column.

3.2. In Vivo Studies: Murine Treatment with High DSF Dose

Based on the above results, we treated *Ctns* knockout (KO) mice with DSF. KO and wild-type (WT) animals received DSF in food from the age of 2 months. Two different concentrations of DSF were initially used, corresponding to an estimated daily dose of 100 (low dose) or 200 (high dose) mg/kg (see methods). We rapidly observed in both WT and KO animals significant growth impairment after DSF treatment, especially at the highest dose (Figures 3A and 4A). We therefore decided to sacrifice animals treated with the 200 mg/kg/day dose for three months (i.e., at 5 months of age). Biochemical and histopathological parameters were evaluated to measure kidneys and liver function.

From the kidney standpoint, untreated KO mice at 5 months of age had more glycosuria compared to WT animals, and developed marked low-molecular weight proteinuria (LMWP) (Table 1). Treatment with high-dose DSF decreased glucose excretion, increased calciuria, and had no impact on low-molecular weight proteinuria (Table 1). Serum creatinine and blood urea nitrogen levels were unchanged (data not shown).

Table 1. Urinary parameters in WT and KO mice treated with high DSF dose for three months.

		WT		KO	
Urine Tests	Measure Unit	Untreated	DSF 200	Untreated	DSF 200
Albumin	µg/mg Creatinine	5.05 [3.49–12.1]	7.66 [6.59–11.1]	8.58 [5.02–9.79]	20.7 [10.5–76.3]
Glucose	mg/mg Creatinine	0.29 [0.26–1.02]	0.34 [0.24–0.78]	7.59 [4.41–16.2] §	0.40 [0.28–1.66] *
LMWP	µg/mg Creatinine	38.2 [13.8–39.5]	37.7 [10.2–69.1]	157 [75.1–447] §	258 [79.6–474]
Calcium	mg/mg Creatinine	0.12 [0.09–0.17]	0.12 [0.09–0.18]	0.21 [0.15–0.26]	1.17 [0.52–3.36] *
Phosphate	mg/mg Creatinine	0.60 [0.14–1.66]	1.51 [0.15–2.88]	0.66 [0.15–1.85]	2.58 [0.99–6.43]

Data are represented as median [interquartile range]; $n = 4$ mice per group. Low molecular weight proteins (LMWP), 200 mg/kg/day DSF dose (DSF 200). § $p < 0.05$ untreated WT mice vs. untreated KO mice; * $p < 0.05$ untreated KO mice vs. treated KO mice.

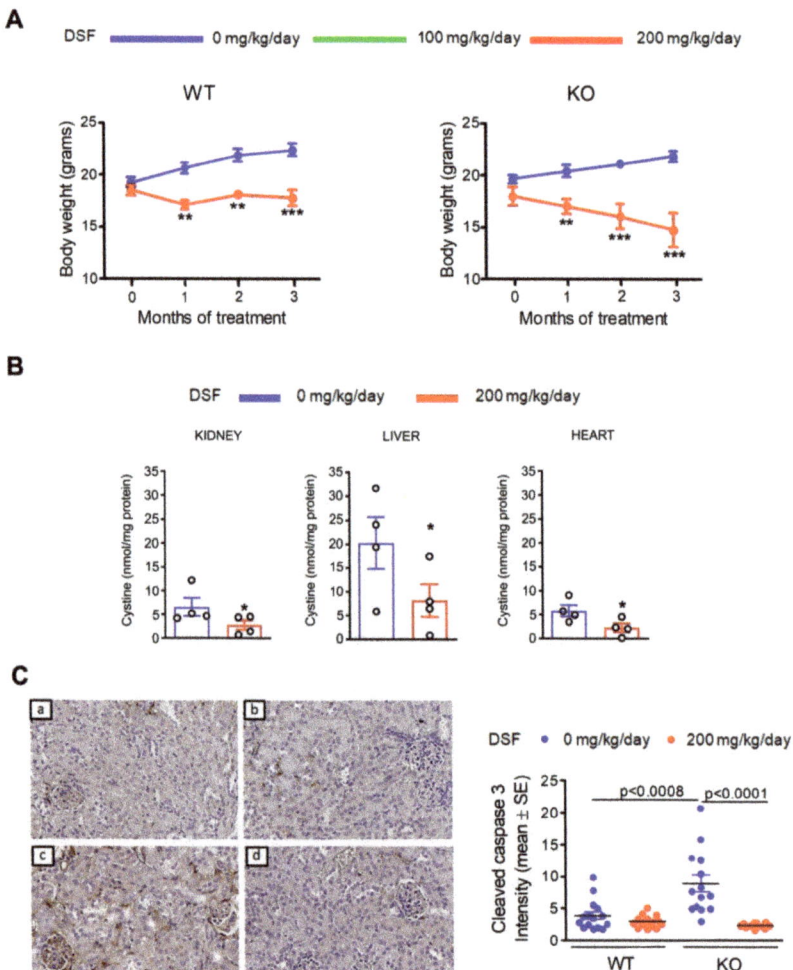

Figure 3. Short-term treatment with high DSF dose. Two-month-old mice were fed on standard or DSF-supplemented diet at an estimated dose of 200 mg/kg of body weight/day. (**A**) Body weight in animals fed on standard or DSF-supplemented diets for three months. Data are shown as mean ± SEM; n = 9 WT and 4 KO mice; ** $p < 0.005$, *** $p < 0.0005$ compared to untreated animals. (**B**) Cystine content in kidneys, liver, and heart of KO animals sacrificed at 5 months of age (n = 4 mice per group). Values are indicated as mean ± SEM; * $p < 0.05$ compared to untreated mice. (**C**) Representative immunohistochemistry images stained with anti-cleaved caspase-3 antibodies in kidneys obtained from WT (**a,b**) and KO (**c,d**) mice that were fed on standard (**a,c**) or DSF-supplemented (**b,d**) diets. Scale bar: 100 µm. The graph shows the mean cleaved caspase-3 intensity measured on five separate slides per animal (n = 3 mice per group).

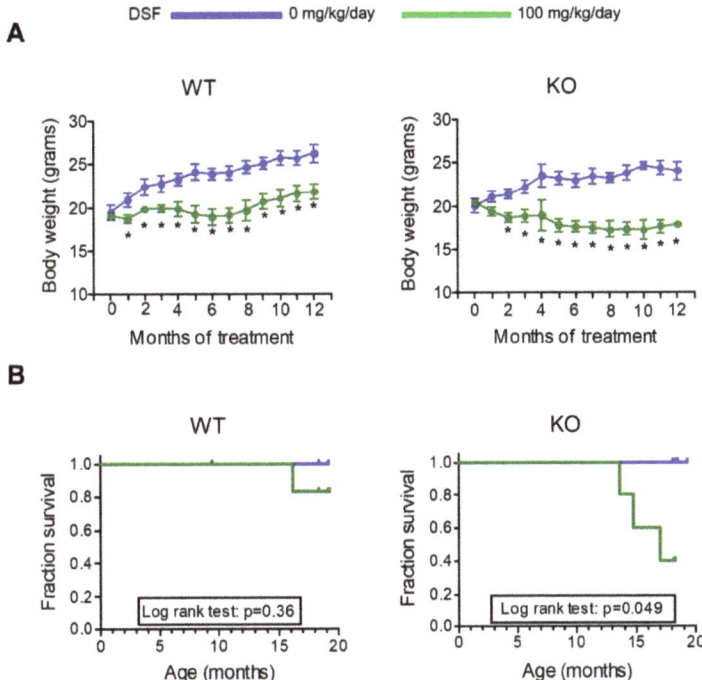

Figure 4. Long-term treatment with low DSF dose. Two-month-old mice were fed on standard or DSF-supplemented diets at an estimated dose of 100 mg/kg/day for 16 months. (**A**) Body weight; data are shown as mean ± SEM; n = 5 mice per group; * $p < 0.05$ compared to untreated animals. (**B**) Kaplan–Meier survival curves in the same animals.

Evaluation of liver function tests revealed increased plasma alkaline phosphatase levels in DSF-treated animals compared to untreated animals, which did not exceed the normal range (Table S1). All other studied markers were unaltered (Table S1). By standard liver histology techniques, we did not observe abnormal changes, including fibrosis, steatosis, inflammation, or signs of hepatocellular damage (data not shown).

After sacrifice, we measured the impact of DSF on cystine accumulation and apoptosis. As shown in Figure 3B, cystine content was decreased in the kidneys, liver, and heart of DSF-treated KO mice. Kidney histology did not show pathological changes, including tubular atrophy, interstitial fibrosis, mesangial expansion, or glomerular damage in both DSF-treated and untreated KO animals (data not shown). However, an increased number of apoptotic cells was observed in untreated cystinotic kidneys (Figure 3C), but not in kidneys from KO animals treated with high-dose DSF (Figure 3C), confirming the in vitro observations (Figure 2B).

3.3. In Vivo Studies: Murine Treatment with Low DSF Dose

Animals receiving 100 mg/kg/day DSF dose were monitored for 18 months. Urine parameters were available every 2 months, until the age of 1 year. Intermediate results are illustrated in Figure S1; results at 12 months are detailed in Table 2. At 1 year of age, KO mice had markedly more albuminuria, low-molecular weight proteinuria, and diuresis compared to WT mice. DSF treatment failed to improve urinary parameters.

Table 2. Urinary parameters in WT and KO mice at 12 months of age, after 10 months of treatment with DSF.

		WT		KO	
Urine Tests	Measure Unit	Untreated	DSF 100	Untreated	DSF 100
Albumin	μg/mg Creatinine	5.05 [4.26–6.40]	11.5 [5.68–13.8]	15.1 [14.4–36.2] [§]	19.0 [17.9–36.8] [*]
Glucose	mg/mg Creatinine	0.18 [0.08–0.84]	0.42 [0.19–1.12]	2.71 [1.34–3.85] [§]	9.00 [4.21–29.4] [*]
LMWP	μg/mg Creatinine	16.4 [5.30–26.6]	35.4 [26.8–63.2]	1939 [985–4353] [§]	5758 [1434–13972] [*]
Calcium	mg/mg Creatinine	0.30 [0.25–0.35]	0.26 [0.22–0.35]	0.32 [0.30–0.57]	0.42 [0.21–0.54]
Phosphate	mg/mg Creatinine	2.08 [0.70–2.77]	1.74 [0.17–2.50]	2.93 [1.47–3.56]	2.62 [1.03–3.53]
Diuresis	ml	1.20 [0.75–2.10]	1.75 [1.62–2.00]	3.05 [2.32–3.25] [§]	3.00 [1.60–3.25]

Data are represented as median [interquartile range]; $n = 5$ mice per group. Low molecular weight proteins (LMWP), 100 mg/kg/day DSF dose (DSF 100). [§] $p < 0.05$ untreated WT mice vs. untreated KO mice; [*] $p < 0.05$ untreated WT mice vs. treated KO mice.

On average, body weight of mice treated with DSF was lower compared to untreated animals (Figure 4A). After the age of 12 months, mice were followed until death or sacrificed at 18 months. As shown in Figure 4B, treatment with DSF decreased survival only in KO animals ($p = 0.049$).

During the initial dose-testing assays, we also tested a pilot cohort of five KO mice treated with a DSF dose of ~50 mg/kg/day. Of these, three animals died between 16 and 18 months. Since most animals treated with the 100 mg/kg/day dose had died before the age of 18 months, we pooled together the data of four surviving KO animals treated with either 50 or 100 mg/kg/day of DSF. These results are shown in Table S2 and Supplementary Figure S2. We observed no significant differences between treated and untreated animals. In particular, we failed to observe a decrease in tissue cystine content, unlike what we observed at 5 months in animals treated with the 200 mg/kg/day dose. This was not related to decreased food intake, which was monitored, and is further substantiated by high DDC levels in tissues obtained from treated animals (Figure S2).

3.4. In Vivo Studies: Zebrafish Embryos and Larvae

In parallel to murine studies, we performed assays on cystinotic (KO) zebrafish to assess DSF safety. WT and KO zebrafish embryos were treated within 1 h after fertilization with different concentrations of DSF. Hatching rates were monitored at 48, 72, and 96 h post-fertilization (hpf) and dysmorphic features were analyzed at 96 hpf. Embryos were monitored for mortality rates at different time points (6, 12, 24, 48, 72, and 96 hpf). As shown in Figure 5A, the mortality rate was higher in untreated KO larvae than in untreated WT larvae ($p < 0.007$). Larvae mortality increased very rapidly with increasing doses of DSF in KO fishes (Figure 5B). The 50% lethal concentration of DSF (LD50) was 146 μM in WT embryos and 2 μM in KO embryos (96 hpf).

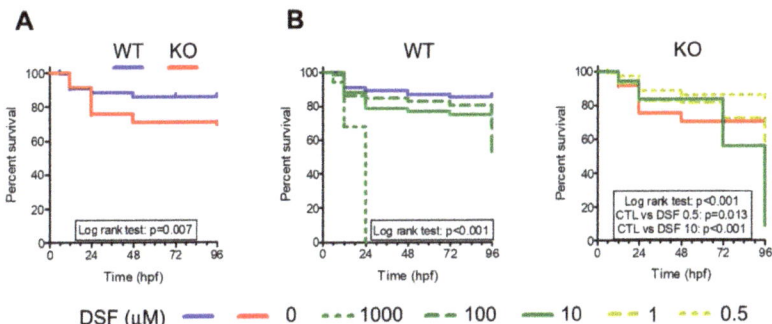

Figure 5. Effect of DSF on survival in wild-type (WT) and cystinotic (KO) zebrafish embryos and larvae. (**A**) Survival curves of untreated KO ($n = 82$) and WT ($n = 126$) embryos and larvae. (**B**) Survival curves of WT and KO embryos treated with different DSF concentrations as indicated in the figure legend. All curves are obtained from at least 100 larvae. Survival was monitored for 96 h post-fertilization (hpf).

Similarly, hatching was delayed and larval malformations were significantly more frequent in zebrafish treated with DSF (Figure 6A–C). These effects were observed at very low DSF concentrations (0.5 µM) in KO larvae, and were remarkably less pronounced in WT larvae, indicating increased sensitivity to DSF in cystinotic larvae. The average cystine levels after exposure of KO larvae to 1 µM DSF for 120 h was 2.4 ± 0.87 and 3.7 ± 0.54 nM cystine/mg protein in untreated ($n = 11$) and treated ($n = 3$) larval homogenates, respectively. At these DSF concentrations, the drug had no apparent cystine lowering effect. At higher concentrations, DSF was too toxic. Taken together, the above results suggest that DSF has a specific toxicity in cystinotic zebrafish.

3.5. N-Acetyl Cysteine Can Rescue Disulfiram Toxicity in Cystinotic Cells

Based on our in vivo results, we hypothesized that DSF reacts with free cellular thiols, oxidizing the cells (Figure 7).

We therefore measured in vitro the redox status in cystinotic ciPTEC treated with 10 µM DSF for 24 h. This dose was shown to decrease cystine accumulation and apoptosis in vitro (Figure 2). Under these conditions, the levels of reactive oxygen species (ROS) remained stable (0.99 ± 0.003 vs. 0.79 ± 0.07; $p = 0.09$, in untreated and treated cells, respectively), while the GSH/GSSG ratio decreased by more than 50% (127 ± 3 vs. 59 ± 10; $p < 0.02$ in untreated and treated cells, respectively). In addition, we also confirmed higher cell mortality in cystinotic cells exposed to DSF (LD50: 107 µM in cystinotic cells vs. 275 µM in wild-type cells) (Figure 8A). Cystinotic-specific DSF toxicity was completely abolished when cells were cultured with L-Cysteine or with N-acetyl cysteine (Figure 8B,C).

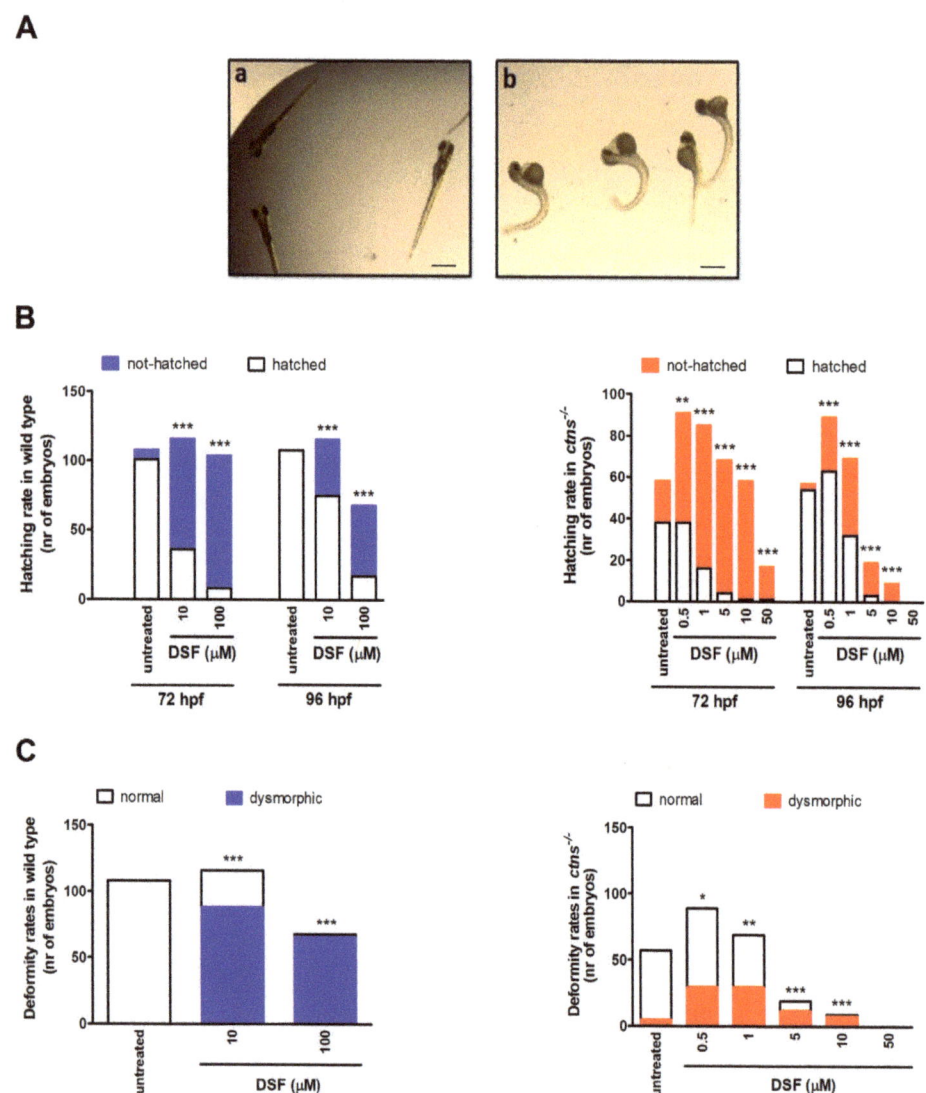

Figure 6. Effect of DSF on hatching and deformity rate in wild-type (WT) and cystinotic (KO) zebrafish embryos and larvae. (**A**) Representative microscopy image of WT (a) and KO (b) zebrafish embryos. Scale bar: 1 mm. (**B**,**C**) Hatching and deformity rates in embryos and larvae treated with different doses of DSF (WT: n = 116 and 104 at 10 and 100 µM, respectively; KO: n = 91, 85, 68, 58, and 17, at 0.5, 1, 5, 10, and 50 µM, respectively). Deformity rates were evaluated after 96 hpf. * p < 0.05, ** p < 0.01, *** p < 0.001 compared to untreated embryos or larvae.

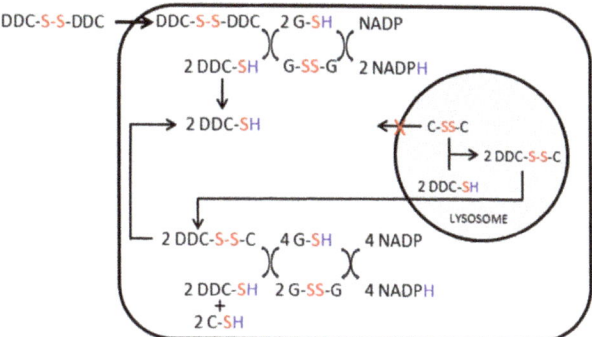

Figure 7. A hypothetical model illustrating the effects of DSF in cystinotic cells. DSF (DDC-S-S-DDC) is a disulfide that is reduced to diethyldithiocarbamate (DDC) in the cytosol, consuming GSH and other free thiols. Consequently, cells are more exposed to free radicals, causing oxidative cell damage and death. Similarly to cysteamine, reduced DDC can react with cystine (C-SS-C) in lysosomes, forming a mixed disulfide (DDC-S-S-C) that allows clearance of cystine.

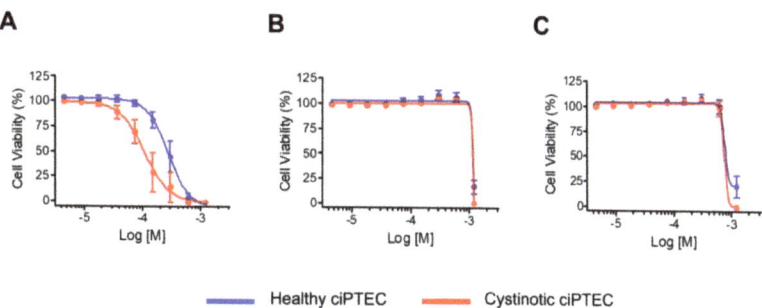

Figure 8. DSF toxicity in cystinotic cells. (**A**) Cell viability was measured in healthy and cystinotic ciPTEC after incubation with increasing DSF doses (from 4.5 µM to 1.2 mM). (**B**,**C**) The same experiment was repeated after incubation with L-cysteine (1.8 mM) or N-acetyl cysteine (1.8 mM) for 24 h.

4. Discussion

Cystinosis is a severe metabolic disease causing cystine accumulation in most tissues. Currently, the disease is treated with cysteamine. This treatment improves clinical outcome, but progression of chronic kidney failure cannot be prevented and other long-term complications still develop in many patients. Our study aimed at identifying new treatments for cystinosis. To this end, we screened a compound library using two characteristic phenotypes of cystinotic cells, namely cystine accumulation and high propensity to undergo apoptosis [9]. Among the compounds that we identified, we selected DSF as a potential molecule for drug repositioning.

DSF is a synthetic molecule that was produced by the German chemist M. Grodzki in 1881 [16]. It was initially used in the rubber industry and was subsequently investigated for clinical use. In the early 1940s, DSF was proposed for treating scabies and worm infections, based on its copper chelating activity. These clinical assays revealed the potential use of DSF to treat alcohol abuse [16]. DSF diffuses rapidly in most tissues [17], where it interacts with sulfhydryl residues of proteins [18,19]. In particular, DSF inhibits acetaldehyde dehydrogenase in the liver, and renders subjects intolerant to alcohol. Recently, DSF has been reported to have in vitro and in vivo anti-inflammatory properties [20], which may be relevant in cystinosis, since cystine crystals cause inflammation [21,22].

Our data show that DSF decreases cystine accumulation and increases resistance of cystinotic cells to apoptosis in vitro. Apoptosis of cystinotic cells has been attributed to cysteinylation of protein kinase C delta [23] and/or to oxidative damage of mitochondria [24].

DSF appeared particularly interesting because it has been used for more than 50 years in humans for various clinical purposes. It has a relatively good safety profile in subjects treated for alcohol abuse, and has a very low cost, which would be extremely valuable in low-income countries. To our knowledge, DSF has never been used in cystinosis. Unfortunately, our results show that prolonged exposure to DSF is toxic to mice, and that toxicity is markedly increased in cystinotic animals. Higher toxicity was also confirmed in zebrafish harboring a nonsense mutation in exon 8 of the *ctns* orthologue gene. In this model, we observed increased lethality and severe developmental abnormalities at early embryonic stages. We did not observe a cystine-depleting effect, unlike what has been reported with cysteamine [14], probably because larvae died at cystine-lowering concentrations. Although disappointing, these results demonstrate the importance of a thorough drug evaluation, even when using a drug repositioning approach based on molecules where extensive clinical data are available. Of note, we cannot exclude that an intermittent treatment would have produced positive results with fewer side effects.

The murine cystinotic model that was used in these studies reproduces only in part the human disease. Similarly to humans, mice accumulate large amounts of intracellular cystine, but kidney disease develops later, and many long-term complications of cystinosis are not observed. From the renal standpoint, the phenotype is characterized by progressive development of low molecular weight proteinuria from three months of age, followed by albuminuria around 6 months of age, and chronic renal failure around one year of age. Glycosuria has a biphasic evolution. It increases from 3 to 6 months and regress around the age of 10 months. This trend has been observed in different laboratories using the same mouse model and has no clear explanation. It is remarkable that glycosuria regressed faster in animals treated with DSF, which may be related to the hypoglycemic effect of DSF. This has been shown in obese mice treated with similar doses of DSF [25]. Remarkably, the authors of this latter study observed that DSF increases energy expenditure and causes weight loss [26], which may explain, at least in part, poor animal growth in our study.

The reasons for the observed increased mortality in DSF-treated KO mice remains an open question. The zebrafish data point to a specific toxic effect of DSF on cystinotic larvae. In other cell models, oxidative stress has been proposed to be the main mechanism of DSF-mediated cell toxicity [27–29]. Cystinotic cells have relative glutathione deficiency and produce more ROS when exposed to oxidative stress [30–32]. Cell oxidation can also cause apoptosis. The anti-oxidative proprieties of cysteamine may explain the anti-apoptotic effects of this drug [24,33]. In addition, antioxidant treatment has been shown to protect proximal tubular cells in the same cystinotic mouse model [34,35]. Further supporting the role of pathogenic oxidation in cystinosis, we observed that N-acetylcysteine and L-cysteine restore cell viability of cystinotic cells treated with DSF.

We also observed the formation of mixed disulfides of DDC with cysteine, similarly to what has been described with cysteamine. This finding supports the cystine-lowering effect of DSF, but also proves that DSF is reduced to DDC in cells, which can severely oxidize cells, as illustrated in Figure 6. Conversely, DSF may have positive effects. In particular, it may prevent apoptosis by forming mixed disulfides with caspase-3, which inhibits the enzymatic activation of the apoptosis cascade [36,37]. Our results show, however, that the net balance between these opposite effects is unfavorable in cystinotic cells.

Supplementary Materials: The following are available online at https://www.mdpi.com/article/10.3390/cells10123294/s1, Figure S1: Urine parameters in mice: long-term treatment with low dose DSF. Wild-type (dashed line) and cystinotic (continuous line) mice were fed on standard (blue line) or DSF-supplemented- diet (100 mg/kg/day, green line). Urine was collected every two months. Data are reported as median values; $n = 5$ mice per group. Figure S2: Cystine and diethyldithiocarbamate (DDC) in 18-month-old mice treated with low DSF doses. WT and KO mice were fed on standard diet or DSF supplemented diets at 50 (square green dots) and 100 (round green dots) mg/kg/day.

Cystine (A) and DDC (B) content in kidneys, liver and heart. Each dot represents the mean cystine values measured on two aliquots of tissue per animal; n = 4 or 5 per group. * $p < 0.05$, ** $p < 0.01$, *** $p < 0.001$. Table S1: Hepatotoxicity parameters measured in plasma of WT and KO mice treated with disulfiram (DSF) for three months. Table S2: Hepatotoxicity and urinary parameters in WT and KO mice at 18 months of age, after 16 months of treatment with disulfiram (DSF).

Author Contributions: Conceptualization, F.E.; methodology, A.T. and M.A.E.; validation, B.M.G.; formal analysis, M.C.; investigation, A.T., M.A.E., F.B., E.D.L., S.B., M.J.J., A.J., S.C., A.P., C.D.S., L.R.R., I.G. and P.F.; resources, L.P.v.d.H., C.D.-V. and B.M.G.; writing—original draft preparation, A.T. and F.E.; project administration, A.T., E.L. and R.M.; funding acquisition, F.E., E.L. and R.M. All authors have read and agreed to the published version of the manuscript.

Funding: This research was funded by the Cystinosis Research Foundation (grant no. CRFS-2014), the Italian Ministry of Health (Ricerca Corrente grant no. RC2015), E-rare European Union (grant no. E-Rare-2 JTC 2014), and the Foundation of Scientific Research Flanders (award 11Y5216N).

Institutional Review Board Statement: The study was conducted in accordance with the European 2010/63/EU directive on the protection of animals used for scientific purposes, and authorized by the Italian Ministry of Health (authorization number 230/2015-PR).

Conflicts of Interest: The authors declare no conflict of interest.

References

1. Elmonem, M.A.; Veys, K.R.; Soliman, N.A.; van Dyck, M.; van den Heuvel, L.P.; Levtchenko, E. Cystinosis: A review. *Orphanet J. Rare Dis.* **2016**, *11*, 47. [CrossRef]
2. Emma, F.; Nesterova, G.; Langman, C.; Labbe, A.; Cherqui, S.; Goodyer, P.; Janssen, M.C.; Greco, M.; Topaloglu, R.; Elenberg, E.; et al. Nephropathic cystinosis: An international consensus document. *Nephrol. Dial. Transplant.* **2014**, *29* (Suppl. 4), iv87–iv94. [CrossRef] [PubMed]
3. Kasimer, R.N.; Langman, C.B. Adult complications of nephropathic cystinosis: A systematic review. *Pediatr. Nephrol.* **2021**, *36*, 223–236. [CrossRef]
4. Gaide Chevronnay, H.P.; Janssens, V.; Van Der Smissen, P.; N'Kuli, F.; Nevo, N.; Guiot, Y.; Levtchenko, E.; Marbaix, E.; Pierreux, C.E.; Cherqui, S.; et al. Time course of pathogenic and adaptation mechanisms in cystinotic mouse kidneys. *J. Am. Soc. Nephrol.* **2014**, *25*, 1256–1269. [CrossRef]
5. Park, M.; Helip-Wooley, A.; Thoene, J. Lysosomal cystine storage augments apoptosis in cultured human fibroblasts and renal tubular epithelial cells. *J. Am. Soc. Nephrol.* **2002**, *13*, 2878–2887. [CrossRef] [PubMed]
6. Taranta, A.; Bellomo, F.; Petrini, S.; Polishchuk, E.; De Leo, E.; Rega, L.R.; Pastore, A.; Polishchuk, R.; De Matteis, M.A.; Emma, F. Cystinosin-LKG rescues cystine accumulation and decreases apoptosis rate in cystinotic proximal tubular epithelial cells. *Pediatr. Res.* **2017**, *81*, 113–119. [CrossRef]
7. Jezegou, A.; Llinares, E.; Anne, C.; Kieffer-Jaquinod, S.; O'Regan, S.; Aupetit, J.; Chabli, A.; Sagne, C.; Debacker, C.; Chadefaux-Vekemans, B.; et al. Heptahelical protein PQLC2 is a lysosomal cationic amino acid exporter underlying the action of cysteamine in cystinosis therapy. *Proc. Natl. Acad. Sci. USA* **2012**, *109*, E3434–E3443. [CrossRef]
8. Emma, F.; Hoff, W.V.; Hohenfellner, K.; Topaloglu, R.; Greco, M.; Ariceta, G.; Bettini, C.; Bockenhauer, D.; Veys, K.; Pape, L.; et al. An international cohort study spanning five decades assessed outcomes of nephropathic cystinosis. *Kidney Int.* **2021**, *100*, 1112–1123. [CrossRef] [PubMed]
9. Bellomo, F.; De Leo, E.; Taranta, A.; Giaquinto, L.; Di Giovamberardino, G.; Montefusco, S.; Rega, L.R.; Pastore, A.; Medina, D.L.; Di Bernardo, D.; et al. Drug repurposing in rare diseases: An integrative study of drug screening and transcriptomic analysis in nephropathic cystinosis. *Int. J. Mol. Sci.* **2021**. Submitted.
10. Wilmer, M.J.; Saleem, M.A.; Masereeuw, R.; Ni, L.; van der Velden, T.J.; Russel, F.G.; Mathieson, P.W.; Monnens, L.A.; van den Heuvel, L.P.; Levtchenko, E.N. Novel conditionally immortalized human proximal tubule cell line expressing functional influx and efflux transporters. *Cell Tissue Res.* **2010**, *339*, 449–457. [CrossRef] [PubMed]
11. Pastore, A.; Lo Russo, A.; Greco, M.; Rizzoni, G.; Federici, G. Semiautomated method for determination of cystine concentration in polymorphonuclear leukocytes. *Clin. Chem.* **2000**, *46*, 574–576. [CrossRef] [PubMed]
12. Jamalpoor, A.; van Gelder, C.A.; Yousef Yengej, F.A.; Zaal, E.A.; Berlingerio, S.P.; Veys, K.R.; Pou Casellas, C.; Voskuil, K.; Essa, K.; Ammerlaan, C.M.; et al. Cysteamine-bicalutamide combination therapy corrects proximal tubule phenotype in cystinosis. *EMBO Mol. Med.* **2021**, *13*, e13067. [CrossRef] [PubMed]
13. Nevo, N.; Chol, M.; Bailleux, A.; Kalatzis, V.; Morisset, L.; Devuyst, O.; Gubler, M.C.; Antignac, C. Renal phenotype of the cystinosis mouse model is dependent upon genetic background. *Nephrol. Dial. Transplant.* **2010**, *25*, 1059–1066. [CrossRef]
14. Elmonem, M.A.; Khalil, R.; Khodaparast, L.; Khodaparast, L.; Arcolino, F.O.; Morgan, J.; Pastore, A.; Tylzanowski, P.; Ny, A.; Lowe, M.; et al. Cystinosis (ctns) zebrafish mutant shows pronephric glomerular and tubular dysfunction. *Sci. Rep.* **2017**, *7*, 42583. [CrossRef]
15. Harper, C.; Lawrence, C. *The Laboratory Zebrafish*, 1st ed.; CRC Press: Boca Raton, FL, USA, 2011; pp. 1–274.

16. Kragh, H. From disulfiram to antabuse: The invention of a drug. *Bull. Hist. Chem.* **2008**, *33*, 82–88.
17. Johansson, B. A review of the pharmacokinetics and pharmacodynamics of disulfiram and its metabolites. *Acta Psychiatr. Scand.* **1992**, *369*, 15–26. [CrossRef]
18. Lipsky, J.J.; Shen, M.L.; Naylor, S. In vivo inhibition of aldehyde dehydrogenase by disulfiram. *Chem. Biol. Interact.* **2001**, *130–132*, 93–102. [CrossRef]
19. Vallari, R.C.; Pietruszko, R. Human aldehyde dehydrogenase: Mechanism of inhibition of disulfiram. *Science* **1982**, *216*, 637–639. [CrossRef]
20. Deng, W.; Yang, Z.; Yue, H.; Ou, Y.; Hu, W.; Sun, P. Disulfiram suppresses NLRP3 inflammasome activation to treat peritoneal and gouty inflammation. *Free Radic. Biol. Med.* **2020**, *152*, 8–17. [CrossRef] [PubMed]
21. Prencipe, G.; Caiello, I.; Cherqui, S.; Whisenant, T.; Petrini, S.; Emma, F.; De Benedetti, F. Inflammasome activation by cystine crystals: Implications for the pathogenesis of cystinosis. *J. Am. Soc. Nephrol.* **2014**, *25*, 1163–1169. [CrossRef] [PubMed]
22. Elmonem, M.A.; Makar, S.H.; van den Heuvel, L.; Abdelaziz, H.; Abdelrahman, S.M.; Bossuyt, X.; Janssen, M.C.; Cornelissen, E.A.; Lefeber, D.J.; Joosten, L.A.; et al. Clinical utility of chitotriosidase enzyme activity in nephropathic cystinosis. *Orphanet J. Rare Dis.* **2014**, *9*, 155. [CrossRef]
23. Park, M.A.; Pejovic, V.; Kerisit, K.G.; Junius, S.; Thoene, J.G. Increased apoptosis in cystinotic fibroblasts and renal proximal tubule epithelial cells results from cysteinylation of protein kinase Cdelta. *J. Am. Soc. Nephrol.* **2006**, *17*, 3167–3175. [CrossRef]
24. De Rasmo, D.; Signorile, A.; De Leo, E.; Polishchuk, E.V.; Ferretta, A.; Raso, R.; Russo, S.; Polishchuk, R.; Emma, F.; Bellomo, F. Mitochondrial Dynamics of Proximal Tubular Epithelial Cells in Nephropathic Cystinosis. *Int. J. Mol. Sci.* **2019**, *21*, 192. [CrossRef] [PubMed]
25. Bernier, M.; Mitchell, S.J.; Wahl, D.; Diaz, A.; Singh, A.; Seo, W.; Wang, M.; Ali, A.; Kaiser, T.; Price, N.L.; et al. Disulfiram Treatment Normalizes Body Weight in Obese Mice. *Cell Metab.* **2020**, *32*, 203–214.e4. [CrossRef] [PubMed]
26. Bernier, M.; Harney, D.; Koay, Y.C.; Diaz, A.; Singh, A.; Wahl, D.; Pulpitel, T.; Ali, A.; Guiterrez, V.; Mitchell, S.J.; et al. Elucidating the mechanisms by which disulfiram protects against obesity and metabolic syndrome. *NPJ Aging Mech. Dis.* **2020**, *6*, 8. [CrossRef] [PubMed]
27. Hothi, P.; Martins, T.J.; Chen, L.; Deleyrolle, L.; Yoon, J.G.; Reynolds, B.; Foltz, G. High-throughput chemical screens identify disulfiram as an inhibitor of human glioblastoma stem cells. *Oncotarget* **2012**, *3*, 1124–1136. [CrossRef] [PubMed]
28. Allensworth, J.L.; Evans, M.K.; Bertucci, F.; Aldrich, A.J.; Festa, R.A.; Finetti, P.; Ueno, N.T.; Safi, R.; McDonnell, D.P.; Thiele, D.J.; et al. Disulfiram (DSF) acts as a copper ionophore to induce copper-dependent oxidative stress and mediate anti-tumor efficacy in inflammatory breast cancer. *Mol. Oncol.* **2015**, *9*, 1155–1168. [CrossRef]
29. Falls-Hubert, K.C.; Butler, A.L.; Gui, K.; Anderson, M.; Li, M.; Stolwijk, J.M.; Rodman, S.N., III; Solst, S.R.; Tomanek-Chalkley, A.; Searby, C.C.; et al. Disulfiram causes selective hypoxic cancer cell toxicity and radio-chemo-sensitization via redox cycling of copper. *Free Radic. Biol. Med.* **2020**, *150*, 1–11. [CrossRef] [PubMed]
30. Mannucci, L.; Pastore, A.; Rizzo, C.; Piemonte, F.; Rizzoni, G.; Emma, F. Impaired activity of the gamma-glutamyl cycle in nephropathic cystinosis fibroblasts. *Pediatr. Res.* **2006**, *59*, 332–335. [CrossRef] [PubMed]
31. Levtchenko, E.; de Graaf-Hess, A.; Wilmer, M.; van den Heuvel, L.; Monnens, L.; Blom, H. Altered status of glutathione and its metabolites in cystinotic cells. *Nephrol. Dial. Transplant.* **2005**, *20*, 1828–1832. [CrossRef]
32. Cherqui, S.; Courtoy, P.J. The renal Fanconi syndrome in cystinosis: Pathogenic insights and therapeutic perspectives. *Nat. Rev. Nephrol.* **2017**, *13*, 115–131. [CrossRef] [PubMed]
33. Bellomo, F.; Signorile, A.; Tamma, G.; Ranieri, M.; Emma, F.; De Rasmo, D. Impact of atypical mitochondrial cyclic-AMP level in nephropathic cystinosis. *Cell Mol. Life Sci.* **2018**, *75*, 3411–3422. [CrossRef]
34. Galarreta, C.I.; Forbes, M.S.; Thornhill, B.A.; Antignac, C.; Gubler, M.C.; Nevo, N.; Murphy, M.P.; Chevalier, R.L. The swan-neck lesion: Proximal tubular adaptation to oxidative stress in nephropathic cystinosis. *Am. J. Physiol. Renal. Physiol.* **2015**, *308*, F1155–F1166. [CrossRef] [PubMed]
35. Festa, B.P.; Chen, Z.; Berquez, M.; Debaix, H.; Tokonami, N.; Prange, J.A.; Hoek, G.V.; Alessio, C.; Raimondi, A.; Nevo, N.; et al. Impaired autophagy bridges lysosomal storage disease and epithelial dysfunction in the kidney. *Nat. Commun.* **2018**, *9*, 161. [CrossRef]
36. Nobel, C.S.; Kimland, M.; Nicholson, D.W.; Orrenius, S.; Slater, A.F. Disulfiram is a potent inhibitor of proteases of the caspase family. *Chem. Res. Toxicol.* **1997**, *10*, 1319–1324. [CrossRef] [PubMed]
37. Nobel, C.S.; Burgess, D.H.; Zhivotovsky, B.; Burkitt, M.J.; Orrenius, S.; Slater, A.F. Mechanism of dithiocarbamate inhibition of apoptosis: Thiol oxidation by dithiocarbamate disulfides directly inhibits processing of the caspase-3 proenzyme. *Chem. Res. Toxicol.* **1997**, *10*, 636–643. [CrossRef] [PubMed]

MDPI
St. Alban-Anlage 66
4052 Basel
Switzerland
Tel. +41 61 683 77 34
Fax +41 61 302 89 18
www.mdpi.com

Cells Editorial Office
E-mail: cells@mdpi.com
www.mdpi.com/journal/cells

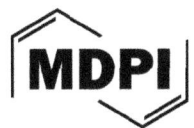

www.ingramcontent.com/pod-product-compliance
Lightning Source LLC
LaVergne TN
LVHW070414100526
838202LV00014B/1453